SP.

txk

Gen.

2/48

RECENT ADVANCES IN CANCER AND RADIOTHERAPEUTICS

Recent Advances in
CANCER and
RADIOTHERAPEUTICS:
CLINICAL ONCOLOGY

Edited by

KEITH E. HALNAN
MA, MD, MRCP, FFR

Director, Glasgow Institute of Radiotherapeutics,
Royal and Western Infirmaries,
Honorary Clinical Lecturer, University of Glasgow

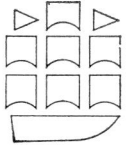

1972
CHURCHILL LIVINGSTONE
EDINBURGH AND LONDON

First Published 1972

International Standard Book Number
0 443 00834 5

© Longman Group Ltd. 1972

Any correspondence relating to this volume should be
directed to the publishers at
104 Gloucester Place, London, W1H 4AE.

Printed in Great Britain by
The Whitefriars Press Ltd., London and Tonbridge

Introduction

It is now a well known truism that one in five of all of us will develop some form of cancer before we die, often a long time before! This may well be an understatement since the death rate from infections continues to fall. However, the management of human cancer is now at a highly interesting phase of development, and it seemed well worthwhile reviewing some of the more interesting topics in a selective rather than a comprehensive way. The chapters are intended to be readable and critical surveys and are written by authors actively working in these fields. They are designed for undergraduate and postgraduate students as well as consultants and general medical and scientific readers; they are not just for specialists. Clinical management of cancer, neoplasia, or 'oncology' is beginning to coalesce in the English-speaking countries. In many others, especially in Europe, there are already Institutes and Departments of Oncology. It may be a sign of the times that in Britain an Association of Head and Neck Oncologists is now flourishing, and that the Royal Society of Medicine has a newly formed section of Oncology.

A striking recent feature of clinical work in cancer has been the increasing number of valuable clinical trials undertaken, especially in breast cancer. The first chapter is by Robert McWhirter—himself responsible for stimulating these advances—who reviews and cogently criticises current treatment; much of this chapter can be applied to the orthodox treatment of other tumours.

Many people think of chemotherapy as the future treatment of cancer. Chemotherapy has been used since the early nineteen forties, and is now beginning to make a substantial impact on the clinical problem; new and valuable compounds continue to appear. The outstanding success of chemotherapy in the control of the rare disease, choriocarcinoma, is an inspiration to us all. One of the main fields in which chemotherapy has been applied with valuable though still limited success is leukaemia in children. The clinician himself continues to make important contributions, and the recognition of Burkitt's lymphoma has been one of the major milestones of the last decade, The common lethal varieties of human cancer may seem less interesting but they remain vitally important to their human hosts—our patients— and breast cancer especially is one of these.

For many years excisional surgery was the only sure method of cure for cancer. The major current advance in surgery itself is the possibility of successful organ transplantation. This may not yet be of substantial value for treatment of cancer, but it leads to evaluation and investigation of many intriguing secondary problems. Immunology is one of these which itself is beginning to develop advances in clinical treatment, in leukaemia especially.

Radiotherapy has become the second major method of cure, and over the last 50 years has achieved perhaps the first place for palliative treatment of human cancer. There are at present several highly promising technological advances—'growth points'—in radiotherapeutics. The use of computers is one obvious example. Others depend upon radiobiology, which has taken on a new rational and scientific lease of life. The 'oxygen-effect' (a probable cause of many failures of conventional X-ray therapy) is one of the more important aspects, leading to the exploration of treatment in hyperbaric oxygen, and by fast neutrons. The easy availability of artificial radioactive nuclides as radiation sources has led to endolymphatic radiotherapy—a possible method for improved treatment of the lymphatic spread of a tumour—and to 'after-loading' methods to overcome the main disadvantages of radium treatment, which has already achieved so much especially in gynaecological cancer.

Many other topics might have been discussed if space and time had been more flexible. Very sincere thanks are due to the distinguished contributors to this volume, all of them extremely busy, and most of them refreshingly punctual with delivery of their chapters. Personal thanks are also due to my secretary, Mrs. Z. Willoughby, to the publishers for all their help, and to my wife and daughters for putting up with so much work at home.

K.E.H.

Contributors

J. MAXWELL ANDERSON, M.B., Ch.B., F.R.C.S.Ed. & Eng.,
Consultant Surgeon, and Director, Wolfson Laboratory, The Royal Infirmary, Glasgow, Scotland.

K. D. BAGSHAWE M.D., F.R.C.P.,
Director, Department of Medical Oncology, Charing Cross (Fulham) Hospital, London, England.

P. R. F. BELL, M.D., F.R.C.S.,
Consultant Surgeon, Western Infirmary, Glasgow, Scotland.

N. M. BLEEHEN, M.A., B.Sc., B.M., B.Ch.(Oxf.), M.R.C.P.(Lond.), F.F.R., D.M.R.T.,
Professor of Radiotherapy, The Middlesex Hospital, London, England.

PETER CLIFFORD, M.Ch., M.D.,(h.c., Karol. Inst. Stockholm), F.R.C.S., D.L.O.,
Lately Consultant in Charge, Department of Head & Neck Surgery, Kenyatta Hospital, Nairobi, Kenya, East Africa.

WILLIAM DUNCAN, M.B., Ch.B., M.R.C.P.(Ed.), F.F.R., D.M.R.T.,
Professor of Radiotherapy, University of Edinburgh, Scotland. (Lately Consultant Radiotherapist, Christie Hospital & Holt Radium Institute, Manchester, England).

GERALD E. FLATMAN, M.D., F.R.C.S., F.F.R., D.M.R.T.,
Deputy Director, Glasgow Institute of Radiotherapeutics, Western Infirmary, Glasgow, Scotland.

C. A. JOSLIN, M.B., B.S., F.F.R., D.M.R.T.,
Consultant Radiotherapist, University Hospital of Wales, Clinical Teacher, Welsh National School of Medicine, Cardiff, Wales.

ROBERT McWHIRTER, F.R.S.(Ed.), M.B., Ch.B.,F.R.C.P.(Ed.), F.R.C.S.(Ed.),
D.M.R.E., F.F.R., F.F.R.R.C.S. I., Hon.F.C.R.A.,
Lately Professor of Radiotherapy, University of Edinburgh, Scotland.

SASHA MORRIS, M.B., Ch.B., D.M.R.T.,
Assistant Radiotherapist, Glasgow Institute of Radiotherapeutics,
Western Infirmary, Glasgow, Scotland.

J. STEWART ORR, B.Sc., F.Inst.P.,
Principal Physicist, Institute of Radiotherapeutics and Regional
Department of Clinical Physics and Bio-Engineering, Glasgow,
Scotland.

I. D. H. TODD, M.B., M.R.C.P., F.F.R.,
Consultant Radiotherapist, Christie Hospital & Holt Radium
Institute, Manchester, England.

M. L. N. WILLOUGHBY, M.A., M.D., M.R.C.Path.,
Consultant Haematologist, The Royal Hospital for Sick Children,
Glasgow, Scotland.

Contents

1 An Analysis of the Treatment of Breast Cancer

ROBERT McWHIRTER

Some thirty to forty years ago it appeared as if the treatment of breast cancer had been finalized. There was universal agreement that radical mastectomy was the best method of treatment and, indeed, it was generally regarded as the only method which offered any prospect of cure. The operation was held in such high regard that any suggestion that there might be other methods worthy of consideration was treated almost as heresy and the introduction of new methods was vigorously opposed.

In spite of opposition, many other methods have been introduced with the result that now the conflicting claims put forward by protagonists of each procedure have given rise to great confusion. To add to the confusion it has been stated that the survival rates will be the same whatever method of treatment is employed. It has even been suggested that none of the methods has the slightest influence on the natural course of the disease.

Progress cannot be made if there is unquestioning acceptance of all that has gone before but a state of complete uncertainty is not immediately helpful. In the long run, however, a state of uncertainty may be advantageous because it provokes a critical re-appraisal of:

(A) the treatment methods we employ,
(B) the procedure adopted when we attempt to compare the value of different methods of treatment.

A. REVIEW OF TREATMENT METHODS

With advantage we can begin our appraisal of treatment methods by trying to ascertain just why so many conflicting proposals have come to be made. It soon becomes evident that our inability to determine the precise extent of the disease in any patient is a factor of major importance. Clearly the extent of treatment should be governed by the extent of the disease and it is interesting to reflect that if we could determine with certainty the extent of spread from the primary site, our whole approach to treatment could be rationalized immediately. Patients with distant metastases would be spared the unnecessary discomfort of radical treatment. Assessment of the value of the methods employed in the eradication of local disease would be greatly simplified. Methods of controlling distant metastases could be instituted while the patient's general health was still good and therefore at a stage when some measure of control would be far more likely to be achieved.

Unfortunately we have no means of determining the precise extent of the disease in any patient although, as we shall see presently, some progress has been made in respect of lymph node involvement. We are still a long way however from being able to detect more distant metastases unless of course the involvement is gross. Radiographic examination is still the best method of recognizing metastases in the skeleton and lungs but the method fails to detect early involvement. This is not surprising when we recall that one thousand million cells can fit into a sphere 1 cm. in diameter. A 1 cm. osteolytic deposit in the spine, which is a common site of involvement, is most unlikely to be detected and post-mortem examination shows that deposits of this size in the lungs are not always visible. Radio-isotope bone scans may be of some assistance but they are never a substitute for first class radiographs, and it is important to note that a positive scan does not necessarily indicate the presence of a metastatic deposit. Bone marrow examination is so seldom of value that it has been largely abandoned.

RADICAL MASTECTOMY

When we come to examine the classical Halsted operation in the light of the above remarks we find that frequently the scope of the operation is not commensurate with the extent of the disease. In many it is unnecessarily extensive whereas in others it is inadequate. Thus in patients with negative axillary nodes, dissection of the axilla cannot improve the survival rate and in patients where the disease has spread beyond the axilla there is no possibility of the operation being successful. The percentage of patients in whom axillary dissection may be life-saving is difficult to determine exactly but clearly it must be small. The following calculations give some indication of the proportion of patients in whom cure may depend on axillary dissection. Of the patients nowadays regarded as suitable for radical mastectomy, the axillary nodes are negative in approximately 60%, and in this 60% axillary dissection may be omitted without any disadvantage. In the remaining 40%, the axillary nodes are positive and of these patients some 60% are either dead or have clinical evidence of distant metastases within five years of the operation. The percentage continues to rise in subsequent years and accordingly we can say that in at least 24% (60% of 40%) of the total patients dissection of the axilla fails in its purpose. Combining these observations it may now be stated that in some 84% (60%

plus 24%) of the total patients dissection of the axilla is not a life-saving procedure. Simple mastectomy alone would be just as effective in all but 16% of the patients we regularly treat by radical mastectomy.

The overall survival rates from radical mastectomy have always been encouraging and because of the great importance attached to the dissection of the axilla, it is often assumed that axillary dissection is largely responsible for the success achieved. It is only on closer inspection that it has come to be appreciated that the reputation of the operation has depended, in large measure, on the excellent results in patients with negative nodes. On the basis of the calculations just made and assuming an 80% five year survival rate in patients with negative nodes, the overall survival rate would be 64% (80% of 60% plus 16%) but it will now be evident that in at least three quarters of the survivors axillary dissection played no part in their survival.

Negative nodes are not a test of the value of axillary dissection; the test comes when the nodes are positive and it is in this group of patients that almost every surgeon has expressed disappointment with his results. Handley (1952) has provided one reason why the failure rate is so high in patients with positive axillary nodes. His observations, now amply confirmed by other workers, have shown that by the time the axillary nodes are invaded, the internal mammary nodes are also invaded in approximately 50% of the patients. In addition it has been demonstrated by biopsy of the supraclavicular nodes and by follow up studies after radical mastectomy that the supraclavicular nodes are also commonly involved by the time the axillary nodes are invaded. Both observations help to explain why the survival rates are low in patients with positive axillary nodes.

When the internal mammary and supraclavicular nodes are invaded, standard radical mastectomy does not offer any chance of cure. Recognizing this point, Haagensen (1956) carries out a biopsy of the internal mammary nodes and of the apical axillary nodes before accepting a patient for treatment by radical mastectomy. If the biopsy taken from either site is positive, radical mastectomy is not performed because, as Haagensen rightly says, involvement of these sites places the patient beyond the scope of the operation. In terms of lymph node involvement he has defined very clearly the useful limits of radical mastectomy and his observations are of great importance in the rationalization of treatment. As might be expected from the restriction of the operation to patients with less advanced disease, the survival rates he presents are excellent. Within the limits proposed by Haagensen, radical mastectomy may well remain the best method of treatment.

Our ultimate objective must always be a reduction of the mortality from breast cancer. So far we appear to have failed because the mortality rates, or more correctly the fatality rates, in our national statistics are the same today as they were at the beginning of the century. While we will not reduce the mortality by continuing to perform radical mastectomy in patients beyond the scope of the operation we must, at the same time, note that restriction of the operation to more favourable patients will not save the life of a single additional patient. From all that has been said it would appear that if we are to attempt to reduce the mortality from breast cancer we must examine more extensive methods of treatment capable of application to more patients and in particular capable of application to patients with positive internal mammary and/or supraclavicular nodes.

While a more radical approach may be indicated in some patients the survey also shows that there is a place for more conservative treatment. We have seen that a conservative approach requires consideration in patients with negative axillary nodes and possibly also in patients still in the operable category, but where there is a high probability of distant metastases being present.

Both the more radical approach and the more conservative approach require careful consideration. It is convenient to discuss the more radical approach in the first place.

THE MORE RADICAL APPROACH

As already noted some 50% of the patients in the clinically operable category with positive axillary nodes also have involvement of the internal mammary nodes. Involvement of the internal mammary nodes is comparatively rare in patients with negative axillary nodes but may occur in subareolar tumours and in tumours situated in the medial half of the breast. Supraclavicular involvement is very rare indeed if the axillary nodes are negative but when the axillary nodes are positive, biopsy shows that the supraclavicular nodes may also be invaded in patients ordinarily regarded as operable.

Both surgery and radiotherapy have been employed in the treatment of secondarily involved internal mammary and supraclavicular nodes.

The feasibility of complete surgical excision of the internal mammary and supraclavicular nodes was explored by Wangensteen (1956) but the high morbidity and mortality associated with this extensive operation render it unlikely to become a routine method of treating breast cancer. In an operation associated with little or no morbidity, Urban (1964) has resected the internal mammary nodes in continuity with the breast. The results he has obtained are encouraging and the extension of treatment beyond the scope of the standard radical operation would appear to be worth undertaking.

In patients where standard radical mastectomy has been performed, the scope of treatment may be extended by irradiating, immediately after the operation, the internal mammary and supraclavicular nodes. The value of radiotherapy given immediately after radical mastectomy was examined by Paterson and Russell (1959) who found that the survival rates were no better than those obtained when radiotherapy was given only if and when local recurrence took place. In Edinburgh, from 1935–40, radiotherapy was given routinely immediately after radical mastectomy. The local recurrence rate was markedly reduced but unfortunately there was little improvement in the five year survival rate.

In 1941, following a discussion with the senior surgical staff of Edinburgh Royal Infirmary, it was decided to substitute radiotherapy for surgery in the treatment of all the regional lymph nodes. A clinical trial was proposed but was rejected because in those days any trial involving patients was not considered to be ethical. At a time when radical mastectomy was the unchallenged method of treatment, it was admittedly a bold decision to substitute radiotherapy for surgery in the treatment of all the lymph nodes and some account must be given of the reasons leading up to this decision. Keynes (1937) had shown earlier that radium implantation of the regional nodes yielded results comparable to surgical dissection and it was thought that X-ray treatment might be even more effective because of the much better dose distribution. X-ray treatment had already been shown to be effective in the treatment of local recurrence. Prophylactic radiotherapy given immediately after radical mastectomy had markedly reduced the incidence of recurrences on the chest wall and parasternal masses due to internal mammary node involvement had become exceedingly uncommon. In a small number of patients treated by simple mastectomy and radiotherapy in the period 1935–40, the results were encouraging. The decision had the full support of the late Sir John Fraser (1939) who had recently reviewed the patients he had treated by radical mastectomy and had found that the survival rates, especially in patients with positive nodes, were disappointing. We were also encouraged by the fact that the new method of treatment would offer exactly the same prospect of cure as radical mastectomy if the axillary nodes were negative. The decision to continue to remove the breast before irradiating the nodes was based on the findings in patients with advanced disease who had been treated entirely by radiotherapy. In these patients the response in the nodes was always much better than in the breast and, indeed, it was only rarely that the primary tumour disappeared entirely.

With few exceptions (axillary tail tumours, lymph nodes in continuity with the primary tumour, patients with pulmonary tuberculosis and patients with severe peripheral vascular disease of the arm) it was found that simple mastectomy and radiotherapy could be undertaken in all patients suitable for the standard radical operation. Table I shows the

TABLE I
ALL PATIENTS UNDER 65 YEARS OF AGE TREATED BY SIMPLE MASTECTOMY
AND RADIOTHERAPY.
INTERNATIONAL STAGING.

		No. of Patients	Percentage Alive		
			5 yrs	10 yrs	15 yrs
Stage I	T.1 N.O	206	79	64	47
	T.2 N.O	394	68	48	40
	Total	600	72	54	43
Stage II	T.1 N.1	116	67	51	43
	T.2 N.1	375	55	41	32
	Total	491	58	43	35
Stage III	Total	690	37	24	17

No correction made for deaths from intercurrent disease.

crude survival rates of all patients treated by simple mastectomy and radiotherapy. The patients have been classified according to the international form of staging adopted in 1960. The analysis has been confined to patients under 65 years of age so as to lessen the effect of death from intercurrent disease on the long term survival rates.

The Table shows the survival rates to be expected when all the regional lymph nodes are treated entirely by radiotherapy. The results in Stages I and II appear to be comparable to those obtained by radical mastectomy but a clinical trial is obviously essential before a decision can be reached regarding the relative value of surgery and radiotherapy in the treatment of lymph nodes. The findings in the more advanced patients in Stage III will be discussed later.

It is important before going further to try to decide if the extension of treatment to the internal mammary and supraclavicular nodes is likely to be of any value. There is plenty of evidence to show that as the extent of the local disease increases the frequency of distant metastases increases. Thus it is well known that distant metastases are relatively infrequent in patients with negative axillary nodes but are common in patients with positive nodes. It has also been shown that the frequency of distant metastases increases as the number of nodes involved increases. If it could be shown that distant metastases are present in all patients with positive internal mammary and/or supraclavicular nodes then the development of more extensive methods of treatment would not be worth attempting. The following evidence appears to support the view that the attempt should be made.

As already stated, Urban (1964) has demonstrated that positive internal mammary nodes may be successfully removed by surgery. In a clinically operable series of 86 patients with histologically proven metastases in the internal mammary nodes he obtained a five year survival rate of 46·5% and a recurrence free rate of 40%.

In another clinically operable series of 123 patients with histologically proven metastases in the nodes at the apex of the axilla or in the internal mammary nodes, Guttmann (1966), employing two million volt X-ray therapy as the sole means of treatment, obtained a five year survival rate of 52%.

Even in patients with more advanced disease full treatment of all the regional lymph node areas would still appear to be indicated. It may be presumed that a high proportion of Stage III patients have internal mammary node involvement. (It is interesting that there is rarely clinical evidence of this pre-operatively and that parasternal masses indicative of extracapsular spread from the internal mammary nodes are almost entirely confined to patients who have been surgically treated). In many of the Stage III patients in Table I the axillary nodes were fixed and in some the supraclavicular nodes were enlarged. Fortunately fixation of the axillary nodes and enlargement of the supraclavicular nodes do not interfere with full radical treatment by radiotherapy and all patients placed in Stage III have been included provided always that simple mastectomy could be performed without cutting through obvious disease. It will be noted from Table I that the five year survival rate for this group of patients was 37%.

In an analysis confined to patients with enlarged supraclavicular nodes (and often with fixed axillary nodes in addition) a five year survival rate of 17% was obtained in Edinburgh following treatment of all the regional nodes by radiotherapy (McWhirter, 1964).

These findings suggest that distant metastases may not be present in all patients with internal mammary and supraclavicular node involvement, and that more extensive treatment appears to be worth attempting not only in patients who are clinically operable but also in patients who are inoperable because of the presence of gross local disease.

THE MORE CONSERVATIVE APPROACH

We must now turn from these more extensive methods of treatment and examine the conservative approach to the management of breast cancer. More conservative measures have been advocated for many years but they have often been dismissed as a form of treatment to be used only in patients unsuitable for radical mastectomy. Thirty years ago Fitzwilliams (1940) in this country advocated the adoption of conservative surgery in patients with disease of limited extent but, in spite of the results he was able to present, his work received little support from his surgical colleagues. Surprised by the good survival rates obtained in patients they had treated conservatively, other surgeons went to considerable length to explain them away, so firmly did they believe that radical mastectomy was the only method by which breast cancer might be cured.

A number of workers have maintained that small tumours can be treated adequately by local excision and radiotherapy. In addition to advising that the regional lymph nodes be treated by radium implantation, Keynes (1957) also advised that small primaries should be treated by local excision and that the whole breast should be removed only if the tumour was large. Mustakallio (1954) for many years has treated small breast cancers by local excision followed by X-ray therapy to the breast and lymph nodes, and in a series of 127 patients he obtained a five year survival rate of 84% and a ten year survival rate of 72%. Porritt (1964) advised that the breast should not be removed if the primary tumour was small and showed that his results from local excision followed by radiotherapy, when this appeared to be indicated, were superior to those he obtained by radical mastectomy. Hedley Atkins has set up a clinical trial to compare local excision and radiotherapy with radical mastectomy in the treatment of tumours of limited extent. His findings are awaited with great interest.

When radical mastectomy was being discussed we noted in patients with negative nodes that dissection of the axilla was unnecessary. We also noted that spread beyond the axilla could be presumed in more than half the remaining patients with positive axillary nodes and that axillary dissection in these patients could not be curative. It was then estimated that the same survival rates would have been obtained in some 84% of the patients if they had been treated by simple mastectomy alone. If now conservative measures (simple mastectomy or even only local excision of the tumour) are restricted to patients with very early disease it should not occasion surprise if the survival rates are found to be identical or almost identical to those obtained by radical mastectomy.

The comments just made in respect of radical mastectomy apply with equal force to the routine use of the still more radical forms of treatment discussed earlier. These methods will not be any more effective when all the regional lymph nodes are negative and will still fail if distant metastases are already present.

In spite of the fact that distant metastases to the skeleton and elsewhere may not be detected pre-operatively, it is the presence or absence of distant spread which largely determines the outcome of treatment. When metastases are present the length of survival will depend on the sites involved, the extent of metastatic spread at the time of operation and very importantly, on the rate of growth of the tumour. As a general rule, tumours which are well-differentiated grow slowly and tumours which are undifferentiated grow rapidly. In addition to these inherent or intrinsic factors there is now increasing evidence that the reaction of the host to the tumour may exert an important controlling influence.

The fact that tumours continue to grow after the aetiological factors have ceased to act, and the ability of cells to maintain their identity as malignant cells through many cell divisions, is strong evidence in favour of the somatic mutation theory of the origin of tumours. Chromosomal aberrations have been identified in many tumours and if it is ultimately established that malignant cells are genetically different from the host cells of origin, it would not be surprising if tumours did excite an immunological response similar to that encountered when a tissue transplant has been performed. Good evidence of an immunological response has certainly been found in experimental animals and the presence of tumour antibodies has now been firmly established.

Crile (1967) has stressed the possible importance of the host reaction in the treatment of breast cancer and his stimulating observations have gained increasing support as our knowledge of tissue and organ transplantation has extended. In his laboratory studies on mice, he has shown the important role which the regional lymph nodes play in the development of systemic immunity to tumour cells, and how this immunity may be lost if the regional lymph nodes are removed. This experience has led him to advise against the removal of uninvolved axillary nodes. He states "Since systemic immunity to the spread of small cancers may reside largely in the regional lymph nodes, such cancers should probably be treated first by local excision or local radiation, sparing the nodes. Perhaps it is only in the treatment of large and advanced cancers that lymph nodes, involved or uninvolved, can be removed with impunity. In such circumstances, as much of the tumour as possible should be removed or destroyed in the hope that the host might regain immunologic competence against the tumour".

Recognizing the unreliability of clinical examination in the determination of the state of the axillary nodes, Crile inserts a finger into the axilla at the time of the operation and has shown that the error rate in assessing the state of the nodes, as judged by the appearance of enlarged nodes subsequent to treatment, is reduced to 8%. If the nodes seem to be uninvolved, the axilla is not dissected and only a simple mastectomy is performed. If and when enlarged nodes are discovered, they are removed and this delayed removal does not appear to impair the patient's prognosis. If the nodes are found to be involved and are still operable a modified radical mastectomy is performed with preservation of the pectoral muscle. The axillary dissection is deliberately less extensive than that usually performed in the standard radical operation and does not extend to the apex of the axilla because Crile believes, as Haagensen (1956) does, that axillary dissection will fail if the nodes are invaded. If the nodes are inoperable, he advises simple mastectomy with radiotherapy to the axilla. If there is any reason to suspect that the internal mammary nodes may be involved, they are treated by radiotherapy. The five year survival rate he obtained in a series of 256 patients in the operable Stages I and II was 70%.

It will be noted that Crile's approach is carefully (and by digital examination of the axilla fairly accurately) graded to the extent of the lymph node involvement. There is therefore much that can be said in favour of the policy he has advocated and this may still be the best line to pursue, even if it should be shown that the immunological response is not important in the control of distant metastases. If, however, it is established that a cancer specific antigen is produced in human breast cancer, and if the body is capable of an efficient response, it would be of the greatest importance to try to develop this response to its fullest extent. If the defence mechanism could be stimulated sufficiently to lead to the destruction of all tumour cells, this would be ideal. Even if we fall short of this ideal and succeed only in establishing some control over the growth of metastases, a very great advance would still have been made. Thus, if we could detect metastases at the pre-symptomatic stage and so control them that the patient remained asymptomatic for a period of several years this would, in many instances, be as effective as the admittedly more satisfying academic goal of complete destruction of all tumour cells. Every patient must die sooner or later and if we enable a patient to escape death from breast cancer, even if cancer cells are present at the time of death, then we would be quite entitled to claim that the breast cancer had been successfully treated.

As already stated, there is now abundant evidence to show that an immunological response does develop in certain tumours in experimental animals, and probably also in some human tumours. In human breast cancer however, the evidence in favour of an efficient response is still in doubt and we must recognize that all breast cancers may not evoke a response.

Quite apart from some self-induced change in the hormone status of the patient, spontaneous regression of clinically evident breast cancer must be exceedingly rare, if indeed it occurs at all. The only "spontaneous" regression in my personal experience of several thousand patients with breast cancer, was a pre-menopausal patient who showed a remarkable improvement in general health and in the metastases in her skeleton following extensive metastatic destruction of her ovaries.

We know too that many years usually elapse before breast cancer attains a size at which it may be recognized. Throughout this long period the host response has clearly been inadequate to prevent its continued growth. It has been suggested that the immunological response always lags behind the growth of the tumour and if the bulk of the tumour is removed, the balance could be so upset that the immunological response would then be adequate to control any residual tumour, at least for a period of time. It has also been suggested that if only a few malignant cells are left behind after the operation these cells could be overwhelmed and destroyed completely—a statement so easily made but so difficult to prove!

The lymphocyte reaction around tumours and the regional lymph node enlargement due to sinus histiocytosis are often quoted as evidence of a cancer specific response. Similar reactions however can be found in the absence of cancer (e.g. following the rupture of a cyst or of a duct) and we must interpret this finding with caution.

The success which may be obtained by simple mastectomy alone has sometimes been attributed to the fact that limited treatment does not interfere with the host reaction and that any residual cells are destroyed by this means. Limited forms of treatment are, as a rule, undertaken in selected patients with small tumours and therefore in circumstances where the prognosis is in any case favourable. We have become so conditioned to more radical treatment that we are immediately surprised if limited, but as we have seen, adequate treatment should prove successful.

The delay in the appearance of local recurrences or distant metastases has often been quoted in favour of the existence of some immunological control. We must note that tumour deposits grow at different rates and as Willis (1934) has pointed out so admirably in his book "The Spread of Tumours in the Human Body" the environment exerts a marked influence on tumour cells and even determines whether metastatic cells will grow or not. An unsuitable environment combined with a poor blood supply may be sufficient to explain many of these late metastases. We must note too that the delay in the appearance of metastases may be due to the simple fact that the natural rate of growth of the tumour is slow, as it is in differentiated tumours where the majority of the cells differentiate and few remain to continue the growth of the tumour.

While not intending to deny the existence of immunological control over tumour growth enough has now been said to show that we must not be too ready to accept as supporting evidence findings which may have an alternative and often simpler explanation.

Before leaving the conservative approach, reference must be made to the belief expressed from time to time that none of the methods of treatment we employ have any effect on the natural progress of breast cancer.

Lees and Park (1951) examined the influence of delay on the survival rates of patients whose mastectomy specimens had been sent to their laboratory. They found that there was no material difference between the survival rates of patients who sought advice quickly and the survival rates of patients who had delayed for many months. Since it did not appear to matter when the operation was performed they concluded that the operation had no influence on the survival rates and that it could be regarded as nothing more than an incident in the course of the disease.

Rapid growth of a tumour alarms a patient and stimulates her to seek advice quickly. It should also be noted that patients with rapidly growing tumours who delay for any length of time are automatically excluded from investigations of this type because they either become inoperable or die before reaching hospital. On the other hand the patient with a slowly growing tumour with little change in size from month to month, often delays in seeking advice and if she does, she is likely to remain operable and therefore eligible for inclusion in the analysis. As delay increases the proportion of less favourable tumours falls and the proportion of more favourable tumours increases, and accordingly it is not surprising that the survival rate is maintained in spite of the adverse influence of delay. The observation made by Lees and Park is quite correct and it is true in all sites. Indeed in some sites (e.g. thyroid) it will be found that the survival rates are much higher in patients who delay and that where long delay occurs nearly all the patients have well-differentiated tumours. It is unfortunate that Lees and Park interpreted their findings incorrectly because it is still stated from time to time that there is no advantage in early treatment.

Bond's (1968) observations have led him to believe that breast cancer is incurable, that metastases occur at a very early stage and that radiotherapy to patients with negative nodes may worsen the survival rate. The communication has attracted considerable attention and merits discussion in some detail.

Firstly he examined the ratio of cancer deaths to deaths from other causes. In a series of 3,665 patients in Manchester Stages I and II who had died from 1 to 25 years after treatment, he concluded that ". . . the disease is disseminated in all cases before a curative attempt was made, and that the disease is in fact incurable". The analysis shows that the proportion of deaths from other causes increases progressively in the following manner:

20% of the deaths in the 5th year were due to other causes.
50%   ,,   ,,   13th year   ,,   ,,
80%   ,,   ,,   25th year   ,,   ,,

In other words the longer the patient survived the greater was the chance of escaping death from breast cancer. As already noted every patient must die from some cause sooner or later and the patients who escape death from breast cancer can be regarded as having been successfully treated and in fact cured in the only practical sense of the term. Breast cancer could be regarded as incurable only if treatment endowed patients with an immunity to death from any other cause (and provided of course they did not achieve immortality!) It has long been known that patients may die from breast cancer many years after treatment and that the proportion who die from this cause depends on the extent of the disease at the time of treatment. Manchester Stages I and II are more advanced than International Stages I and II and include large primary tumours, tumours which have ulcerated and a higher proportion with secondarily involved nodes. In less advanced cancers the chance of dying after the 7th year from any cause may be no greater than in patients of the same age without breast cancer and when this stage is reached we are entitled to claim that treatment was successful.

Secondly Bond has concluded from a series of observations that metastatic spread occurs at a very early stage in the disease and he states ". . . that the first daughter cell from the first division may be the first metastasis". The conclusion is based on the extraordinarily variable accounts given by patients of the interval which has elapsed since they first noted the tumour. Patients not only vary greatly in their ability to recognize a mass in the breast but often have great difficulty in recalling when they first noticed it. Thus one patient may state that she has been aware of a 1 cm diameter tumour for over a year, while the next, presenting with a 10 cm tumour about to ulcerate through the skin, may claim that she only noted the swelling yesterday! This information of very doubtful value has been correlated with the size of the primary tumour. The communication does not reveal how the tumour size was determined. Measurements made by the pathologist would be reliable but if the size was based on the usual ward record where, as often as not, the house surgeon likens the tumour to various types of fruit, eggs and vegetables, then it would be as unwise to base a conclusion on tumour size as it would be to draw any deduction from the statements made by patients concerning delay. Nevertheless from such inaccurate information and from a relatively few observations plotted on semi-logarithmic paper Bond proceeds to extrapolate his graph backwards over a long period of time and claims that he has thereby established in virtually all cases ". . . that within a very few doubling times metastases must have occurred."

Thirdly Bond states "but when supplementary radiation is given in the node negative cases, for both radical and local mastectomy, there is a highly significant fall of 9% in the 5 year survival rate". Throughout his paper Bond stresses the importance of the regional nodes in the mediation of antibody response and where nodes do not appear to be involved he concludes ". . . it is clearly essential to maintain the viability of the nodes so that even node biopsy is impermissible" and goes on to state that "radiation is totally contra-indicated when the nodes are not involved clinically".

In the absence of a uniformly agreed policy, the treatment which any patient receives is a matter of individual judgement but when the methods employed in any one centre are analysed, certain trends can usually be distinguished. It is common to find that more extensive methods tend to be employed in patients with more extensive disease. It is important to examine the data in Bond's paper to see if this tendency exists.

First of all we may note that the 4,113 patients with negative nodes are equally distributed between the two surgical methods of treatment (50% radical mastectomy and 50% local mastectomy) but when the 2,366 patients with positive nodes are examined we find that three times as many were treated by radical mastectomy (74% compared with 26%). Analysed according to the clinical extent of the disease, we find that twice as many Stage II patients were treated by radical mastectomy (66% by radical mastectomy and 34% by local mastectomy). It is therefore obvious that patients with more extensive disease tended to be treated by more extensive surgery.

Interest centres on the use of radiotherapy and the overall position is set out in the following table (taken from Bond's Table III)

TABLE II

ALL PATIENTS IN STAGES I AND II

Operation	Radiotherapy	% of Patients in Stage II	% of Patients with positive nodes
Local Mastectomy	No R.T.	21	11
	R.T.	35	28
Radical Mastectomy	No R.T.	31	24
	R.T.	48	55

Following both operations it will be seen that radiotherapy was given more often to patients with more extensive disease as determined either by clinical examination or by the state of the nodes.

Turning now to the use of radiotherapy after local mastectomy in patients with negative nodes, the first question which arises is—why was radiotherapy given to 68% of the patients and why was it withheld in the remaining 32%? In view of the general trend just demonstrated it is difficult to avoid the conclusion that radiotherapy was given to patients with more extensive disease. The conclusion finds further support from within the present group of patients. We are told (Table III, Bond) that nodes were excised in only 24·6% of patients not given radiotherapy and in only 21·1% of those given radiotherapy. Thus, of the 2,669 patients treated by local mastectomy, nodes were excised in only 589 patients. In the remaining 2,080 patients the state of the nodes appears to have been assessed from the clinical findings. Since the above numbers approximate very closely to the numbers of patients stated to have positive and negative nodes it is highly probable that nodes were removed only when they were thought to be positive.

TABLE III

ALL PATIENTS TREATED BY LOCAL MASTECTOMY

	No. of Patients		No. of Patients
Nodes excised	589	Nodes stated to be Positive	618
Nodes not excised	2080	Nodes stated to be Negative	2051
Total	2669	Total	2669

Clinical assessment of the state of the nodes is unreliable. The percentage of positive nodes can be seriously underestimated in patients who do not have palpable nodes. The following table (taken from Table III, Bond) comes as no surprise:

TABLE IV

ALL PATIENTS IN STAGES I AND II

PERCENTAGE WITH POSITIVE NODES

	Stage I	Stage II	Total
	%	%	%
Local Mastectomy	12	47	23
Radical Mastectomy	31	66	46

As expected the discrepancy is most marked in Stage I patients and there can be little doubt that many of the local mastectomy patients assigned to the 'negative' node category did in fact have positive nodes. This point appears to have been appreciated at the time of treatment because the proportion of 'negative' node patients given radiotherapy was higher in the local mastectomy group (68% compared with 57%) and it would seem reasonable to presume that radiotherapy was given whenever there was any doubt about the state of the nodes and that it was withheld only where there was no reason to suspect node involvement. The high survival rate (Table V, Bond) in the patients where radiotherapy was withheld would be difficult to explain on any other basis.

Bond states that the odds are 10,000,000 to 1 against the difference of 9% being a chance observation and concludes ". . . we must accept the reduced survival as resulting from the use of radiation". When a difference of this order is found we are entitled to assume that *some factor* has almost certainly been responsible for the difference—but it does not follow that it must be the factor we would like it to be. We must examine the data very carefully and look for the most probable explanation. As we have seen the difference could be very easily explained by the inclusion of patients with positive nodes in the irradiated group.

It should be noted that no evidence is presented in support of the statement that ". . . even lymph node biopsy is impermissible"—the complete surgical removal of the axillary nodes has no adverse effect on the age corrected five year survival rate (Table V, Bond).

Speaking about antibody production in the regional lymph nodes, Bond (1968) also states "Their retention for a period following mastectomy might reduce local recurrence. . . ." In his Table VII the total local recurrence rate in unirradiated node negative patients is 15% (4·1% plus 10·9%) in the local mastectomy group and 8·9% (2·9% plus 6·0%) in the radical mastectomy patients—i.e. the local recurrence rate is almost halved in the patients in whom the nodes were removed!

Having removed the all important regional nodes from the axilla it is also difficult to see how radiation following radical mastectomy could have an adverse effect. The remaining nodes in the internal mammary and supraclavicular regions are all relatively small and few in number.

At a time when extravagant claims were being advanced in support of the value of the cancer campaigns launched upon the public, McKinnon (1954) drew attention to the fact that none of these measures had brought about a reduction in the national death rate from breast cancer. The pathologist nowadays is often called upon to examine tissue removed from breasts where there was only a minor degree of induration. At times he may have considerable difficulty in reaching a decision and there is no doubt that he now reports many more borderline malignancies. These borderline cases contribute to better survival rates but their treatment does not influence the national death rate, because as McKinnon pointed out, many of these lesions would not have proved fatal if they had been left untreated.

The improvement in the survival rates of treated patients is also due to the more careful selection of patients for treatment and the fact that the proportion of patients with positive nodes has fallen from 60% to 40% is good evidence that fewer advanced patients are now being treated. The interesting point is the fact that this more careful selection has not led to fewer patients being treated. Indeed the reverse is the case. Many more patients now seek advice at an earlier stage so that a higher fraction of the total patients satisfy the more strict criteria of operability. But if higher survival rates are being obtained in a larger fraction of the total patients the national death rate from breast cancer should fall. The paradox may be explained by a rising incidence of breast cancer but since we refuse to accept compulsory registration of cancer we cannot be sure that this is so. The adoption of a complete cancer registration scheme is clearly required so that we may find out what progress, if any, is being made.

OTHER FORMS OF THERAPY

Endocrine therapy may bring about such a striking improvement in some patients that the hope was entertained at one time that it might be possible by this means to achieve permanent control over the disease or even its complete eradication. Endocrine therapy remains a very valuable means of palliation but unfortunately the benefit conferred is always temporary. As in every other type of cancer, the value of cytotoxic drugs has been extensively investigated but compared with endocrine therapy, palliation is obtained less often, any improvement which does occur is of shorter duration and the side effects are such that this form of treatment is falling into disfavour.

TREATMENT POLICY PROPOSED

Surgery and radiotherapy thus remain the only two methods of treatment whereby cure may be obtained but in their application our outlook may be beginning to change.

As we have seen, one of the most interesting developments in the treatment of breast cancer in recent years is the possibility of being able to control the disease by immunological means. The work of Crile (1967) in this field is outstanding and his observations should be studied in full. If it can be shown that a cancer specific antigen is produced in human breast cancer, and if the body is capable of an efficient response, not only would his conservative approach be fully justified but the further exploitation of this field might well revolutionize our whole approach to breast cancer. However, until further evidence becomes available it is important that we should not attribute to a tumour host reaction, findings which could well be explained on some other basis. As Crile (1967) himself points out a clinical trial is required for the more complete evaluation of the role of immunology in the control of breast cancer.

We saw that the extent of treatment should be determined by the extent of the disease and if we had the ability to detect the precise extent of disease in every patient our problems in respect of treatment would be largely resolved. A good case can be made out for more conservative treatment in many patients whereas in others more radical treatment must be adopted if the patients are to be offered any prospect of cure. Ability to detect small metastatic foci in distant sites is still a long way off and we have no option but to continue to offer full treatment to all patients in whom distant metastases cannot be demonstrated. Fortunately considerable progress has been made in the detection of spread to the regional lymph nodes. Accordingly, following the usual clinical and radiographic investigations, the state of the regional lymph nodes must, for the time being, be our guide to the extent of treatment. The state of the axillary nodes may be ascertained by digital examination as Crile (1967) advises, or by removing the lower nodes and submitting them to immediate histological examination. In the detection of spread to the internal mammary nodes and to the nodes at the apex of the axilla, the technique adopted by Haagensen (1956) would appear to be most appropriate.

Investigation of the state of the lymph nodes will prolong the time taken for the operation but the advantages are considerable. In approximately half the patients in whom radical mastectomy is currently performed it should be possible to reduce treatment to simple mastectomy alone. It is worth pointing out that some of these negative node patients will die from distant metastases because blood spread can occur before the regional nodes are invaded. The important point which must be noted is that more extensive treatment could not be any more effective and might even be harmful in patients whose tumours are under immunological control. By investigating the nodes in the manner described the more extensive methods of treatment could be reserved for patients beyond the scope of radical mastectomy.

The policy just outlined can be illustrated in a little more detail as follows. (It has been assumed in all patients that the disease within the breast is operable.)

1A. *Axillary Nodes Negative.* Primary tumour in lateral half of breast
      No further node biopsy required
      Simple mastectomy alone

1B. *Axillary Nodes Negative.* Primary tumour in medial half of breast or subareolar.

    Biopsy internal mammary nodes
- (a) If internal mammary nodes negative
  Simple mastectomy alone
- (b) If internal mammary nodes positive
  Simple mastectomy and radiotherapy or Urban operation.

2. *Axillary Nodes Positive and Mobile*
    Biopsy internal mammary and apical axillary nodes
- (a) If internal mammary and apical axillary nodes negative
  Patey or Halsted operation
- (b) If internal mammary nodes positive and apical axillary nodes negative
  Simple mastectomy and radiotherapy or Urban operation
- (c) If internal mammary nodes negative or positive and apical axillary nodes positive
  Simple mastectomy and radiotherapy

3. *Axillary Nodes Fixed and/or Supraclavicular Nodes Enlarged.*
    Simple mastectomy and radiotherapy

Before long this or any other scheme of treatment based on the state of the regional nodes could provide information of considerable interest. Subdivision of patients in this manner could also be of great value when different methods of treatment are being compared.

B. COMPARISON OF THE VALUE OF DIFFERENT METHODS OF TREATMENT

In the policy just outlined different methods of treatment were proposed. Others could be suggested. It is important to find out which method is best.

At first sight it might appear that the best method of treatment could be recognized without difficulty from an examination of the survival rates. There would indeed be no difficulty if survival rates were determined entirely by the method of treatment. Unfortunately this is not so. Many factors influence survival rates; treatment is only one factor and is not necessarily the most important.

Some of the more important factors influencing survival rates are as follows: the age and general health of the patient; the proportion of undifferentiated cells and the rate of growth of the tumour; the size of the primary tumour and the extent to which spread has occurred, to adjacent structures, to the regional lymph nodes, and to more distant sites.

If no treatment is given the shape of the survival curve is determined by the combined influence of these factors and will vary according to the influence exerted by each factor. Thus in respect of the rate of growth, the shape of the curve for slowly growing tumours will be quite different from that of rapidly growing tumours. This curve, obtained in the absence of treatment, might, for convenience, be labelled the 'basic survival curve'.

When treatment is given these factors continue to exert their influence and the 'basic survival curve' is modified only if treatment is effective and only in so far as treatment can exert an effect. The first point is self evident; the second requires some elaboration. Effective treatment will modify the 'basic survival curve' if in the majority of patients, the tumour is small and the disease is confined to the primary site. On the other hand the shape of the 'basic survival curve' may not be modified appreciably if in the majority of patients, the disease has already spread to distant sites.

When two different methods of treatment are being compared our difficulties would disappear if we had the ability to form groups of patients with identical 'basic survival curves'. When a clinical trial is undertaken we try to get as near to these ideal conditions as it is possible to do so. Conscious selection of the treatment method is avoided by allocating treatment on a randomized basis. We rely on the assignment of adequate numbers to each of the two methods to ensure that the two groups of patients will be as nearly comparable as it is possible to make them. Adequate numbers are therefore essential if one of the main requirements of a trial is to be satisfied. When, however, do the numbers become adequate?

ADEQUATE NUMBERS

If all the patients entering a trial had much the same life expectancy or 'basic survival curve' then relatively small numbers should suffice to ensure comparability. This fortunate state of affairs might obtain in a trial involving healthy mice all of the same age and all derived from the same inbred strain. In a clinical trial involving breast cancer the position is quite different. There is marked variation in age, extent of disease, rate of growth of the tumour and indeed, in every one of the factors which affect the 'basic survival rate'. In these circumstances the numbers required to ensure comparability will be much higher and probably considerably higher than has been appreciated hitherto. Some indication of the numbers required could be gained by treating the two groups of patients in a trial, not by different methods but by the same method. If the numbers are adequate the survival rates should be the same. Clinical trials involving the same method of treatment could be organized very easily. No ethical problems would arise and the results would be of considerable interest.

This test of adequacy of numbers can be incorporated within a trial designed to compare the value of two different methods of treatment. Having formed the two main groups in the usual way, each group is then divided by a second random procedure into two sub-groups. The sub-groups can be identified by a suitable symbol and the trial then proceeds in the ordinary way but we now have two groups of patients treated by one method and two groups treated by the other. This in fact is what has been done in a clinical trial at present being undertaken in Edinburgh.

The trial, in which radical mastectomy is compared with simple mastectomy and radiotherapy, was commenced in 1964 and up until the end of March 1969 the total number of patients entered was 396. It is much too soon to attempt a complete analysis but the four year survival rates, obtained by actuarial or life table analysis, are of interest in relation to the problem of adequacy of numbers. Subgroups R.1 and R.2 were treated by radical mastectomy and subgroups S.1 and S.2 were treated by simple mastectomy and radiotherapy.

TABLE V

TOTAL PATIENTS

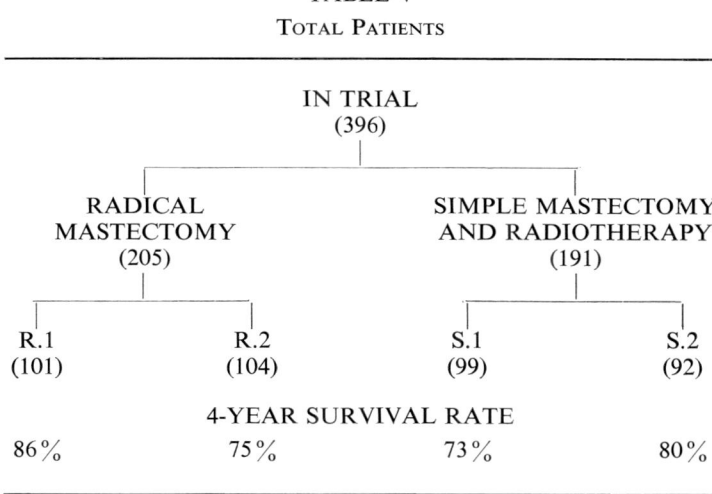

IN TRIAL (396)			
RADICAL MASTECTOMY (205)		SIMPLE MASTECTOMY AND RADIOTHERAPY (191)	
R.1 (101)	R.2 (104)	S.1 (99)	S.2 (92)
4-YEAR SURVIVAL RATE			
86%	75%	73%	80%

The difference in the survival rates of the patients treated by the same method is of particular interest. The difference in the survival rates of the R.1 and R.2 patients is 11% and is just on the borderline of being statistically significant (2 S.E.D. $= 11\cdot3$). The finding illustrates the importance of the numbers being adequate to ensure comparability.

If R.1 and R.2 patients had been treated by different methods it might have been concluded that the method employed in R.1 patients was superior to that by which R.2 patients had been treated!

SUBSEQUENT TREATMENT

In any trial involving patients subsequent treatment must never be withheld even although it should complicate the assessment of the results.

Subsequent treatment may be required when the original method fails and if completely or even only partially successful the survival rates will no longer reflect the true value of the original method. Recurrence-free rates may be a better basis of assessment.

In the Edinburgh Trial a number of patients in the radical mastectomy series received radiotherapy for recurrences. In some, the treatment was at least temporarily successful. In the simple mastectomy series further radiotherapy could not be given and local recurrences were rarely excisable.

TABLE VI

SURVIVAL RATES AND RECURRENCE-FREE RATES

	Radical Mastectomy	Simple Mastectomy and Radiotherapy
No. of Deaths	29	36
4-year Survival Rates	80%	76%
No. Alive but Recurrent*	21	10
Total Dead or Recurrent	50	46
4-year Recurrent-Free Rates	69%	72%

* Includes patients whose recurrence had been apparently successfully treated and who were free from disease at the time of the assessment.

Subsequent treatment is usually only temporarily successful and, as a rule, has little influence on ten year survival rates. When the assessment is made at an earlier date, say at the end of five years, recurrence-free rates should be presented.

DIFFERENCES CONFINED TO A SMALL FRACTION

A trial is ethical only if those taking part in it are completely satisfied beforehand that they do not know whether one method of treatment is better than the other. It follows that the survival rates of the methods compared are unlikely to differ greatly from one another.

In trials involving methods which have in common the removal of the breast by surgery, any difference in the survival rates will be limited to a small fraction of the total patients. Whatever additional treatment is given, it will have no influence on the survival rates of patients with negative nodes or patients with distant metastases. We saw previously that these two groups account for some 84% of the operable patients. Accordingly additional methods of treatment cannot influence the outcome in more than 16 out of every 100 patients treated. If, for example, a trial were undertaken to compare axillary dissection extending to the apical nodes with some less extensive surgical procedure or to compare surgery with radiotherapy in the treatment of axillary nodes, then the difference in the overall survival rates could not exceed 16%. Indeed the difference is likely to be much less, because a difference of 16% could arise only if all 16 patients treated by one method survived and all 16 patients treated by the other method died. A small difference in a small fraction of the total patients may not produce a statistically significant difference in the overall survival rates and it is therefore not surprising that in most of the trials already completed it has been reported that the methods compared, appeared to be of equal value.

Subdivision of the patients (or stratification as it is sometimes called) according to the state of the regional nodes is clearly essential for the identification of the subgroup (or subgroups) in which one method may be better than any other.

CONCLUSIONS

From all that has been said it will now be obvious that in the design and interpretation of clinical trials the clinician and the statistician have each an important role to play.

When a statistically significant difference is found in the survival rates, the clinician must examine the data very carefully to determine which factor (or factors) is most likely to be responsible. He must not be too ready to conclude that the factor responsible is the one he would like it to be.

It is important to bear in mind that survival rates are not determined entirely by treatment. The two groups of patients must be comparable in all material respects before a difference in the survival rates can be attributed to a difference in value of the methods of treatment employed. We rely on the allocation of adequate numbers to each group to ensure comparability and we have seen that the numbers required in clinical trials may be much higher than has been appreciated hitherto.

Subsequent treatment may distort the earlier survival rates and if the analysis is undertaken in less than ten years, recurrence-free rates should also be presented.

The ethical requirements of a trial render it unlikely that there will be a marked difference in the survival rates. When methods do differ in value, the difference will almost certainly be limited to a small fraction of the total patients.

In conclusion it may be stated that while clinical trials undoubtedly afford the best means of comparing the value of different methods of treatment they must never be regarded as a simple means of solving our problems.

REFERENCES

BOND, W. H. (1968). The influence of various treatments on survival rates in cancer of the breast. In 'Proceedings of a Symposium on the Treatment of Carcinoma of the Breast', Jarrett, A. S. (Ed.). Amsterdam: Excerpta Medica Foundation, 24.

CRILE, G., Jr. (1967). A Biological Consideration of Treatment of Breast Cancer. Illinois: Charles C. Thomas.

FITZWILLIAMS, D. C. L. (1940). A plea for a more local operation in really early breast carcinoma. Br. med. J., ii, 405.

FRASER, Sir J. (1939). Some reflections on the pathogenesis and treatment of cancer of the breast. Edinburgh Post-Graduate Lectures in Medicine. Vol. 1. Edinburgh: Oliver and Boyd.

GUTTMANN, R. J. (1962). Survival and results after 2 million volt irradiation in the treatment of primary operable carcinoma of the breast with proved positive internal mammary and/or highest axillary nodes. Cancer, 15, 383.

HAAGENSEN, C. D. (1956). Disease of the Breast. Philadelphia: W. B. Saunders Co.

HANDLEY, R. S. (1952). Further observations of internal mammary lymph chain in carcinoma of breast. Proc. R. Soc. Med., 45, 565.

KEYNES, G. (1937). Conservative treatment of cancer of breast. Br. med. J., ii, 643.

McKINNON, N. E. (1954). Control of cancer mortality. Lancet, i, 251.

McWHIRTER, R. (1964). Should more radical treatment be attempted in breast cancer? Am. J. Roentg., 92, 3.

MUSTAKALLIO, S. (1954). Treatment of breast cancer by tumour extirpation and roentgen therapy instead of radical operations. J. Fac. Radiol., 6, 23.

PARK, W. W. & LEES, J. C. (1951). The absolute curability of cancer of breast. Surgery, Gynec. Obstet., 93, 129.

PATERSON, R. & RUSSELL, M. H. (1959). Clinical trials in malignant disease. Part III. Breast cancer: evaluation of post-operative radiotherapy. J. Fac. Radiol., 10, 175.

PORRITT, A. (1964). Early carcinoma of the breast. Br. J. Surg., 51, 214.

URBAN, J. A. (1964). Surgical excision of internal mammary nodes for breast cancer. Br. J. Surg., 51, 209.

WANGENSTEEN, O. H., LEWIS, F. J., & ARHELGER, S. W. (1956). Extended or superradical mastectomy for carcinoma of breast. Surg. Clins N. Am., 36, 1051.

WILLIS, R. A. (1934). The Spread of Tumours in the Human Body. London: J. & A. Churchill.

2 Cancer Chemotherapy— The Present Position

I. D. H. TODD

This chapter excludes the chemotherapy of choriocarcinoma and of the acute leukaemias since these are dealt with in Chapters 3 and 4. It deals mainly with the chemotherapy of the lymphomas and, to a lesser extent, of the solid tumours. Special reference is made to combination therapy using radiotherapy with cytotoxic drugs.

INTRODUCTION

The chemotherapy of malignant disease has now been practised for over twenty five years. Special interest during this period has always been given to newly developed drugs, especially when these are in a different class from the existing agents. During the past decade or so, a number of new agents have come into use and, of those which are likely to remain in use, one must mention the vinca alkaloids, vinblastine and vincristine, the methyl-hydrazine derivative procarbazine, actinomycin D and cyclophosphamide. Many other agents have been tried and particular interest has been aroused by hydroxyurea and asparaginase though neither drug is really outstanding in the type of disease considered in this chapter. Whilst one always hopes for brilliant new drugs one cannot count on their arrival, so much effort has been put into studying the most effective uses of the present agents. This has often entailed using a combined approach, either two or more cytotoxic drugs, a cytotoxic drug with a hormone, or drugs in association with radiotherapy. The number of variables in these studies is so high, when account is taken of the pattern of the diseases under consideration and the almost limitless possibilities of permutating drugs and doses, that final answers will be a long time in coming. However, safe combinations and some impressive results have been achieved and will be mentioned in due course.

A number of general texts have been published on cancer chemotherapy. With regard to pharmacology the chapter in Goodman and

Gilman (Calabresi and Welch, 1965) is very good and the article by Oliverio and Zubrod (1965) in the Annual Review of Pharmacology is also helpful. With regard to the clinical aspects, both for the specialist and for the non-specialist, the following two books can be unreservedly recommended: *Cancer Chemotherapy* by Greenwald (1967) and *Cytotoxic Drugs in the Treatment of Cancer* by Boesen and Davis (1969).

HODGKIN'S DISEASE AND MALIGNANT LYMPHOMA

Most workers find that Hodgkin's disease is more responsive to chemotherapy than the other varieties of lymphoma, but even though this be accepted it is often worthwhile attempting chemotherapy for malignant lymphoma in the same way as for Hodgkin's disease itself. Many alkylating agents have been used in the treatment of Hodgkin's disease and have proved to be effective but those in most widespread use at present are probably mustine, chlorambucil and cyclophosphamide. The response rate to any one of these agents, when used as the first cytotoxic agent, is about 60% but the duration of response tends to be short (e.g. Karnofsky, Miller and Phillips report 6–10 weeks duration on average), although Scott (1963) does claim that the period can be extended by the use of chlorambucil. In his series the average duration of response with mustine is 12 weeks and this is extended to 36 weeks by the use of chlorambucil as a maintenance agent. In the author's experience (Todd, 1970) maintenance therapy does not prolong the duration of remission in the case of cyclophosphamide nor of chlorambucil used alone but he is unaware of a published series precisely similar to that of Scott.

When relapse occurs and a second treatment is required the response rate in the case of mustine falls to about 30%. In fact, it is also of this order if an alternative alkylating agent such as cyclophosphamide is used, indicating some degree of cross resistance. Fortunately certain new drugs have been introduced which, whilst producing the same order of response rate as the alkylating agents, do not show cross resistance to them.

The first of these is vinblastine, which became widely available about 1960 and now has a firmly established place. The earlier dose schedules for vinblastine were presented on a weight basis but the present tendency, where the drug is being used alone in the treatment of an adult, is to give it as a standard weekly intravenous dose of 10 mg, dropping the dose or extending the interval between doses once response has occurred. On this regime it is necessary to give at least 40 mg before it can be decided that the patient is not going to respond. Given adequate dosage the response rate is high; Armstrong (1966), from the pooled results of fifteen North American papers, quotes 72% and Jelliffe (1969), in a series of 126 patients, quotes 74%. In order to avoid the inconvenience of regular intravenous injections, although as these can be administered to outpatients the disadvantage is less than with mustine, attempts have been made to give vinblastine by mouth (Bond, Rohn, Bates, and Hodes, 1966; Macdonald and Lacher, 1966) but were abandoned due to uncertainty of absorption and gastrointestinal complications. Vinblastine has been compared directly with alkylating agents. For example, in papers from Roswell Park, Stutzman, Ezdinli and Stutzman (1966) and Ezdinli and Stutzman (1968), vinblastine is compared with cyclophosphamide and mustine, and the conclusion is drawn that vinblastine is superior to cyclophosphamide but that there is no significant difference between vinblastine and mustine in the ability to induce a remission. They also suggest that the sequence *mustine – vinblastine* is superior to *vinblastine – mustine*.

The second agent is procarbazine (formerly known as ibenzmethyzin) which first became available for clinical trial in 1963. This drug is given by mouth in a dose of up to 300 mg daily. Its main disadvantage is a tendency to cause nausea and vomiting in about 30% of patients although this can often be controlled by an antiemetic such as chlorpromazine and tends to diminish or disappear if the drug induces a remission. Procarbazine also has the less common side effect of incompatibility with alcohol so patients must be warned of this possibility. Much useful information on this drug, including evidence for its lack of cross resistance with the alkylating agents and vinblastine, is available in *Natulan* edited by Jelliffe and Marks (1965).

There is, at present, growing enthusiasm for various combinations of chemotherapeutic agents in the primary treatment of advanced Hodgkin's disease (the use of radiotherapy for the primary treatment of Stages 1 and 2 Hodgkin's disease is undisputed). The use of combination treatment has received impetus from the successes achieved in the palliation of acute leukaemia in childhood. Reports by Frei, DeVita, Moxley and Carbone (1966) and by Carbone (1967) outline certain combinations and their early results. They use the following two programmes:—

A

Cyclophosphamide	600 mg/m²	Days 1 and 7 i.v.
Vincristine	1·2 mg/m²	Days 1 and 7 i.v.
Methotrexate	30 mg/m²	every 4 days i.v.
Prednisone	60 mg/m²	daily p.o.

Each course to last 14 days. Three courses in all.

B

Nitrogen mustard	6 mg/m²	Days 1 and 7 i.v.
Vincristine	1·4 mg/m²	Days 1 and 7 i.v.
Procarbazine	100 mg/m²	daily p.o.
Prednisone	40 mg/m²	daily p.o.
		courses 1 and 4

Each course to last 14 days. Six courses in all.

Rest periods of 14 days or longer are allowed between courses. Using this type of treatment they claim 80% complete, with an additional 10% partial, remissions in previously untreated patients. They also claim the average duration of unmaintained remission to be in excess of 10 months. These results are impressive and are supported by work from other centres, e.g. Nicholson and colleagues (1970), but there are as yet no published results to compare this type of regime with the more conventional sequential chemotherapy. It also appears that quadruple chemotherapy is much less effective and less well tolerated in patients who have had previous chemotherapy or previous extensive radiotherapy. There is now considerable evidence, especially from Kaplan (e.g. Kaplan and Rosenberg, 1966) that aggressive radiotherapy to all standard lymph node regions leads to more prolonged and better quality remissions than are obtained with shorter courses and lighter dosage. Trials are now under way, in several areas, to compare radiotherapy of the Kaplan type with quadruple chemotherapy (using, usually, a modification of programme B above) in the primary treatment of advanced Hodgkin's disease.

CHRONIC MYELOID LEUKAEMIA

The most important recent publication in the U.K. on this disease is that on the *Comparison of Radiotherapy and Busulphan Therapy* by the Medical Research Council's Working Party for Therapeutic Trials in Leukaemia (1968). This was a random trial involving 102 previously untreated patients; 48 were started with busulphan and 54 with radiotherapy, usually X-ray treatment to the spleen. Three features were taken into particular account during assessment of the patients: survival, control of spleen size, and efficiency in restoring and maintaining satisfactory levels of haemoglobin concentration. The latter two features were used to give an objective value for the quality of survival.

In terms of survival and maintenance of haemoglobin concentration the busulphan group showed a definite superiority, and in control of spleen size it was also superior though to a lesser extent. From this trial it is clear that chemotherapy using busulphan is the better form of management although the trial is open to the criticism that a regime using a continuous treatment, busulphan, is compared with an intermittent regime using radiotherapy, and in some cases the relapse after one course of radiotherapy had been allowed to progress to an advanced stage before a further course was begun. Unfortunately the rate of response to the two forms of treatment is not recorded, so one cannot test the impression that radiotherapy gives a faster initial response. (If this were the case then the sequential use of splenic irradiation and busulphan may provide the optimum management.) Whilst accepting that busulphan should be the mainstay in managing the patient with chronic myeloid leukaemia, radiotherapy will still have a place in the refractory case and where there is some urgency in obtaining a response.

Apart from the well established risks of excessive marrow depression (much less often seen with low dose schedules of the order of 2–6 mg daily), amenorrhoea in menstruating women, skin pigmentation, and occasional gastrointestinal toxicity, Kyle, Schwartz, Oliver and Dameshek (1961) also draw attention to the rarer complications seen with busulphan therapy. These include testicular atrophy, hyperuricaemia, a syndrome clinically suggesting adrenal cortical insufficiency, and pulmonary fibrosis. The syndrome suggesting adrenal cortical insufficiency includes skin pigmentation, weakness, anorexia and loss of weight, although laboratory investigations do not show evidence of adrenal failure. The pulmonary fibrosis may respond to steroid therapy (Neu, 1962).

Whilst busulphan remains the standard drug for the management of chronic myeloid leukaemia, claims have been made for other agents. For example, dibromomannitol has been put forward by Eckhardt, Sellei, Horvath, and Institoris (1963) and appears to be effective. Experience with this drug is limited outside Hungary, but Ramanan and Israëls (1969) have treated 13 patients and consider the drug to be effective but to have no advantages over busulphan. Wilson, Monto, Pisciotta, Rohn and Louis (1969) describe the use of piposulfan and state: "The therapeutic effectiveness of this agent appears to be similar to that for busulphan". Hydroxyurea has also received considerable attention recently (Symposia on Hydroxyurea, 1964 and 1967) and is of proven effectiveness in chronic myeloid leukaemia both in the chronic phase and in the blastic phase, although in the latter state, the response tends to be very short lived. This drug is probably best held in reserve until conventional treatment fails.

POLYCYTHAEMIA VERA

During the past twenty years, radiophosphorus treatment has been generally accepted as providing the best long-term management of polycythaemia. However, this view was challenged by Perkins, Israëls and Wilkinson (1964) who suggested that the disease could equally well be managed by drugs and, furthermore, that the risk of terminal acute leukaemia was less (no such case occurred in the 127 patients they reported). The drugs used include thiotepa, pyrimethamine, mustine, busulphan, naphthyl-chloroethylamine, triethylenemelamine, mannomustine, uracil mustard and acetylphenylhydrazine. Venesection was used in most patients at some time and a few had no specific therapy. The authors kindly supplied their full data to Halnan and Russell (1965) who were able to compare a series of 107 patients treated during approximately the same period and in the same city but using

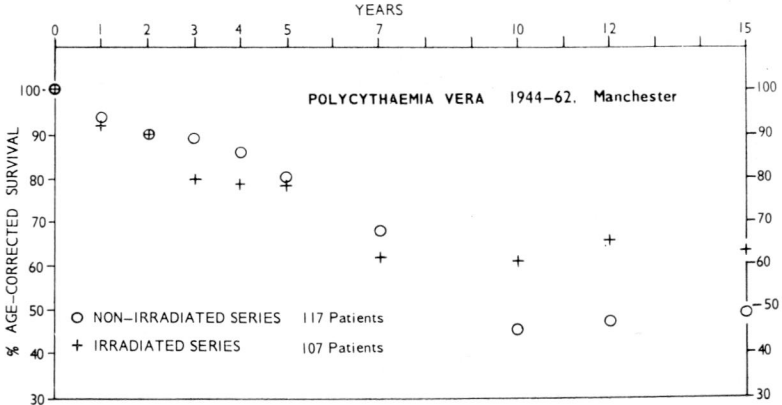

FIG. 2.1. This is taken from Halnan and Russell (1965). It shows how the survival rates for the series of irradiated and non-irradiated patients are closely similar, there being no significant difference between them.

radiotherapy as the principle treatment. No case of leukaemia was recorded in their series and there was no significant difference in the survival rates (Fig. 1). Watkins, Fairley and Scott (1967) have published a series of 81 patients, the great majority of whom were managed with radiophosphorus, in which one case of acute leukaemia and one of acute erythraemic myelosis occurred, and in which the survival rate is similar to that presented by Perkins *et al* and by Halnan and Russell. If it is accepted that the survival rates are the same, then other factors such as convenience to the patient and ease of surveillance will determine the best form of management. In the majority, radiophosphorus does provide a very convenient form of management although it is reassuring to know that, in other respects, chemotherapy is not inferior and can be used with confidence where necessary.

MULTIPLE MYELOMA

It is now clear that survival rates have been substantially improved since the introduction of melphalan and cyclophosphamide in the treatment of myeloma. For example, Bergsagel, Sprague, Austin and Griffith (1962), and Speed, Galton and Swan (1964) have demonstrated the effectiveness of melphalan, and Rivers, Whittington and Patno (1963) that of cyclophosphamide. In most series, the survival times have been doubled or trebled in the responders. About 50% of the patients treated appear to respond but there is general agreement that, in the non-responders, the drugs should be abandoned in order to conserve the marrow.

Cyclophosphamide and melphalan have been compared (Galton and Peto, 1968; Rivers and Patno, 1969 and Medical Research Council's Working Party for Therapeutic Trials in Leukaemia 1971), in the management of myelomatosis and appear to be equally effective. These drugs are usually given in a low dose maintenance regime, although there are proponents for regimes using higher but intermittent dosage. Hoogstraten, Costa, Cuttner, Forcier, Leone, Harley and Gildewell (1969), who have used intermittent therapy, find that it is less effective than continuous maintenance therapy for the control of pain.

It must not be forgotten that corticosteroids also have a specific effect in myelomatosis. Alexanian, Haut, Khan, Lane, McKelvey, Migliore, Stuckey and Wilson (1969) show that the "median survival for patients treated with melphalan–prednisone was about six months longer than the survival of patients treated with melphalan alone". Salmon, Shadduck and Schilling (1967) in a small series suggest that the best method of giving prednisone may be in a dosage of 200 mg every other morning, but this awaits confirmation.

At present the optimum method of managing myelomatosis would appear to be by continuous low doses of cyclophosphamide or melphalan. If no response occurs, the drug should be abandoned and prednisone substituted. If response is established on the chosen alkylating agent, then prednisone may also be added to the regime (the delay in adding prednisone being to ensure that patients do not have prolonged fruitless treatment with a cytotoxic agent). Radiotherapy would still be available for the non-responder and, in particular, for relief of local bone pain.

SOLID TUMOURS

When a new agent is introduced it is customary to try it in a wide variety of solid tumours but there are few enough drugs of sufficient value to be used routinely in the management of tumours in such sites as breast, bronchus, ovary, testis, colon and in malignant melanoma. Cyclophosphamide is probably the most generally useful cytotoxic drug in conditions such as carcinoma of the breast or carcinoma of the bronchus because it has a wide margin of safety in its dosage (cf. thiotepa) and can be given by mouth. Its major complication is the high incidence of partial epilation and this complication cannot be avoided— it was once considered that a scalp tourniquet applied before an injection of the drug would offer protection but a trial of this device showed it to be a failure. (Cole, M. P., Jackson, A. W. and Todd, I. D. H. in a series of 37 patients treated in the Christie Hospital, Manchester, found an epilation rate of the same order as that obtained with the oral routine and no tourniquet. Further when cyclophosphamide, tagged with radiophosphorous, was used a similar count rate was recorded above and below the tourniquet, indicating the ineffectiveness of this procedure). Brock (1967) has since published clear evidence that cyclophosphamide is activated in the liver; although apparently only 10% of the drug is so activated it accounts for almost all of the drug's activity.

In carcinoma of the breast about one third of the patients with advanced malignancy may be expected to respond to cyclophosphamide or an alternative agent such as thiotepa. Attempts have been made to improve the response rate and to diminish the degree of marrow depression by combining the cytotoxic drug with testosterone (Watson and Turner, 1959) or with an alternative anabolic steroid such as nandrolone.

Fluorouracil was synthesized in 1957 and was soon brought into clinical use (Curreri, Ansfield, McIver, Waisman and Heidelberger, 1958). In a review of a substantial series, such as the 594 cases described by Brennan, Talley, San Diego, Burrows, O'Bryan, Vaitkevicius and Horeglad (1964), the authors record a 20% response rate for carcinoma of colon, rectum, stomach and breast and rather less good results for cancer of the head and neck, ovary, cervix, liver and gall bladder. One of the disadvantages of fluorouracil therapy is that the standard course of treatment does require admission to hospital for about two weeks but methods have been developed which are suitable for outpatient treatment; for example Jacobs, Luce and Wood (1968) describe a method using rapid intravenous injections weekly.

One very new drug that should be mentioned is Bleomycin (Clinical Screening Group of E.O.R.T.C., 1970). This Japanese antibiotic appears particularly interesting since it is claimed to be selectively effective upon well differentiated squamous cell carcinoma, to have little or no effect upon the blood, and yet potentially capable of lethal side effects in the lungs, in the form of pneumonitis or fibrosis, possibly similar to 'busulphan lung'.

One new compound, I.C.R.F. 159, has recently shown to be selectively effective in mice in inhibiting metastatic spread (Salsbury, Burrage and Hellmann 1970). Only very preliminary work has so far been undertaken in man.

Intra-arterial chemotherapy was developed from 1950 onwards as an attempt to concentrate the cytotoxic drug in the tumour and, at the same time, reduce systemic toxic effects. It found its main application in the management of solid tumours as most of these are relatively resistant to the available drugs administered systemically. The initial uncritical enthusiasm for this procedure has evaporated and it is now reserved mainly for uncontrolled malignant melanoma confined to a limb (Creech and Krementz, 1964). In particular the once widely practised treatment of head and neck tumours by this method has been virtually abandoned because of the high incidence of complications. As one of the contraindications to the method is previous radiotherapy, it may still find a place in areas where radiotherapy is not available.

The ultimate form of intra-arterial chemotherapy was the development of a technique for occlusion of the aorta in mid-torso to permit relative sparing of the marrow above or below the occlusion (Miller Lawrence, Kim, Dorrenchamp and Randall, 1962) and this method was applied in Kenya by Clifford, Oettgen, Beecher, Brown, Harries and Lawes (1963). The non-availability of radiotherapy in Kenya at the time was the main justification for employing the technique and may still provide a reason for using intra-arterial methods in certain areas.

SKIN CANCER

The chemotherapy of skin cancer using crude caustics has a very long history but, with the advent of scientific surgery and later radiotherapy, fell into disuse until recently. Belisario (1959) describes an effective method for dealing with very early malignancies in which electrocautery under local anaesthesia is followed by the application of a paint made up of 20% podophyllin in compound tincture of benzoin, reapplied on two successive days. Of more general interest is the method developed by Klein and his colleagues (e.g. Klein, Stoll, Milgrom, Trenkle, Graham and Helm, 1966, which can be used as a source for earlier references) and by Goldman (1963). In this method, a preparation consisting of 5% or 20% fluorouracil in hydrophilic base is applied sparingly to the tumour which is then covered with an occlusive dressing of plastic film. This is repeated daily for up to a month and gives rise to a reaction which closely mimics a radiation reaction. It appears to be effective in two-thirds to three-quarters of superficial basal cell carcinomata. It is not suggested that this treatment should supplant standard surgical and radiotherapeutic techniques but it is a very useful method to have in reserve for multiple tumours (intraepidermal carcinoma as well as basal cell carcinoma), especially in the elderly and for the tumour which is recurrent after standard procedures. It also seems possible, in some cases, to give effective re-treatments when the tumour recurs after initially effective treatment with this cream.

Immunotherapy. Williams and Klein (1970) also describe the use of immunotherapy in skin cancer. Certain agents, which produce contact dermatitis of the delayed hypersensitivity type, are found to give rise to more intense immune reactions in skin tumours than in normal skin. The reaction is sufficient to destroy the tumours with "resolution of more than 95% of multiple superficial basal cell carcinomas tested for observation periods of up to five years". Two compounds, 2,3,5 – triethylene-imino-benzoquinine (TEIB) and dinitrochloro-benzene (DNCB), have been used and the technique is described in the paper quoted above. This use of immunotherapy is of great interest although the technique is too time-consuming for routine use.

COMBINED TREATMENTS

Stimulated by the advances achieved in the control of the acute leukaemias by the use of combination regimes clinicians have explored the possibilities of such regimes in other tumours using combinations of drugs with radiotherapy, drugs with hormones or drugs with drugs.

CYTOTOXIC DRUGS WITH RADIOTHERAPY

The addition of a cytotoxic drug or drugs to the radiation treatment might be expected to improve results:—

(a) By causing an increase in effectiveness of the radiation treatment
(b) By sensitizing the tumour to radiation more than the surrounding tissue
(c) By eradication of metastases
(d) In an emergency situation, when the combined effect will be quicker than that of radiation alone.

If a drug increases the effectiveness of radiation without a differential effect on tumour as compared with normal tissue, it is unlikely to be of direct value. A drug which possibly comes into this class is synkavit. The drug itself has no tumour inhibitory effect, but it does seem to potentiate the effect of radiation within certain limits. In animal work Marrian, Marshall and Mitchell (1961) show how, in the Walker tumour, synkavit improves the control achieved although the same effect could largely, but not entirely, be obtained by an 80% addition to the radiation dose level quoted. It was Mitchell's work which stimulated Edith Paterson and the late H. C. Warrington to mount a trial to evaluate the effect of adding synkavit to the standard radio-therapeutic techniques for bronchial carcinoma. The results of this trial were published by Evans and Todd (1969). During the four year period 1963 to 1967 all cases of bronchial carcinoma accepted for radio-therapy were entered into the trial and were divided at random into

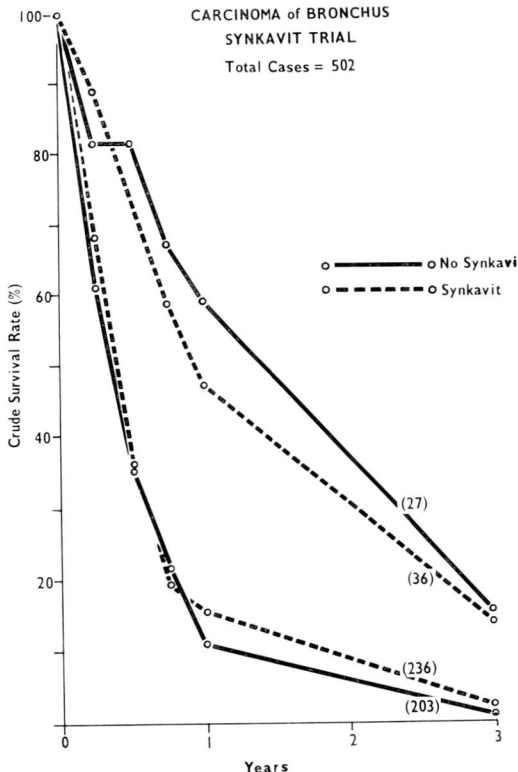

FIG. 2.2. This is taken from Evans and Todd (1969). The upper two curves are for patients with early bronchial carcinoma and the lower two curves are for patients with late bronchial carcinoma. In neither case is there a significant difference between those who did and those who did not receive synkavit.

two groups. One group received radiotherapy alone and the other groups received synkavit in addition. As can be seen from Fig. 2, under the conditions of this trial, synkavit conferred no benefit.

Even if there is not true synergism between a drug and radiation it has been argued that, by the preliminary use of a cytotoxic drug and the subsequent reduction of tumour size, with alteration in vascularity and reduction in the number of hypoxic cells, the response to radiation may be enhanced and there might be improvement in cure rates (Kramer, 1969). At first, Friedman and Daly (1967) treated head and neck cancer with methotrexate and followed on with a 'sublethal' dose of radiation, but latterly (Friedman, 1969; Kramer, 1969) the methotrexate has been followed by a full course of radiotherapy. About 75% of the primary tumours and a rather lower percentage of secondarily involved nodes show a favourable response to the preliminary treatment with methotrexate and Friedman's impression is that his best results are achieved in those cases with advanced primary tumour but without node involvement.

Vermund, Gollin and Ansfield (1969) describe a series of random trials using combined treatment in the form of fluorouracil and radiotherapy, compared with radiotherapy alone. The following tumours are included: inoperable bronchogenic carcinoma, advanced carcinoma of the oral cavity, oral pharynx, laryngopharynx, nasopharynx and paranasal sinuses, bladder, glioblastoma multiforme, inoperable carcinoma of the breast, stage IV cancer of the ovary and stage III cancer of the uterine cervix. Their preliminary results suggest improvement in local tumour control and in survival rate after combined treatment in patients with cancer of the oral cavity and oropharynx. There were 60 and 24 patients respectively in these two groups. Although these numbers are far from negligible, Kramer (1969) considers that, in the multi-institutional trial centred on the Jefferson Medical Centre, which is at present being run to compare methotrexate and radiotherapy with radiotherapy alone, a total of 1,200 cases will be required if a statistically valid 10% difference in results is to be demonstrated. If this estimate is correct, it goes far to explain why so much uncertainty bedevils the interpretation of the results of trials to test combined treatments.

Of more than usual interest in this context is a trial carried out by Fletcher, Suit, Howe, Samuels, Jesse and Villareal (1963) in which patients with head and neck cancer were admitted under two physicians who divided the patients at random into two groups. One group received a course of fluorouracil and the other group had inert intravenous infusions. Both groups had routine radiotherapy with weekly assessment by the radiotherapists who did not know which patients were receiving the cytotoxic drug. After 6,000 rads in six weeks, the radiotherapists were informed of the patients who had not had the fluorouracil and these patients were given supplementary radiation of up to 1,500 rads. Fletcher and his colleagues concluded that the use of the cytotoxic agent may have been associated with more rapid regression of the primary, but that this was not followed by an increase in 'permanency of control'. They emphasized the need for controls in this type of study and also the necessity to analyse, separately, tumours which originate in different anatomical sites.

Another trial conducted by Moertel and colleagues (1969) at the Mayo Clinic, is producing highly suggestive evidence that the combination of 5-fluorouracil and radiotherapy is particularly useful and effective for inoperable gastro-intestinal adenocarcinoma.

If, when irradiating a tumour, the addition of a drug would permit the same effect on the tumour but reduce troublesome side effects, then a gain would be registered. It is this type of consideration which led to the introduction of tretamine in combination with radiotherapy for bilateral retinoblastoma. A succession of papers, Reese, Hyman, Tapley and Forrest (1958), Reese and Ellsworth (1963), and Tapley (1964), has been published on this subject and the story unfolds as follows: In 1933 a technique was developed for irradiating tumour in the second eye. At a dose range of 7,000 to 17,000 rads this was quite effective, as far as control of tumour and survival were concerned, but there was a high incidence of loss of vision ascribed to radiation effects (these complications were, most important, vitreous haemorrhage, but also haemorrhagic retinitis, retinal detachment, acute glaucoma, atrophy of the retina, phthisis bulbi and cataract). There was also radiation necrosis in the orbit, requiring surgery, and even a few cases of radiation induced sarcomas and carcinomas. Kupfer (1953) showed that mustine could influence retinoblastoma; so, at that time, the radiation dose was dropped to 3,500 rads in three weeks, or 4,500 rads in four weeks, and, at the same time, tretamine was given in the hope that the tumour could be controlled without troublesome side effects—in particular with preservation of useful vision. This objective was achieved in that the percentage of patients with useful vision rose from 50 to over 70. More recently, however, an alternate series has been running for patients with relatively limited tumour in the second eye (group I and II in Reese's classification) in which one group had irradiation alone and the second group had irradiation with tretamine. Fifty cases were in the trial at the time of reporting by Reese and Ellsworth (1963) and the success rate was over 80% in each group. From this it would appear that the important improvement in the regime has been the reduction in the dose of radiation rather than the addition of the cytotoxic drug, although it is only fair to add that Reese still advocates the addition of tretamine, preferably given intra-arterially, to the more advanced cases.

When a cytotoxic agent is added to radiotherapy in the hope that microscopic metastases will be eradicated by the drug, whilst the radiation deals with the primary mass, it is logical, if the intention is cure, to regard the cytotoxic drug as the main treatment. However, there are few enough tumours where chemotherapy has proven potential to cure, so in most cases a combination treatment of this type will be designed simply to achieve better palliation. The use of actinomycin D in Wilms' tumour deserves special consideration. The potentiation of the radiation effects, which has been pointed out by D'Angio, Farber, Maddock (1959) and others is, if nothing else, a potentiation of side effects such as cutaneous erythema, so it would be optimistic to look for sensitization of the tumour rather than of the surrounding tissues. However, actinomycin D has undoubtedly been shown to have a marked effect on some deposits of Wilms' tumour so, if it is to be of benefit, it should be by virtue of its effect on metastases. That the results of the treatment of Wilms' tumour have improved over the past ten to twenty years is generally accepted. To a certain extent this can be attributed to better surgery, including the tendency to concentrate experience of this tumour in the hands of a few expert surgeons, and to more effective radiotherapy, but several recent claims have been made for the introduction of actinomycin D; Fernbach and Martyn (1966) claim an improvement in the two year survival rate from 43% (6/14) to 92% (12/13). Burgert and Glidewell (1967) claim an improvement from 52% to 78% emphasizing that the drug should be given early at about the time of the nephrectomy. Colebatch, Howard, Williams, Kussle and Clark claim an improvement in one year survival rate from 22% to 70%. Not all reports are so enthusiastic. For example Maier and Horshaw (1967) state that their survival rate of 44% at two years remained unchanged (51 patients) and Reiquan, Prosper, Akers, Allen, and Beatty (1965) although impressed with the temporary effect of actinomycin D did not find that it increased the survival rate. Obviously factors of selection come into these studies and the data is not often presented in such a fashion that results can readily be compared. However at least it is clear that the introduction of this drug has not been associated with a deterioration in survival rate (a few years ago many radiotherapists were seriously concerned lest, by marrow depression, the actinomycin D would prejudice the necessary radiotherapy). If the drug were to delay the growth of metastases, then the two year figures could be improved without a change in the long term results, so that the possibility of the drug improving cure rates remains unproven but, short of cure, it could still be of value in prolonging survival.

Many papers have been published on the combination of radiotherapy with cytotoxic agents in the treatment of bronchial carcinoma. Typical is one by Gollin, Ansfield, Curreri, Heidleberger and Vermund (1962) who, using fluorouracil, claim that this drug lengthens the survival period and that, under the same conditions, a similar improvement is not seen with cyclophosphamide. More recently Horwitz, Wright, Perry and Bassett (1965) have published a trial on the use of chlorambucil in this disease. They claim to have shown that the routine use of this drug, after appropriate radiotherapy, increases the mean survival time by 50% but the number of patients in their trial (30) is rather small. With the drugs at present available it hardly seems likely that one could eradicate metastases and thus influence long term survival rates but, if their development can be delayed for a few months, as Horwitz suggests, and if the side effects of the drug used are minimal, then this approach may have some palliative value.

As there is now a range of drugs of proven potency in Hodgkin's disease, it would seem possible that, if the main mass of disease were to be eradicated by radiotherapy, microscopic foci might be controlled by appropriate chemotherapy. Paterson (1958) published a trial in which patients with early Hodgkin's disease confined to the neck were treated on the one hand by radiotherapy alone and, on the other, by a combination of radiotherapy and mustine. The results at five years showed no significant difference. Halnan (1964) published the results of this trial at ten years when again there was no difference between the two groups. This trial along with nine others published series is discussed by Miller (1966). In each of these series radiotherapy alone is compared with a combined treatment using radiotherapy plus an alkylating agent. Miller observes "the differing opinions are fairly well balanced between affirmative and negative views". He also points out that none of the series was randomized. Hancock and Ledlie (1967) and Pike, Hancock and Ledlie (1967) describe a random trial of radiotherapy alone, compared with the combination of radiotherapy and a single injection of mustine in stage I and stage II Hodgkin's disease. Their results are preliminary but they maintain that, by statistical manipulation using the Wilcoxon rank test, they may be "regarded as substantive". Their results do appear to favour the combined treatment although one must be excused for preferring to wait until the trial matures before fully accepting this finding.

CYTOTOXIC DRUGS WITH HORMONES

Cytotoxic drugs have usually been combined with hormones in the treatment of conditions such as carcinoma of the breast where the hormone is likely to have specific activity. An example is the combination of thiotepa and testosterone advocated by Watson and Turner (1959), and another favoured combination is cyclophosphamide with nandrolone, both combinations being used in cancer of the breast. Apart from a specific effect on tumour, it is thought that the anabolic steroids may have a protective effect on the bone marrow thus permitting a higher and, presumably, more effective dose of the cytotoxic agents to be given.

The corticosteroids are sometimes given in conjunction with cytotoxic drugs for a number of different reasons, including control of complications such as haemolytic anaemia, reduction of inflammatory reactions around tumour deposits, and simple tonic effect. In some tumours such as myeloma, a steroid such as prednisone has a specific anti-tumour effect (Alexanian, Haut, Khan, Lane, McKelvey, Migliore Stuckey and Wilson, 1969) so it is logical to combine it with other agents for this reason. Little controlled work has been done to assess the combinations of a steroid with a cytotoxic agent in tumours in which there is no expectation of specific effect, but Reitemeir, Moertel and Hahn (1967) do report such a study in which fluoromethalone, fluorouracil or a combination of fluoromethalone and fluorouracil were given on a randomized basis to 112 patients with far advanced gastrointestinal adenocarcinoma. They concluded "fluoromethalone in combination with 5–FU (fluorouracil) does not exceed the palliation obtained from 5–FU alone, nor does it alter the toxicity of 5–FU. An appreciable incidence of gastrointestinal haemorrhage or perforation was associated with the use of fluoromethalone".

COMBINATIONS OF ONE OR MORE CYTOTOXIC DRUGS

The literature on cancer chemotherapy is rich in reports on multiple drug therapy. However, the use of several drugs at a time introduces so many variables in terms of possible combinations and dose schedules that dispassionate assessment becomes very difficult. In the treatment of acute leukaemia regimes using several drugs are now well established and of accepted worth. Some claims are made for the extension of this type of therapy to generalized solid lymphomas such as Hodgkin's disease (e.g. Carbone in Perry, Thomas, Johnson, Carbone and Haynes, 1967) and promising initial results are encouraging more extended trials. However, the effectiveness of such regimes in other solid tumours is more open to question. For example Nathanson, Hall, Dederick, Yount and Miller (1966) report on studies of three separate combinations: (a) cyclophosphamide, fluorouracil and actinomycin D (b) mitomycin C, melphalan and vincristine, and (c) fluorouracil, mercaptopurine and methotrexate. The treatments were given to patients known to have drug resistant tumours and half the conventional dose of each agent was used. They concluded that "The results suggest independent actions with respect to toxicity, but do not indicate that combination therapy caused a greater anti-tumour effect than the effect expected with a single drug".

CONCLUSION

Cancer chemotherapy can, at different levels, result in cure as in choriocarcinoma or Burkitt's lymphoma, high grade palliation as in the acute and chronic leukaemias, or relatively short lived palliation as seen with most solid tumours. It also has a less well defined role in combined treatments. But what is very clear now is that cancer chemotherapy has won for itself an established place in the management of very many forms of malignant disease. It is also a rapidly changing subject with the frequent introduction of new drugs and of new ways of applying old ones, so one can predict with confidence that much of this chapter will be woefully out of date when the contents of other chapters are still fresh.

REFERENCES

ALEXANIAN, R., HAUT, A., KHAN, A. V., LANE, M., MCKELVEY, E. M., MIGLIORE, P. J., STUCKEY, M. J. & WILSON, H. E. (1969). Treatment for multiple myeloma. *J. Am. med. Ass.*, **208**, 1680.

ARMSTRONG, J. G. (1966). Vinblastine in the treatment of cancer—a review. *Clin. Med.*, **73**, 41.

BELISARIO, J. C. (1959). *Cancer of the Skin*. London: Butterworth and Co. Ltd., p. 151.

BERGSAGEL, D. E., SPRAGUE, C. C., AUSTIN, C., & GRIFFITH, K. M. (1962). Evaluation of new chemotherapeutic agents in the treatment of multiple myeloma IV, L-phenyl-alanine mustard. *Cancer Chemother. Rep.*, **21**, 87.

BOESEN, E., & DAVIS, W. (1969). *Cytotoxic Drugs in the Treatment of Cancer*. London: Arnold.

BOND, W. H., ROHN, R. J., BATES, L. H., & HODES, M. E. (1966). Treatment of neoplastic diseases with an improved oral preparation of vinblastine sulphate. *Cancer*, **2**, 213.

BRENNAN, M. J., TALLEY, R. W., SAN DIEGO, E. L., BURROWS, J. J., O'BRYAN, R. M., VAITKEVICIUS, V. K., & HOREGLAD, S. (1964). Critical Analysis of 594 Cancer Patients Treated with 5-Fluorouracil. *Chemotherapy of Cancer*. Plattner, P. A. (Ed.). Amsterdam: Elsevier, p. 118.

BROCK, N. (1967). Pharmacologic characterization of cyclophosphamide (NSC-26271) and cyclophosphamide metabolites. *Cancer Chemother. Rep.*, **51**, 315.

BURGERT, E. O., & GLIDEWELL, O. (1967). Actinomycin in Wilms' tumour. *J. Am. med. Ass.*, **199**, No. 7, 464.

CALABRESI, P., & WELCH, A. D. (1965). Cytotoxic Drugs, Hormones and Radioactive Isotopes. *The Pharmacological Basis of Therapeutics*. Goodman, L. S. and Gilman, A. (Eds.). New York: Macmillan.

CARBONE, P. P. in PERRY, S., THOMAS, L. B., JOHNSON, R. E., CARBONE, P. P., & HAYNES, H. A. (1967). Hodgkin's disease. *Ann. intern. Med.*, **67**, 433.

CLIFFORD, P., OETTGEN, H. F., BEECHER, J. L., BROWN, F. P., HARRIES, J. R., & LAWES, W. E. (1963). Nitrogen mustard therapy with aortic occlusion in nasopharyngeal carcinoma. *Br. med. J.*, **i**, 1256.

Clinical Screening Co-operative Group of the European Organisation for Research on the Treatment of Cancer (1970). Study of the clinical efficiency of bleomycin in human cancer. *Br. med. J.*, **2**, 643.

COLEBATCH, J. H., HOWARD, R., WILLIAMS, A. L., KUSSLE, J. R., & CLARK, A. C. L. (1964). Results of actinomycin D therapy in Wilms' tumours. *Acta Un. int. Cancr.*, **20**, 491.

CREECH, O., & KREMENTZ, E. T. (1964). Regional perfusion in melanoma of limbs. *J. Am. med. Ass.*, **188**, 855.

CURRERI, A. R., ANSFIELD, F. J., MCIVER, F. A., WAISMAN, H. A., & HEIDELBERGER, C. (1958). Clinical studies with 5-fluorouracil. *Cancer Res.*, **18**, 478.

D'ANGIO, G. J., FARBER, S., & MADDOCK, C. L. (1959). Potentiation of X-ray effects by actinomycin D. *Radiology*, **73**, 175.

ECKHARDT, S., SELLEI, C., HORVÁTH, I. P., & INSTITORIS, L., (1963). Effect of 1,6-dibromo-16-dideoxy-D mannitol on chronic granulocytic leukaemia. *Cancer Chemother. Rep.*, **33**, 57.

EVANS, C. M., & TODD, I. D. H. (1969). Synkavit and radiotherapy in the treatment of bronchial carcinoma. A random trial. *Clin. Radiol.*, **20**, No. 2, 228.

EZDINLI, E. Z., & STUTZMAN, L. (1968). Vinblastine sulfate vs. nitrogen mustard therapy of Hodgkin's disease. *Cancer*, **22**, 473.

FERNBACH, D. J., & MARTYN, D. T. (1966). Role of actinomycin in the improved survival of children with Wilms' tumour. *J. Am. med. Ass.*, **195**, No. 12, 1005.

FLETCHER, G. H., SUIT, H. D., HOWE, C. D., SAMUELS, M., JESSE, R. H., & VILLAREAL, R. V. (1963). Clinical method of testing radiation sensitizing agents in squamous cell carcinoma. *Cancer*, **16**, 355.

FREI, E., DE VITA, V. T., MOXLEY, J. H., & CARBONE, P. P. (1966). Approaches to improving the chemotherapy of Hodgkin's disease. *Cancer Res.*, **26**, 1284.

FRIEDMAN, M. (1969). The Treatment of Squamous Cell Carcinoma of the Head and Neck with Combined Methotrexate and Irradiation. *Frontiers of Radiation Therapy and Oncology*. Vaeth, J. M. (Ed.). Basel and New York: Karger.

FRIEDMAN, M., & DALY, J. F. (1967). The treatment of squamous cell carcinoma of the head and neck with methotrexate and irradiation. *Am. J. Roentg.*, **99**, No. 2, 289.

GALTON, D. A. G., & PETO, R. (1968). A progress report on the Medical Research Council's therapeutic trial in myelomatosis. *Br. J. Haemat.*, **15**, 319.

GOLDMAN, L. (1963). The response of skin cancer to topical therapy with 5-fluorouracil. *Cancer Chemother. Rep.*, **28**, 49.

GOLLIN, F. F., ANSFIELD, F. J., CURRERI, A. R., HEIDELBERGER, C., & VERMUND, H. (1962). Combined chemotherapy and irradiation in inoperable bronchogenic carcinoma. *Cancer*, **15**, 1209.

GREENWALD, E. S. (1967). *Cancer Chemotherapy*. London: Heinemann.

HALNAN, K. E. (1964). Long-term results of X-ray treatment in malignant disease of the lympho-reticular system. *Acta Un. int. Cancr.*, **20**, No. 8, 1771.

HALNAN, K. E., & RUSSELL, M. H. (1965). Polycythaemia vera—comparison of survival and causes of death in patients managed with and without radiotherapy. *Lancet*, **ii**, 760.

HANCOCK, P. E. T., & LEDLIE, E. M. (1967). Treatment of early Hodgkin's disease. *Lancet*, **i**, 27.

HOOGSTRATEN, B., COSTA, J., CUTTNER, J., FORCIER, R. J., LEONE, L. A., HARLEY, J. B., & GLIDEWELL, O. J. (1969). Intermittent melphalan therapy in multiple myeloma. *J. Am. med. Ass.*, **209**, 251.

HORWITZ, H., WRIGHT, T. L., PERRY, H., & BARRETT, C. M. (1965). Suppressive chemotherapy in bronchogenic carcinoma. *Am. J. Roentg.*, **93**, 515.

JACOBS, E. M., LUCE, J. K., & WOOD, D. A. (1968). Treatment of cancer with weekly intravenous 5-fluorouracil. *Cancer*, **2**, 1233.

JELLIFFE, A. M. (1969). Vinblastine in the treatment of Hodgkin's disease. *Br. J. Cancer*, **23**, 44.

JELLIFFE, A. M., & MARKS, J. (1965). *Natulan (Ibenzmethyzin)*. Bristol: John Wright and Sons Ltd.

KAPLAN, H. S., & ROSENBERG, S. A. (1966). Extended field radical radiotherapy in advanced Hodgkin's disease: short-term results of 2 randomized clinical trials. *Cancer Res.*, **26**, 1268.

KARNOFSKY, D. A., MILLER, D. J., & PHILLIPS, R. F. (1963). Role of chemotherapy in the management of early Hodgkin's disease. *Am. J. Roentg.*, **90**, 968.

KLEIN, E., STOLL, H. L., MILGROM, H., TRAENKLE, H. L., GRAHAM, S., & HELM, F. (1966). Tumours of the skin. VI. Study on effects of local administration of 5-fluorouracil in basal cell carcinoma. *J. invest. Derm.*, **47**, 22.
KRAMER, S. (1969). Use of Methotrexate and Radiation Therapy for Advanced Cancer of the Head and Neck. *Frontiers of Radiation Therapy and Oncology.* Vaeth, J. M. (Ed.). Basel and New York: Karger.
KUPFER, C. (1953). Retinoblastoma treated with intravenous nitrogen mustard. *Am. J. Ophthalm.*, **36**, 1721.
KYLE, R. A., SCHWARTZ, R. S., OLIVER, H. L., & DAMESHEK, W. (1961). A syndrome resembling adrenal cortical insufficiency associated with long term busulphan (myleran) therapy. *Blood*, **18**, 497.
MACDONALD, C. A., & LACHER, M. J. (1966). Oral vinblastine sulphate in Hodgkin's disease. *Clin. Pharmac. Ther.*, **7**, 534.
MAIER, J. G., & HORSHAW, W. J. (1967). Treatment of and prognosis in Wilms' tumour. *Cancer*, **20**, 96.
MARRIAN, D. H., MARSHALL, B., & MITCHELL, J. S. (1961). Laboratory and clinical studies of some quinal diphosphates and related compounds in chemical radio-sensitizers and the development of a radioactive drug. *Chemotherapia*, **3**, 225.
Medical Research Council's Working Party for Therapeutic Trials in Leukaemia. (1968). Chronic granulocytic leukaemia: comparison of radiotherapy and busulphan therapy. *Br. Med. J.*, **1**, 201.
Medical Research Council's Working Party for Therapeutic Trials in Leukaemia. (1971). Myelomatosis: comparison of melphalan and cyclophosphamide therapy. *Br. Med. J.* **1**, 640.
MILLER, D. G. (1966). Chemotherapy as a primary treatment in Hodgkin's disease. *Cancer Res.*, **26**, 1303.
MILLER, D. G., LAWRENCE, W., KIM, M., DORENCHAMP, D., & RANDALL, H. T. (1962). Midtorso occlusion for regional cancer chemotherapy. *Cancer Chemother. Rep.*, **18**, 43.
MOERTEL, C. G., CHILDS, D. S. Jr., REITEMEIER, R. J., COLBY, M. Y., & HOLBROOK, M. (1969). 5-Fluorouracil and radiotherapy for gastro-intestinal cancer. *Lancet*, **ii**, 865.
NATHANSON, L., HALL, T. C., DEDERICK, M. M., YOUNT, W. J., & MILLER, S. (1966). Initial pharmacologic studies of three types of combination chemotherapy. *Cancer Chemother. Rep.*, **50**, 259.
NICHOLSON, W. M., BEARD, M. E. J., CROWTHER, D., STANSFIELD, A. G., VARTAN, C. P., MALPAS, J. S., FAIRLEY, G. H., & SCOTT, R. B. (1970). Combination chemotherapy in generalised Hodgkin's disease. *Brit. Med. J.* **2**, 7.
NEU, L. T. (1962). Leukaemia complicating pregnancy. *Missouri Med.*, **59**, 220.
OLIVERIO, V. T., & ZUBROD, C. G. (1965). Clinical pharmacology of the effective anti-tumour drugs. *A. Rev. Pharmac.*, **5**, 335.
PATERSON, E. (1958). Evaluation of chemotherapeutic compounds in the reticuloses. *Br. J. Cancer*, **12**, 332.
PERKINS, J., ISRAËLS, M. C. J., & WILKINSON, J. F. (1964). Polycythaemia vera: clinical studies on a series of 127 patients managed without radiation therapy. *Q. Jl Med., New Series*, **33**, No. 132, 499.
PIKE, M. C., HANCOCK, P. E. T., & LEDLIE, E. M. (1967). Treatment of early Hodgkin's disease. *Lancet*, **ii**, 1361.
RAMANAN, C. V., & ISRAËLS, M. C. G. (1969). Treatment of chronic myeloid leukaemia with dibromomannitol. *Lancet*, **ii**, 125.

REESE, A. B., HYMAN, G. A., TAPLEY, N. DU V., & FORREST, A. W. (1958). The treatment of retinoblastoma by X-ray and triethylmelamine. *American Medical Association Archs. Ophthal., Chicago*, **60**, 897.

REESE, A. B., & ELLSWORTH, R. M. (1963). The evaluation and current concept of retinoblastoma therapy. *Trans. Am. Acad. Ophthal. Oto-lar.*, 164.

REIQUAN, C. W., PROSPER, J. C., AKERS, D. R., ALLEN, R. P., & BEATTY, E. C. (1965). Wilms' tumours. *Rocky Mount. med. J.*, **62**, 43.

REITEMEIER, R. J., MOERTEL, C. G., & HAHN, R. G. (1967). Comparative evaluation of palliation with fluoromethalone, 5-fluorouracil and combined fluoromethalone and 5-fluorouracil in advanced gastro-intestinal cancer. *Cancer Chemother. Rep.*, **51**, 77.

RIVERS, S. L., & PATNO, M. E. (1969). Cyclophosphamide versus melphalan in treatment of plasma cell myeloma. *J. Am. med. Ass.*, **207**, 1328.

RIVERS, S., WHITTINGTON, R. M., & PATNO, M. E. (1963). Comparison of effect of cyclophosphamide and a placebo in the therapy of multiple myeloma. *Cancer Chemother. Rep.*, **29**, 115.

SALMON, S. E., SHADDUCK, R. K., & SCHILLING, A. (1967). Intermittent high-dose prednisone (NSC-10023) therapy for multiple myeloma. *Cancer Chemother. Rep.*, **51**, 179.

SALSBURY, A. J., BURRAGE, K., & HELLMANN, K. (1970). Inhibition of metastatic spread by I.C.R.F.159: selective deletion of a malignant characteristic. *Br. med. J.*, **4**, 344.

SCOTT, J. H. (1963). The effect of nitrogen mustard and maintenance chlorambucil in the treatment of advanced Hodgkin's disease. *Cancer Chemother. Rep.*, **27**, 27.

SPEED, D. E., GALTON, D. A. G., & SWAN, A. (1964). Melphalan in the treatment of myelomatosis. *Br. med. J.*, **i**, 1664.

STUTZMAN, L., EZDINLI, E. Z., & STUTZMAN, M. A. (1966). Vinblastine sulfate vs. cyclophosphamide. *J. Am. med. Ass.*, **195**, 173.

Symposium on hydroxyurea. (1964). *Cancer Chemother. Rep.*, **40**, 1.

Symposium on pharmacological and clinical results with hydroxyurea. (1967). *Clin. Trials J.*, 869.

TAPLEY, N. DU V. (1964). The Treatment of Bilateral Retinoblastoma with Radiation and Chemotherapy. *Ocular and Adnexal Tumours*. Boniuk, M. (Ed.). St. Louis: Morsby Co.

TODD, I. D. H. (1970). Chemotherapy of the lymphomas. *Proc. R. Soc. Med.*, **63**, 86.

VERMUND, H., GOLLIN, F., & ANSFIELD, F. J. (1969). Clinical Studies of 5-fluorouracil as Adjuvant to Radiotherapy. *Frontiers of Radiation Therapy and Oncology*, Vaeth, J. M. (Ed.). Basel and New York: Karger.

WATKINS, P. J., FAIRLEY, G. H., & SCOTT, R. B. (1967). Treatment of polycythaemia vera. *Br. med. J.* **2**, 664.

WATSON, G. W., & TURNER, R. L. (1959). Breast cancer: a new approach to therapy. *Br. med. J.*, **i**, 1315.

WILLIAMS, A. C., & KLEIN, E. (1970). Experiences with local chemotherapy and immunotherapy in premalignant and malignant skin lesions. *Cancer*, **25**, 450.

WILSON, H. E., MONTO, R. W., PISCIOTTA, A. V., ROHN, R. J., & LOUIS, J. (1969). Treatment of chronic granulocytic leukaemia with piposulfan (NSC-47774). *Cancer Chemother. Rep.*, **53**, 121.

3 Choriocarcinoma and Trophoblastic Tumours

K. D. BAGSHAWE

INTRODUCTION

Gestational choriocarcinoma is significant because it has certain unique features which can help us to understand various aspects of other, more common, tumours. It is well known that it proved to be the first tumour to be frequently curable by systemically active agents. Also, by virtue of producing chorionic gonadotrophin it provides us with an index which is far more sensitive and precise than that available for any other tumour up to the present time, so it is possible to observe fairly promptly the effect, or lack of effect, of therapeutic agents upon its course. Like the mammalian foetus, it is a highly successful allograft and the mechanisms involved in this success may be shared with the foetus on the one hand and with other antigenic tumours on the other. It thus provides a link between two fields of research into fundamental immunological mechanisms. In addition, as a result of the occurrence of choriocarcinomatous elements in teratomata, we have another link with autochthonous tumours.

Again, its parent tissue, the trophoblast, has certain properties which are usually said to be found only in malignant tissues so that distinction between normal and malignant behaviour is rather finely drawn and gestational choriocarcinoma can therefore be regarded in this context as a naturally occurring, minimal deviation tumour. Clearly, if we are to develop an understanding of this tumour, we cannot ignore the normal trophoblast from which it arises.

NORMAL TROPHOBLAST

The trophoblast is formed from the peripheral cells of the cleaving zygote and this probably represents the first stage of embryonic differentiation. Soon after implantation of the blastocyst in the luteal phase endometrium, on about the seventh day after fertilization, the trophoblast can be seen to consist of two cell types. These are the cytotrophoblast or stem cell component and the syncytiotrophoblast. The syncytiotrophoblast may form a true syncytium in certain situations, or multinucleate giant cells, but both are in effect mature end-stage cells with a life cycle perhaps as short as 48 hours. This is significant because mitosis is virtually never seen in these cells and tritiated thymidine labelling of syncytial nuclei occurs only after some delay (Midgeley *et al*, 1963). Speaking generally, both cytotrophoblast and syncytiotrophoblast are present wherever trophoblast is found, whether the trophoblast is normal or malignant, although fragments of tissue as seen in curettings may contain only one or other type of cell.

Throughout the foeto-maternal interface the syncytium or cytotrophoblast, or both, regularly intervene. Even so, breaks in this barrier undoubtedly occur as evidenced by the finding in later stages of pregnancy of foetal blood cells in the maternal circulation.

In several respects the behaviour of normal trophoblast changes during the course of pregnancy. For present purposes it is probably sufficient to distinguish between early and late trophoblast and to observe that, in the variables so far identified, choriocarcinoma resembles early trophoblast. For instance, the cytotrophoblast cells throughout pregnancy show areas of clear or foamy cytoplasm and densely staining nuclei but multiple nucleoli may be found in early pregnancy as well as in choriocarcinoma. The cytoplasm of syncytial cells, both benign and malignant, shows a coarse endoplasmic reticulum consistent with the active hormone synthesis taking place.

Early trophoblast proliferates rapidly and the cell cycle time may be as short as 22 hours (Bagshawe, 1969). The output of chorionic gonadotrophin in early pregnancy doubles about every 48 hours. Early trophoblast invades the endometrium extensively but only isolated trophoblastic cells are to be found in the myometrium. On the other hand, the foetus can establish itself and grow outside the uterus; early trophoblast can also establish itself and grow successfully when transplanted to a variety of tissues (Kirby, 1965). More important perhaps is the invasion of maternal vascular structures in the form of trophoblastic growth within vessels and embolization of trophoblastic elements, mainly syncytial, to the pulmonary capillaries. This trophoblastic deportation has been recognized principally in the latter part of pregnancy but the time at which this process begins is not yet defined.

The mechanisms employed during trophoblastic invasion are largely unknown and understudied. The capacity of the rabbit conceptus to utilize glycogen (Boving, 1959) calls to mind Warburg's (1956) well known observations on glycogen utilization by cancer cells.

Early trophoblast differs from the late trophoblast in its endocrine repertoire. Chorionic gonadotrophin synthesis appears to commence at about the time of syncytial differentiation and its concentration in placental tissue reaches a peak towards the end of the first trimester, after which the blood and urine concentrations fall. The other hormones known to be synthesized by the placenta, with the exception of renin, increase in concentration in the plasma throughout pregnancy. These include placental lactogen, progesterone and its main metabolic product pregnanediol, and the oestrogens. An alkaline phosphatase isoenzyme, specific for the placenta, also appears in the blood as pregnancy progresses. It is of interest that we have not so far found this enzyme in the sera of patients with choriocarcinoma although it has been found in the sera of about 4% of non-pregnant patients with other forms of cancer (Stolbach et al, 1969).

But normal trophoblast, despite its high growth rate and invasive potential, has only a limited capacity for survival. The cells embolizing to the lungs hardly ever produce symptoms and the mechanism by which they are eliminated has not yet been defined. Those trophoblastic fragments which are retained in the uterine wall and pelvic vessels following parturition appear to die out promptly. Similarly, the trophoblast of extra-uterine abdominal pregnancies dies out within a few weeks of removing the foetus.

CHORIONIC GONADOTROPHIN—A TUMOUR INDEX SUBSTANCE

It has been known for more than 40 years that trophoblastic tumours produce a specific protein which can be used as a guide in diagnosis and management. It is only in the last decade, with the replacement of biological by immunological methods for estimating chorionic gonadotrophin, that the value of a tumour specific index has been realized; and even now the picture is sometimes blurred by the continued application of essentially qualitative methods to a quantitative problem.

Of the numerous techniques which have been evolved to estimate the concentration of this protein in body fluids there is only one method, or group of methods, which provide the sensitivity and precision required for an index to tumour activity. This is the radio immunoassay in one of the several forms which now exist (Bagshawe et al, 1966; Wilde et al, 1967). In essence, these methods employ specific antibodies, which have been raised in other species against the antigen to be measured, to combine with the specific antigen in the sample. Isotopically labelled purified antigen is included in the reaction and this competes with the natural antigen for antibody binding. The antigen bound to the antibody is separated from the free antigen by filtration, centrifugation, or electrophoresis and the radioactivity in one of the separated components is counted. Reactions in which known amounts of the antigen are included provide the reference points of a standard line so that precise estimations of very small amounts of a specific protein in a complex mixture of proteins can be determined.

Specificity is of course a relative matter and in the case of HCG the limiting factor is a cross-reaction with pituitary luteinizing hormone (LH).

In consequence, a tumour can be detected only when it is producing enough HCG to raise the total HCG + LH above the normal pre-menopausal LH range. However, this amount is only about a tenth of the amount necessary to give a positive result by the most sensitive 'pregnancy test' methods and about a hundredth of that required for the less sensitive tests (Fig. 1). It also has to be noted that LH values vary substantially with the menstrual cycle and with the state of gonadal steroidogenesis so that to extract all the information possible from HCG assays the clinician has to familiarize himself with the complexities of LH activity.

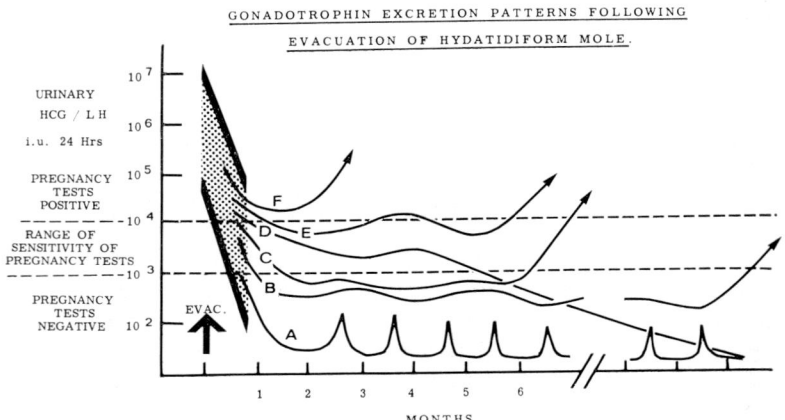

GONADOTROPHIN EXCRETION PATTERNS FOLLOWING

EVACUATION OF HYDATIDIFORM MOLE.

FIG. 3.1. Gonadotrophin excretion patterns following evacuation of hydatidiform mole. Following evacuation of the mole there is a profound fall in the gonado-trophin values. This fall may continue into the normal range, as with example A, and values subsequently show the normal menstrual LH pattern. The rate of fall may slow down but show a gradual and generally progressive reduction (example D). In the other examples (B, C, E, F) active tumour growth occurs after intervals ranging from a few weeks to several years. Pregnancy tests may remain positive as in example F, or be negative for a time as in E, D and C. Although pregnancy tests are negative latent disease can be detected by radioimmunoassay.

The amount of HCG produced by a given number of tumour cells appears to be fairly constant. In 200 cases of trophoblastic tumour seen between 1958–1969, there has been no instance where there was any marked dissociation between the amount of HCG produced and the amount of viable tumour tissue, where this could be assessed. Evidence from a variety of approaches indicates that one tumour cell produces on average about 5×10^{-4} to 5×10^{-5} I.U. HCG/day. Thus a patient excreting 10^6 I.U. HCG/day has about 10^{11} tumour cells. At the point where the tumour HCG is lost in the background of normal LH there are 10^5-10^6 tumour cells. The common notion that choriocarcinomas "always produce a high level of HCG" is quite false and regrettably, is still responsible for delays in diagnosis. (Bagshawe, Golding, Orr, 1969).

By using this index substance, it is frequently possible and necessary to detect a tumour and eliminate it without ever 'seeing it' clinically, histologically or radiologically. During treatment, radiological resolution of tumour masses usually occurs before gonadotrophin excretion reaches normal values if the tumour masses are initially less than about 2 cm in diameter. In the case of larger masses complete radiological resolution may not occur till gonadotrophin excretion has been normal for many weeks or months. Excision of a solitary residual mass from a patient excreting a small excess of gonadotrophin has sometimes

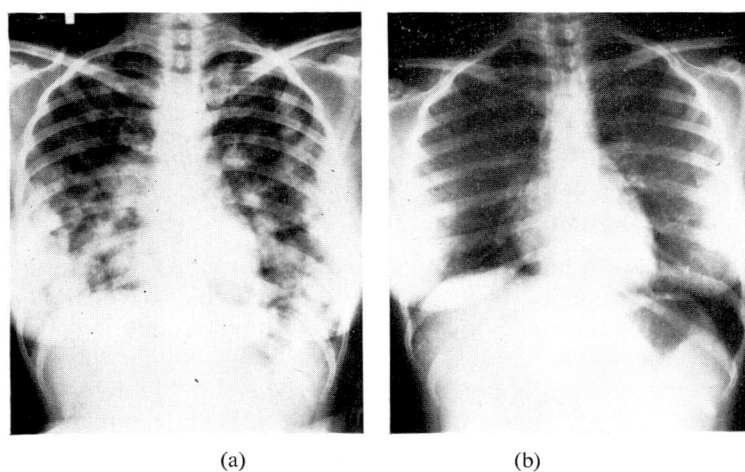

(a)   (b)

Fig. 3.2. (a) Chest radiograph before chemotherapy and (b) 11 months later showing residual solitary metastasis in left upper lobe. Segmental resection of the metastasis produced a transient fall in HCG output consistent with the small amount of viable choriocarcinoma present in the mass, but there proved to be tumour at other sites. (Reproduced by kind permission of Messrs. Edward Arnold from *Choriocarcinoma* by K.D.B.)

revealed a few viable tumour cells but in other instances the mass has proved to be totally necrotic with no viable tumour and the residual tumour has eventually proved to have been elsewhere (Fig. 2a, b).

As well as indicating whether the tumour cell population is increasing or decreasing in size, the rate of alteration of the plasma concentration or urine excretion rate indicates, with certain reservations, the rate of change of cell population size. The rate of clearance of the hormone is close to 1 ml/min so that fluctuations resulting from alterations in synthesis rate are somewhat dampened. Conversely it is possible that some cytotoxic agents interfere with protein metabolism without being lethal to the tumour cells, but on present evidence this is infrequent.

One of the particular advantages of the radioimmunoassay for HCG is that it allows the concentration of the hormone to be measured both in plasma and spinal fluid. This is vitally important in the detection of metastases in the central nervous system and in following the effects of therapy on them. The plasma:CSF ratio is generally greater than 60:1 in the absence of CNS metastases, but in their presence falls to 30:1 or less and sometimes may approach 1:1 (Bagshawe et al, 1968; Rushworth et al, 1968). We have sometimes found evidence of metastases in this way weeks before they were apparent by isotopic scanning, symptomatology or electroencephalographic signs. When the plasma concentration changes rapidly it is to be expected that the plasma: spinal fluid ratio may be disturbed simply because of the slow rate of diffusion of the hormone into and out of the spinal fluid. When making estimations of spinal fluid HCG it is of course essential to take into account any evidence of blood in the spinal fluid. It is not usual to find the total protein content greatly increased in the spinal fluid of these patients.

HYDATIDIFORM MOLE

In hydatidiform mole, the conceptus lacks an intact foetus and shows gross cyst-like swelling of its villi due to accumulation of fluid within the mesenchymal core. Some parts of an embryo may be present, in which case it is described as transitional mole; where the conceptus and placenta are largely normal but some villi show mole-like changes, the term molar-degeneration is applied. Typical molar pregnancies last about 17 weeks and rarely over 30 weeks. In European peoples the incidence of mole is of the order of 1:1000–2000 pregnancies but there are substantial and unexplained geographic variations with an incidence as high as 1:200 pregnancies frequently reported from South-east Asia. The incidence is also age related, being higher in those under 20 and over 40 years of age (Bagshawe, 1969; Smalbraak, 1957).

The majority of moles are female and chromosome patterns are generally, but not always, euploid (Park, 1957). Moles may recur in the same patient and the risk of a second mole may be about four times as high as for a first mole, although a second mole is known to have occurred in only one of the 200 or so cases studied in the Charing Cross (Fulham) series. Mole is accompanied by an increased incidence of toxaemia and often by the formation of large theca lutein cysts which may persist for some time after evacuating the mole and which may give rise to pain. They are sometimes mistaken at laparotomy for metastatic growth.

Distinction between a mole and a normal pregnancy is often difficult but the ultrasonic scan is the most useful means of distinguishing them at present (Donald, 1962). Biochemical methods such as a very high value for HCG production together with a low level of the placental alkaline phosphatase isoenzyme in the serum, or with relatively low steroid values, can be used but are less generally useful. It seems likely, however, that steroid studies will eventually provide a good basis for identifying mole.

Various attempts have been made to use the morphological appearances of hydatidiform moles to predict the likelihood of malignant sequelae but these have not been successful and any correlation which exists is too uncertain to be relied on. A perfectly benign looking mole can give rise to a highly malignant choriocarcinoma and a mole with marked proliferation of its trophoblast can die out (Fig. 3).

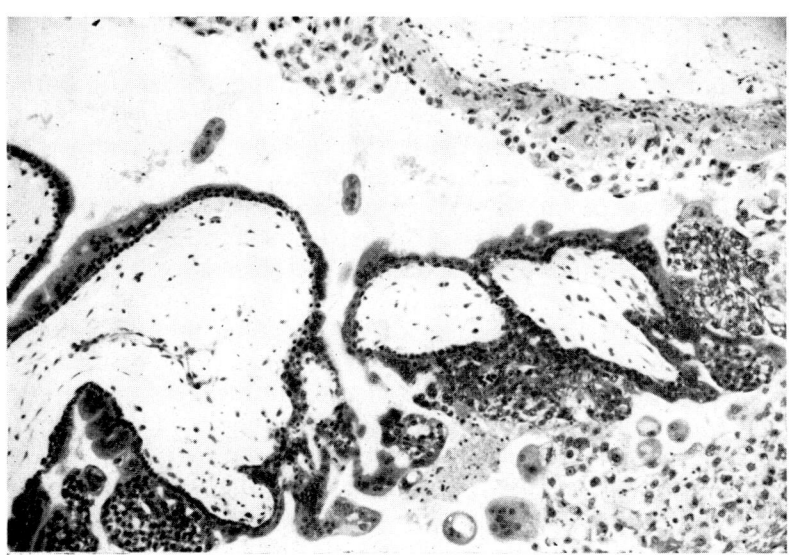

FIG. 3.3. Hydatidiform mole ($\times$ 100) showing quite extensive trophoblastic proliferation with both cytotrophoblast and syncytium in evidence.

It is probably true that molar tissue is deported to the lungs rather more extensively than normal trophoblast, and occasionally deportation occurs on a massive scale causing symptoms and transient radiological opacities. Occasionally this occlusion of the pulmonary vascular tree may be fatal; more commonly it is mistaken for evidence of choriocarcinoma. The distinction between molar deportation which threatens life only by causing vascular occlusion and true metastatic growth has long been recognized although making the distinction may not always be easy. It is also necessary to recognize that true metastases can occur even before a mole has been evacuated. These are commonest in the vagina and lungs and although they may regress spontaneously, this is by no means invariable.

MALIGNANT SEQUELAE OF 'BENIGN' MOLE

The diagnostic confusion which is still commonplace with chorio-carcinoma largely results from its association, in about a half of the cases, with hydatidiform mole. There are several possible sequences which can follow evacuation of a mole and failure to apply our knowledge of these variations in the natural history of the tissue can now be defined as the principal cause of death from choriocarcinoma in the United Kingdom. For this reason I shall try to emphasize this particular problem, for although it is of more direct concern to the gynaecologist than to the oncologist it bears on the general problem of biochemical screening for cancer.

It is unusual, after a term pregnancy or nonmolar abortion, for any trophoblastic remnants to survive more than a day or so. By contrast, the trophoblast remaining in the uterine wall or vessels after evacuation of a mole, generally persists for a time and can be recognized by virtue of its synthesis of chorionic gonadotrophin. The trophoblast may persist only a few days or several years. In most instances it ultimately dies out without sequelae, but so long as it is present there is the possibility of choriocarcinoma appearing and the longer it persists the greater is that risk. The risk of choriocarcinoma after mole in European populations is of the order of 1:30 but an equal proportion may have complications from invasive mole. The main sequences to be observed are illustrated diagrammatically in Fig. 1 although it will be appreciated that numerous variations on these themes can occur.

The amount of trophoblastic tissue which survives, before tumour proliferation is seen, may be very small and its endocrine activity so minimal that normal menstruation may be resumed and pregnancy may occur again before a choriocarcinoma arising from the mole becomes apparent.

The significance of these various post-molar sequelae is greatly increased by the fact that when antitrophoblastic chemotherapy has been initiated within six months of evacuation of a mole, the tumour has, in our series always proved susceptible to chemotherapy and capable of permanent elimination, whereas, when the start of chemotherapy has been deferred beyond this time, some tumours have ultimately proved resistant (Fig. 4). This is not, it may be noted, simply a correlation with the extent of tumour spread or the number of metastases but rather with the age of the tumour, for some 'early' tumours show extensive metastases and are sensitive, whereas other 'late' tumours may have few metastases but prove resistant.

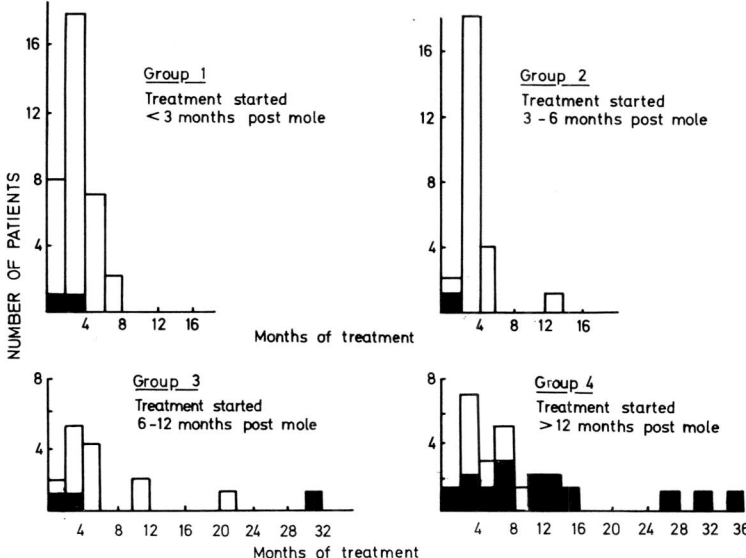

Fɪɢ. 3.4. Relationship between time at which chemotherapy was commenced and duration of chemotherapy. Solid blocks indicate fatal cases. (Reproduced by kind permission of the Editor of the *British Medical Journal*.)

The natural history of hydatidiform mole thus presents us with the dilemma that to treat all or even a high proportion of post-molar trophoblastic proliferations with chemotherapy, as has been suggested, would result in many young women receiving potentially dangerous agents unnecessarily, whereas to withhold chemotherapy until there is unequivocal clinical evidence of an actively growing tumour results in a proportion of them dying from therapeutic failure. How is this problem to be resolved? One solution would be to improve therapy so that it is as effective against 'old' tumours as it already is against 'young' ones. Some progress has been made in this direction, but it is slow and the fact is that present therapy does fail sometimes unless it is started early, and we do not know how long it will be before we can effectively deal with all choriocarcinoma diagnosed at a 'late' stage.

Using present day diagnostic methods and the existing limited therapy, the alternative is to try to ensure that treatment is always initiated sufficiently early. The available data indicate that there are about one thousand patients per year in the United Kingdom with hydatidiform mole. Our evidence indicates that it is possible to select cases for chemotherapy, or where appropriate for surgery, by a careful study of gonadotrophin production as estimated by radioimmunoassay. To ensure that this is done for all patients at risk, some form of notification and use of a centralized or regionalized laboratory service seems necessary. The laboratory can then provide the clinician with a reliable guide to the activity of the persisting trophoblast. Both the technology and the organization necessary to apply it have existed for several years and the cost of providing such a service on a national scale might be less than the cost of treatment and hospital care for patients with advanced disease.

INVASIVE MOLE

This lesion, also known as molar destruens, malignant mole or chorioadenoma destruens, is a common sequel to hydatidiform mole. The frequency with which it is identified depends on the frequency of hysterectomy in the early months after evacuation of moles.

Invasive mole is a trophoblastic proliferation associated with hydropic villous structures and penetration of the myometrium. It may invade blood vessels and cause haemorrhage, or penetrate the serosal surface of the uterus and cause severe abdominal pain; it may metastasize to the vagina and less commonly to the lungs and brain. It may kill, but rarely does so. Part of its importance lies in the difficulty of distinguishing this generally self-limiting condition from choriocarcinoma.

After a mole is evacuated, gonadotrophin values start to fall during the first week (Fig. 1), but it is then common for them to level off well above the normal range, thus indicating the presence of active trophoblast somewhere. When this is found, curettage is indicated and this may reveal some trophoblastic fragments and villi; there may be a further fall in the gonadotrophin levels but only rarely to normal. Obviously, in such cases the trophoblast is elsewhere than in the uterine cavity.

In some patients gonadotrophin production, having levelled off for a while, then shows a progressive fall towards normal. If, whilst the gonadotrophin values are still elevated, pelvic arteriography is performed, a striking abnormality is usually revealed. The uterus (Fig. 5a) is seen to be highly vascular and enlarged and invasive mole is distinguished only with difficulty, if at all, from choriocarcinoma (Cockshott, et al, 1964; Brewis and Bagshawe, 1968). The distinction when it can be made lies in the presence, in invasive mole, of 'punched out areas' corresponding to the avascular villi.

Progressive resolution of these lesions may be followed both by arteriography and, more precisely, by gonadotrophin estimations; and within six months of evacuation the great majority of invasive moles have died out (Bagshawe, 1969).

The difficulty which is critical to the whole problem is that, apart from the small lethal potential of the invasive mole itself, choriocarcinoma can arise well before these six months have passed; it can and

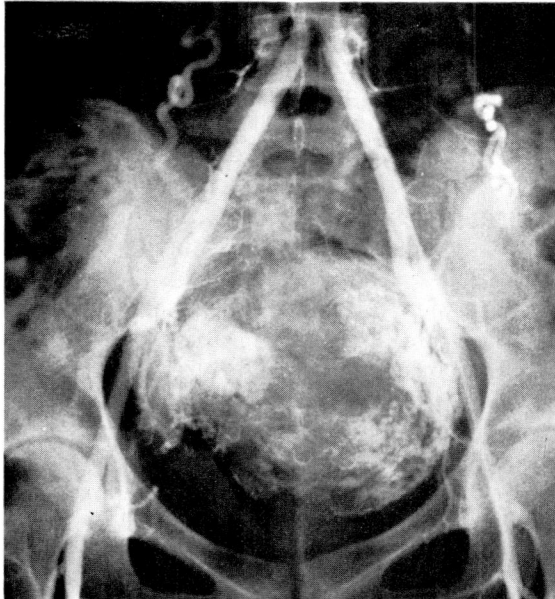

FIG. 3.5a. Pelvic arteriogram 2 years after evacuation of mole. Subsequent hysterectomy revealed choriocarcinoma. Note dilated and tortuous ovarian arteries.

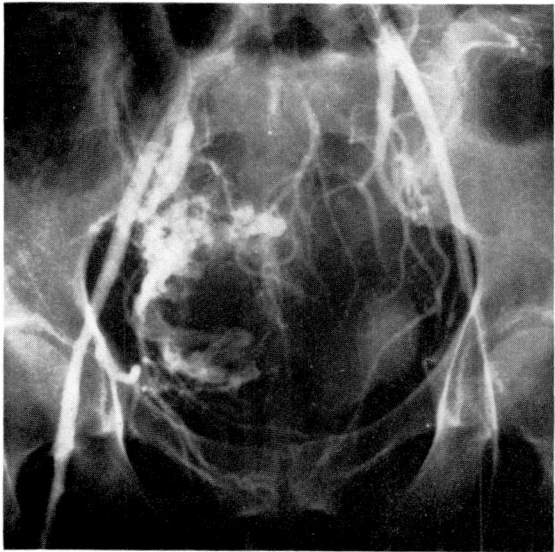

FIG. 3.5b. Arteriogram 1 month after hysterectomy for choriocarcinoma showing extra-uterine arterio-venous fistulae and vaginal metastases.

does kill well within this time and our capacity to eliminate a chorio-carcinoma with certainty depends on starting treatment within this same period.

There is no simple rule of thumb to guide us here. Each case has to be carefully and repeatedly assessed. In fact, by use of radioimmunoassay determinations of hormone activity, radiography, and clinical examination, the selection of cases for treatment can be made with considerable precision. The significance of a particular rate of gonadotrophin excretion is related to the interval since evacuation. Thus a month after evacuation of a mole a gonadotrophin excretion rate equivalent to 5000 I.U./day may merely indicate the need for close surveillance, whereas an excretion rate persisting at about 500 I.U./day six months after evacuation may indicate the need for treatment.

Treatment of Invasive Mole. When morphological examination of curettings reveals molar tissue in the myometrium, and the gonadotrophin excretion rate shows a satisfactory progressive fall, the question of treatment arises. In the absence of symptoms it is usually possible to defer active treatment and the lesion will often regress spontaneously. Active treatment is indicated if the gonadothophin level is not falling, or if it is high, say more than 20,000 I.U. HCG/day and only falling slowly, or if there is pain in the lower abdomen, vaginal metastases which are bleeding, uterine bleeding, dyspnoea, or radiological evidence of pulmonary metastases.

In the absence of pulmonary vascular obstruction by mole, hysterectomy is an effective form of treatment, but in most instances where the patient is young, or has no family, chemotherapy is preferable. Chemotherapy for invasive mole can be comparatively free of unpleasant side effects and of much shorter duration than is normally necessary for choriocarcinoma.

All too often one cannot distinguish invasive mole from post-molar choriocarcinoma, but since both respond to the same chemotherapy it is usually unnecessary to perform hysterectomy for diagnostic reasons.

CHORIOCARCINOMA

The incidence of choriocarcinoma in European population is about 1:40,000 pregnancies whereas it may be 1:6000 pregnancies or more in South-east Asia. About half the cases follow mole, and the remainder follow term deliveries and abortions, with about equal frequency. The three forms of antecedent pregnancy contribute roughly equal numbers of fatal cases, thus reflecting a somewhat better prognosis following mole. The average age of 27 years in European populations is slightly lower than that found in South-east Asia. In the U.S.A. and the U.K.

there appears to be a greater risk of choriocarcinoma following a first than a later pregnancy (Bagshawe, 1969).

The interval between the end of the antecedent pregnancy and diagnosis is partly caused by the difficulties of diagnosis. In our series the mean interval following mole was 8·35 months, following term pregnancy 11·2 months, and following abortion 7·8 months. Instances where the interval is as much as 4 years are uncommon but not exceptional. In some patients who have had a mole, a subsequent normal pregnancy may be followed by choriocarcinoma, and in one of the writer's series the interval between the mole and the normal pregnancy was 13 years. Clearly, patients who have had moles should invariably have gonadotrophin studies after any subsequent pregnancy.

In 4 of 40 patients in the present series hysterectomy revealed no choriocarcinoma, even though there was evidence of active tumour elsewhere. In these cases it must be assumed either that a primary tumour has regressed, or that trophoblast in the extra-uterine pelvic vascular bed or elsewhere in the body has undergone malignant transformation.

Morphology. The characteristic lesion of choriocarcinoma is a reddish purple node with a rim of viable cells surrounding a large necrotic centre. Both cytotrophoblast and syncytium are present in the majority of lesions and sometimes the syncytium is peripherally situated with respect to islands of cytotrophoblast, perhaps as a vestigial tendency towards the organizational form of the primary villus, but the mature villous structure is characteristically absent. In its frequently intravascular sites, the peripheral distribution of living tumour tissue is again observed with the centre of the vessel occupied by thrombus. Blood clot and haemorrhage are to be seen in most lesions and are of course the cause of their colour to the naked eye.

A variety of patterns are formed by the cytotrophoblastic cells. They may be densely packed or rather loose, they may form regular polymorphic masses or trabeculate or foliate arrangements. Cellular polymorphism may be marked, but is found in the trophoblast of the early normal embryo as well as in choriocarcinoma. The cytoplasm is often foamy and the nuclei hyperchromatic and multiple in the syncytial cells (Fig. 6). Mitotic figures are often difficult to identify because of the coarse nuclear chromatin. Leucocytic infiltrations can be identified in association with many tumour masses but are notably variable in extent between patients.

Myometrial invasion is found initially in all cases where there is tumour in the uterus, and it is common for the lesions to reach the serosal surface where it causes pain, or the endometrial surface where it often causes haemorrhage. Clearly the curette can only be of diagnostic help when the lesion is on, or close to, the endometrial surface.

There are two striking features about the spread of this tumour.

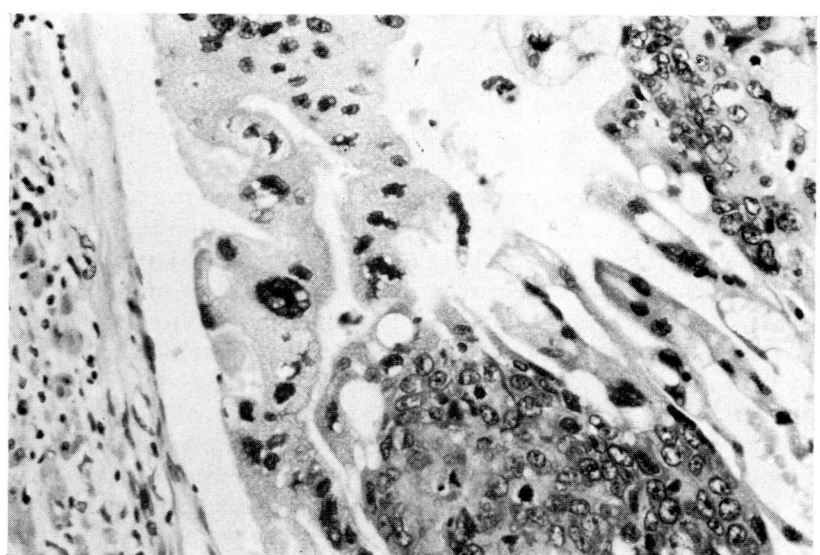

FIG. 3.6. Choriocarcinoma (× 250). Syncytial elements showing coarse endoplasmic reticulum disposed around two areas of cytophoblastic cells.

The first is the great rarity with which it can be found in lymph nodes and bone marrow, and the second is its predilection for spread by the bloodstream and for growth within blood vessels. In the pelvis extra-uterine spread occurs directly and by tracking through vessels which are often pathologically dilated. Fistulae between the vagina and bladder or rectum may occur, and vaginal metastases readily identifiable by pelvic arteriography can cause torrential haemorrhage (Fig. 5b). Within the pelvic veins, large thrombi containing choriocarcinoma are frequent and result in pulmonary embolism. Enlargement of one or both ovaries by lutein cysts is common in both mole and choriocarcinoma, probably due to hormonal factors.

Metastatic spread to the lungs is well recognized and was found radiologically or pathologically in 66% of the author's cases. It may take the form of discrete parenchymal masses, ranging in size from mothballs to cannon-balls, a snowstorm pattern, or an intravascular form, or any combination of these (Figs. 2, 7, 8). The intravascular form is the most likely to cause symptoms but least likely to be recognized radiologically. It presents mainly with exertional dyspnoea and episodic pleuritic pain, and there may be evidence of pulmonary hypertension. The more slowly progressive forms are apt to be mistaken for neurosis until an advanced stage.

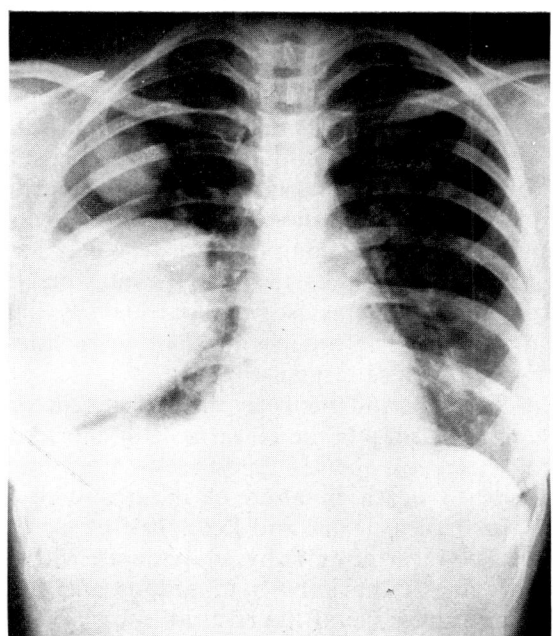

Fig. 3.7. Classical cannon-ball metastases 1 year after delivery by caesarian section. (Reproduced by kind permission of Messrs. Edward Arnold from 'Choriocarcinoma' by K.D.B.)

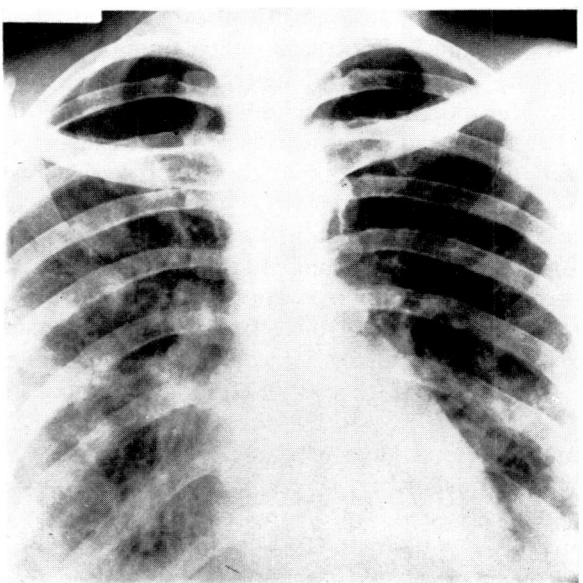

Fig. 3.8. Rapidly growing metastases 8 months after hydatidiform mole. A chest film taken 2 weeks earlier was normal.

Metastases to the brain are common both as a presenting feature and as a complication in the course of treatment. It is exceptional for these to be found in the absence of pulmonary metastases. Intrathecal therapy with methotrexate or cytosine arabinoside can be used successfully but is not without complications. Metastases in the spinal cord may produce complete paraplegia within 2–3 days of the onset of symptoms, yet if treatment is initiated promptly complete recovery may be achieved.

The other common sites of metastases are the intestinal tract, kidneys, liver and omentum. Gut metastases are particularly liable to bleed. They may also perforate before chemotherapy or during the early stages of treatment, or cause intussusception.

Although the latent period between the antecedent pregnancy and the onset of symptoms may be quite variable in choriocarcinoma, the course of the disease subsequently tends to be more uniform so that, untreated, it leads to death in about 4 months with survival only rarely for more than a year (Park and Lees, 1950).

Arteriography. Pelvic arteriography in patients with trophoblastic tumours often provides remarkable radiographs and has contributed significantly to our knowledge of the natural history of the sequelae to hydatidiform mole and particularly to our knowledge of the vascularity of these tumours. It can be used to distinguish mole from normal pregnancy but in clinical practice, if it is known that a patient has a mole, arteriography is unnecessary and, if it is not certain, then the radiation hazard to a normal conceptus may be prohibitive. Nor does the presence of a vascular abnormality persisting after a mole preclude the possibility that the lesion will regress spontaneously. It was also hoped that arteriography would provide a ready means of distinguishing between invasive mole and choriocarcinoma, but except in a few cases where 'punched out' areas can be attributed to vesicles causing filling defects, this is not usually possible.

Despite these limitations pelvic arteriography has a place. It is for instance useful to have visual confirmation of a pathological process which might otherwise be known to exist only from hormonal evidence. It can define the risk of haemorrhage from vaginal metastases and the presence of extra-uterine masses. It can also provide a guide to the safety of hysterectomy, or to the likelihood of uncontrollable haemorrhage.

Where fistulous lesions have been present in the pelvic vasculature at the time of diagnosis, then subsequent arteriography can confirm resolution or persistence. Quite gross lesions have been observed to resolve completely, but aneurysmal dilations resembling mycotic aneurysm have been observed to persist.

Probably the most useful application of arteriography occurs quite commonly in choriocarcinoma patients whose treatment has started comparatively late. A typical patient has pulmonary metastases and a uterine mass initially, and after some months of chemotherapy the lungs have cleared and the uterus is almost normal in size, but gonado-trophin studies indicate persistent tumour activity somewhere. Arterio-graphy at this time may show whether or not there is a residual lesion in the uterus, and therefore whether hysterectomy will be useful.

Immunological Factors in Choriocarcinoma. Ever since it was recogni-zed that gestational choriocarcinoma is a foetal tumour which invades the maternal host there has been a strong suspicion that immunological factors may be involved. If tumours are antigenic the immune response 'ought' to eliminate them when they are insignificant in size. Another anomaly has been that antigenic tissues are destroyed by immune processes and yet the mammalian foetus escapes. Choriocarcinoma seems involved in both anomalies, and both need resolution.

Interest in choriocarcinoma focussed at first on the suggestion that its antigenicity might include not only supposedly weak tumour specific antigens but also supposedly strong transplantation antigens, controlled by genes inherited from the male. It was next pointed out that not all mating pairs in an outbred population such as man are antigenically distinct, and that perhaps choriocarcinoma only occurs where antigenic differences between the parents are minimal, so that the foetus lacks few, if any, antigens not present on maternal cells.

The evidence for an immune reaction against choriocarcinoma may then be summarized as follows: (1) Histological examinations of choriocarcinoma shows, in variable degree, the presence of clusters of mononuclear cells in the tissues adjacent to choriocarcinomatous masses. The presence of a well marked cellular reaction is associated with a better prognosis (Elston, 1969) (2) There are in the sera of many choriocarcinoma patients, antibodies to transplantation antigens which are lacking from their own cells but present on the cells of their respec-tive husbands and, by inference, on the choriocarcinoma cells. This evidence is open to criticism in that such antibodies are known to arise in the course of normal pregnancy and after blood transfusions. Nevertheless, the frequency with which they are found in relation to the number of previous transfusions and pregnancies is such that it seems likely that the antibodies are invoked by antigens on the tumour cells. (3) Evidence has slowly accumulated which indicates that the distribu-tion of the ABO blood groups in patients, and in their husbands, deviates from that of the general population. There is a shift away from Group O in the patients (Scott 1962) and a shift towards Group O in their husbands. More particularly, study of the ABO groups of children resulting from pregnancies from which have arisen choriocarcinoma, have revealed fewer instances than expected in which the child is ABO incompatible with its mother. The most remarkable finding has been that Group A women married to Group O males have almost 10 times more risk of getting choriocarcinoma than Group A women married to Group A males. Moreover, present evidence indicates that Group AB women have a bad prognosis (Bagshawe, Rawlins, Pike, Lawler 1971). We do not yet know the significance of these findings but although they suggest the operation of strong antigenic influences they are not wholly consistent with current immunological concepts.

Evidence from the so-called leucocyte antigen systems is more complex. The leucocytes of children from choriocarcinoma pregnancies in the present series have been studied by Dr. Sylvia Lawler and they have frequently shown antigenic differences from their mothers' cells. Although these antigens are regarded as strong transplantation antigens, it would seem from this that they are notably weaker than ABO factors and that choriocarcinoma is able to grow and to kill in the face of the immune response which they evoke.

It would not be possible to discuss here all the various factors which appear to operate and which may contribute to the success of the foetus as an allograft but they have been reviewed elsewhere (Currie, 1969; Bagshawe, 1969). Suffice it to say that the surface characteristics of trophoblastic cells which form the foetomaternal interface appear to be specially adapted to meet the requirements. They do not, it seems, lack paternally derived transplantation antigens, but certain molecular configurations in the cell periphery appear to mask the antigenic sites (Currie, van Doorninck, and Bagshawe, 1968). This masking is unlikely to be absolute. Indeed, women become immunized against antigens derived from their husband during the course of pregnancy perhaps due to trophoblast in part and also to leakages of leucocytes from the foetus into the maternal circulation. It is also probable that maternal antibody combines with exposed antigen sites on trophoblast and, because these sites are few in number, the antibody fails to be cytolytic to trophoblast. By doing this the antibody also acts as a masking agent and thus hides otherwise exposed antigenic sites from maternal lymphocytes.

The operation of such factors in the growth of experimental tumours has been described as enhancement (Kaliss, 1962) and the antigenic foetus and antigenic tumours may owe their success to similar mechanisms. The escape of antigenic tissues, such as the normal trophoblast and tumour tissues, from destruction possibly owes less to the host's failure to develop an immune reaction than to their non-susceptibility to the reaction which develops.

If this is so, the common proposition that we should endeavour to provoke an immune response against choriocarcinoma and other tumours is open to question. It would perhaps be more pertinent and, no doubt, far more difficult to increase the susceptibility of the target tissue. In the case of choriocarcinoma it is indeed easy to establish a strong immune response, if one is not already detectable against paternal antigens, by injecting the patient with leucocytes or by grafting with skin from the husband. This has been done in some 20 patients in our series but the benefits attributed to this have been marginal. Non-specific immunological stimulation with BCG has also been performed in a number of patients but has frequently failed when combined with concurrent chemotherapy. The possibility that it may be useful

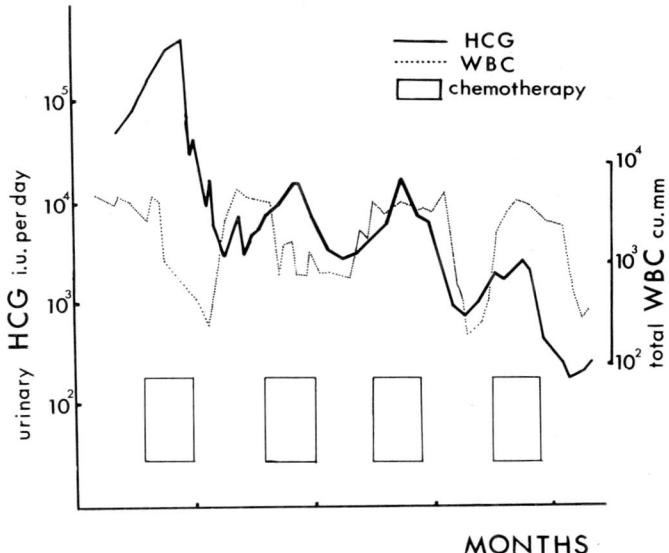

Fig. 3.9. Gonadotrophin excretion and total WBC count during four courses of chemotherapy. The number of surviving tumour cells approximates to the HCG output multiplied by 10^5.

to apply immunisation procedures after chemotherapy has reduced the tumour cell population to a small number does, however, remain.

Chemotherapy should be regarded as the principal form of treatment for choriocarcinoma and invasive mole, but integrated with surgery and radiotherapy in the most effective sequence for the individual patient. Treatment of these tumours is complex and it is difficult to reduce it to a few simple generalizations.

Study of the use of cytotoxic agents in patients with choriocarcinoma has moreover provided evidence which seems relevant to other forms of cancer which lack the special characteristics of this tumour. The evidence is certainly open to different interpretations and it would not be possible to discuss all these here but the interpretations which will be discussed may at least prove provocative.

Starting with the phenomenon of hormone production by these tumours, it is observed that the amount of hormone produced correlates adequately with such other evidence of total tumour mass as may be available and when the total viable tumour mass can be assessed the correlation is closer still. Alterations in HCG production (Fig. 9) can therefore be interpreted as evidence of a parallel alteration in viable tumour. Owing to the cross reaction between LH and HCG, we lose track of the tumour against the background LH when the tumour cell population is about $10^5 - 10^6$ cells, which is about 0·1 cu cm of viable tumour mass. During treatment we witness a progressive reduction in the tumour cell population from perhaps $10^{11} - 10^{12}$ cells down to this level. If treatment is discontinued before normal HCG levels are reached, gonadotrophin production soon starts to increase again and tumour growth can be inferred. As might be expected, if treatment is discontinued as soon as gonadotrophin excretion is normal the same sequence occurs, for there are likely to be at least 10^5 cells ready to start the whole process off again. Treatment has to be continued long beyond attaining normal gonadotrophin values in most patients with choriocarcinoma. It is possible to obtain some idea of how long to go on by plotting the rate of response and by extrapolating this line to the zero cell level. Unfortunately the rate of response in the 'visible' range is not always sustained in the sub-visible range, so successful treatment may take even longer.

Having such a valuable parameter of tumour growth prompts a consideration of what is meant by 'tumour growth'. Tumours generally kill by virtue of the volume they occupy, either in the general sense or in specific anatomical locations. Clinical concepts of tumour growth generally relate to volume. But growth at a cellular level means an increase in the number of tumour cells and we have to inquire into the relationship between tumour volume and cell numbers. Tumours are complex structures and for the most part they do not consist wholly and exclusively of living tumour cells. Many tumour masses, and this includes choriocarcinoma, consist of dead tissue. Many tumour cells die without dividing, so it is necessary to distinguish between the potential growth rate of the population, that is the rate at which it would grow in the absence of losses, and the actual growth rate. The difference between the actual and potential growth rates is the rate of spontaneous cell loss.

An analysis of the data from choriocarcinoma and a consideration of the action of antimitotic agents on an expanding population has led to the proposition that agents which kill cells in mitosis non-selectively only have the ability to achieve a progressive reduction in a tumour population when the rate of spontaneous cell death in the population exceeds a critical value (Bagshawe, 1968). A reduction in the spontaneous cell death rate during therapy could account for the observation that resistance to one agent is generally accompanied by the development of resistance to other agents which operate on other biochemical pathways. Conventional resistance developing through the classical mechanisms of selection and adaptation does, no doubt, operate but it fails to account for many of the resistance phenomena encountered in clinical practice. In this regard it is notable that the three malignant processes which respond most dramatically to chemo-therapy-choriocarcinoma, Burkitt's lymphoma and acute lympho-blastic leukaemia in children—show evidence of very high rates of spontaneous cell death during phases when they are most sensitive to antimitotic agents. Also, at this time, these malignancies are susceptible to a wide variety of antimitotic agents.

Spontaneous cell death within a tumour cell population results from many different mechanisms. Some of these 'losses' occur when cells leave the tumour mass by any route, some occur at the tumour-host interface and are immunologically mediated, others occur within the cell mass and are a consequence of nutritional and genetic factors. It seems to be vitally important that we should define as precisely as we are able, the limits and potentialities of each therapeutic approach to cancer. It is remarkable that the present substantial array of agents, whose essential action is to kill cells engaged in mitotic or pre-mitotic processes, should be employed without defining such parameters much more carefully than is customary at present.

Such matters as these, which arise naturally from a consideration of the response of choriocarcinoma to cytotoxic agents, have of course, much wider significance than the techniques of day-to-day management of choriocarcinoma. But in the context of the individual patient the techniques employed can make life or death differences.

SUMMARY OF TREATMENT METHODS

Workers at the National Institutes of Health, Bethesda, were responsible for the introduction of three valuable agents into the treatment of choriocarcinoma. These were methotrexate (Li, Hertz, Spencer, 1956), vinblastine (Hertz, Lipsett, Moy, 1960) and actinomycin-D (Hertz, 1967). In general, it seems to take many years of systematic study to determine how best to use a particular drug in the treatment of a particular tumour. This process continues in the case of these drugs in choriocarcinoma and so far it has been possible to introduce some marginal improvement in treatment methods every few months.

Present therapy can be summarized as follows. With the preliminary investigations completed and the diagnosis established chemotherapy should be delayed only if there is infection, or if the patient is post-operative, or if the patient is going to be transferred to a unit elsewhere within a few days. Hysterectomy should not be performed as an initial procedure except in menopausal or multiparous subjects, and then only if they have a circumscribed lesion in the uterus identified arterio-graphically with no evidence of distant metastases.

Treatment should be carried out under the conditions most favourable to the avoidance of infection. Blood should be cross-matched. A routine weekly bacteriological examination of the patient's skin, mucosal and intestinal flora is valuable. It is essential to monitor renal and hepatic function as well as the peripheral blood count and gonadotrophin production. Without attention to these a patient with early disease may still be treated successfully but her statistical chances of success are greatly reduced and if the disease has been diagnosed late, the chances of success are small.

Methotrexate used with folinic acid now provides the main line of treatment. It is perhaps a little less effective than methotrexate by it-self in some patients but it has the substantial advantage that it does not cause much loss of intestinal mucosa nor stomatitis, nor alopecia. Properly used it achieves permanent remissions in most cases of early choriocarcinoma as well as invasive mole. The route of administration determines the optimum time relationship between methotrexate and folinic acid and deviation from this can result in loss of therapeutic effect as well as loss of toxicity.

One regime consists of giving methotrexate (25 mg/24 hours) at a constant rate, by intravenous or intra-arterial infusion, together with folinic acid (6 mg) every 12 hours for the period of the infusion. The infusion may be continued for 7 days in most but not in all patients and the next course should begin after a rest period of 7 days. If pro-found leucopenia or thrombocytopenia persists the rest period may have to be extended.

Alternatively, methotrexate (50 mg) is given intramuscularly every 48 hours, with folinic acid (5 mg) by oral route 30 hours after each injection of methotrexate. A total of 4 injections of methotrexate constitutes a complete course which must again be followed by a rest period of one week.

If the response to methotrexate-folinic acid is seen to be tailing off, actinomycin-D is given and sometimes it appears to produce an increased rate of tumour destruction. However, a tumour which has shown resistance to methotrexate is likely to show resistance to actino-mycin-D before long and it is therefore advantageous to give vinblastine also. Actinomycin-D (0·5 mg or 0·01 mg/kg) is given daily for 5–7 days and vinblastine 10 mg is given on the 2nd and 4th days. Individual tolerance is, however, very variable and it must be individually adjusted. Cumulative toxicity tends to occur with actinomycin-D. Vinblastine, by itself, has not proved effective in our hands, nor has vincristine (Bagshawe, 1968).

Where these regimes fail to eradicate the tumour, combinations of methotrexate, folinic acid, actinomycin-D and vinblastine have occasionally produced remissions. 6-Azauridine, an agent which blocks the action of orotodylic decarboxylase in the pyrimidine pathways, may also prove to be of value in the management of choriocarcinoma and although this is a relatively non-toxic drug its use is attended by some unusual pitfalls.

As soon as evidence of drug resistance appears the possibility of surgical intervention should be considered. Hysterectomy may be useful if there is a persisting uterine lesion and a segmental resection or lobectomy has sometimes successfully removed the last remaining pulmonary metastasis.

Unfortunately, many of the finer points in the management of choriocarcinoma cannot be put briefly into words and this is particularly true of the interpretation of the results of gonadotrophin assays, on which so much depends.

Also, it would not be possible to refer in this chapter to choriocarcinoma in ovarian and testicular teratomata in any detail. Ovarian choriocarcinoma has responded in some instances as well as the gestational form. Advanced testicular choriocarcinoma generally responds up to a point; metastases can be reduced or may even disappear altogether, but in the majority of instances complete elimination of the tumour is not achieved. However, sustained remissions have occasionally been obtained in patients with advanced disease. In early cases, where the only evidence of metastatic spread is HCG production after orchidectomy, the few cases seen by this writer have been highly sensitive to chemotherapy and it seems advantageous to use this approach as soon as the diagnosis is established without waiting for metastases to appear.

Units which specialize in the treatment of choriocarcinoma have become familiar with what must be, at the present time, one of the most harrowing experiences in medical practice. A young person is admitted with advanced metastatic disease perhaps including brain metastases, perhaps in coma or with intestinal obstruction. With considerable effort sustained over several months the patient recovers to a state of normal well-being and full function. But in some patients radioimmunoassay indicates that somewhere there is still some residual tumour. Treatment is continued but too often there is a slow and inexorable progression; the gonadotrophins increase, metastases reappear and the tumour finally has the last word. The number of such failures is being reduced gradually by therapeutic advances but the tragedy is that although most of these patients seek medical advice early in their disease, and although the methods needed to establish the diagnosis are readily available, they are not always used early enough.

REFERENCES

BAGSHAWE, K. D. (1968a). Some Immunological Aspects of Choriocarcinoma. *Biology and Surgery of Tissue Transplantation*. Maxwell Anderson, J. (Ed.). Glasgow: Blackwell Scientific Publications.

BAGSHAWE, K. D. (1968b). Tumour growth and antimitotic action. *Br. J. Cancer*, **22**, 698.

BAGSHAWE, K. D. (1968c). Vinca Alkaloids in the Treatment of Gestational Choriocarcinoma. *The Vinca Alkaloids in the Chemotherapy of Malignant Disease*. Sheddar, W. I. H. (Ed.). Ann. Eli Lilly Symposium (1968).

BAGSHAWE, K. D. (1969). *Choriocarcinoma: The Clinical Biology of the Trophoblast and its Tumours*. London: Edward Arnold.

BAGSHAWE, K. D., GOLDING, P. R., & ORR, A. H. (1969). Choriocarcinoma after hydatidiform mole. Studies related to effectiveness of follow-up practice after hydatidiform mole. *Br. med. J.*, **3**, 733.

BAGSHAWE, K. D., ORR, A. H., & RUSHWORTH, A. G. J. (1968). Relationship between concentrations of human chorionic gonadotrophin in plasma and cerebrospinal fluid. *Nature, Lond.*, **217**, 950.

BAGSHAWE, K. D., WILDE, C. E., & ORR, A. H. (1966). Radioimmunoassay for human chorionic gonadotrophin and luteinising hormone. *Lancet*, **i**, 1118.

BAGSHAWE, K. D., RAWLINS, G., PIKE, M. C., LAWLER, S. (1971). ABO Blood-groups in Trophoblastic Neoplasia. *Lancet.*, **i**, 553.

BÖVING, B. G. (1959). The biology of trophoblast. *Ann. N. Y. Acad. Sci.*, **80**, 21.

BREWIS, R. A. L., & BAGSHAWE, K. D. (1968). Pelvic arteriography in invasive trophoblastic neoplasia. *Br. J. Radiol.*, **41**, 481.

COCKSHOTT, W. P., EVANS, K. T., & HENDRICKSE, J. P. de V. (1964). Arteriography of trophoblastic tumours. *Clin. Radiol.*, **15**, 1.

CURRIE, G. A. (1969). The foetus as an allograft: the role of maternal unresponsiveness to paternally derived foetal antigens. Ciba Foundation Symposium on Foetal Autonomy. p. 32. Wolstenholme, G. E. W., & O'Connor, M. (Eds.).

CURRIE, G. A., VAN DOORNINCK, W., & BAGSHAWE, K. D. (1968). Effect of neuraminidase on the immunogenicity of early mouse trophoblast. *Nature, Lond.*, **219**, 191.

DONALD, I. (1962a). 'Sonar': a new diagnostic echo-sounding technique in obstetrics and gynaecology. *Proc. R. Soc. Med.*, **55**, 637.

DONALD, I. (1962b). Clinical application of ultrasonic techniques in obstetrics and gynaecological diagnosis. *J. Obstet. Gynaec. Br. Commonw.*, **69**, 1039.

ELSTON, C. W. (1969). Cellular reaction to choriocarcinoma. *J. Path.*, **97**, 261.

HERTZ, R., LIPSETT, M. B., & MOY, R. H. (1960). Effect of vincaleukoblastine on metastatic choriocarcinoma and related trophoblastic tumours in women. *Cancer Res.*, **20**, 1050.

HERTZ, R., LIPSETT, M. B., & MOY, R. H. (1967). Eight Years Experience with the Chemotherapy of Choriocarcinoma and Related Trophoblastic Tumours in Women. *Choriocarcinoma: Transactions of a Conference of the International Union Against Cancer*. Holland, J. F. and Hreshchyshyn, M. M. (Eds.). p. 66. Berlin: Springer-Verlag.

KALISS, N. (1962). Elements of immunologic enhancement: considerations of mechanism. *Ann. N.Y. Acad. Sci.*, **101**, 64.

KIRBY, D. R. S. (1965). The 'Invasiveness' of the Trophoblast. The Early Conceptus, Normal and Abnormal. *Papers and Discussions Presented at a Symposium Held at Queen's College, Dundee, September 1964.* Park, W. W. (Ed.). p. 68. Edinburgh: Livingstone.

LI, M. C., HERTZ, R., & SPENCER, D. B. (1956). Effect of methotrexate therapy upon choriocarcinoma and chorioadenoma. *Proc. Soc. exp. Biol. Med.*, **93**, 361.

MIDGLEY, A. R. Jr., PIERCE, G. B. Jr., DENEAU, G. A., & GOSLING, J. R. G. (1963). Morphogenesis of syncytiotrophoblast *in vivo*: an autoradiographic demonstration. *Science*, **141**, 349.

PARK, W. W. (1957). The occurrence of sex chromatin in chorionepitheliomas and hydatidiform moles. *J. Path. Bact.*, **74**, 197.

PARK, W. W., & LEES, J. C. (1950). Choriocarcinoma: a general review, with analysis of 516 cases. *Arch. Path.*, **49**, 73, 205, 361.

RUSHWORTH, A. G. J., ORR, A. H., & BAGSHAWE, K. D. (1968). The concentration of HCG in the plasma and spinal fluid of patients with trophoblastic tumours in the central nervous system. *Br. J. Cancer*, **22**, 253.

SCOTT, J. S. (1962). Choriocarcinoma: observations on the etiology. *Am. J. Obstet. Gynec.*, **83**, 195.

SMALBRAAK, J. (1957). *Trophoblastic Growths: A Clinical, Hormonal and Histopathologic Study of Hydatidiform Mole and Chorionepithelioma.* Amsterdam: Elsevier.

STOLBACH, L. I., KRANT, M. J., & FISHMAN, W. H. (1969). Ectopic production of an alkaline phosphatase isoenzyme in patients with cancer. *New Engl. J. Med.*, **281**, 757.

WARBURG, O. (1956). On the origin of cancer cells. *Science*, **123**, 309.

WILDE, C. E., ORR, A. H., & BAGSHAWE, K. D. (1967). A sensitive radioimmunoassay for human chorionic gonadotrophin and luteinising hormone. *J. Endocr.*, **27**, 23.

4 Management of Childhood Leukaemia

M. L. N. WILLOUGHBY

INTRODUCTION

The aim of therapy in acute leukaemia is first to obtain a complete remission and secondly to maintain this state of remission for as long as possible. A third, but at present still elusive objective would be to achieve permanent cure in a significant proportion of patients.

Management of the disease entails not only the selection of appropriate anti-leukaemic therapy but also the use of supportive measures, to correct or compensate for the deficiencies of haemopoietic and immunological function that may be caused either by the leukaemic process or by its therapy. It also involves an element of personal support for the patient and their family throughout what is usually a protracted period of several years.

REMISSION INDUCTION

The adoption of relatively uniform criteria for complete remission has permitted quantitative comparisons between different drug schedules used for the purpose of remission induction. The usual sequence of changes in clinical and haematological manifestations of the disease during initial therapy are shown in Fig. 1.

A state of complete remission is reached when there are:

1. no symptoms attributable to the disease;

2. no hepatosplenomegaly, lymphadenopathy or other clinical evidence of residual leukaemic tissue infiltration;

3. a normal peripheral blood picture with granulocytes 1,500/cu mm or over, platelets 150,000/cu mm or over, haemoglobin 12 G/100 ml or over and with no blast cells seen in the peripheral blood film;

4. a marrow smear of normal cellularity showing predominantly granulocytic and erythroid precursors together with adequate megakaryocytes and less than 5% blast cells, none possessing frankly leukaemic features ('Al Marrow Status'). Such features would include giant nucleoli, nuclear clefts (Reider-Cells), Sudan-Black Positive auer

71

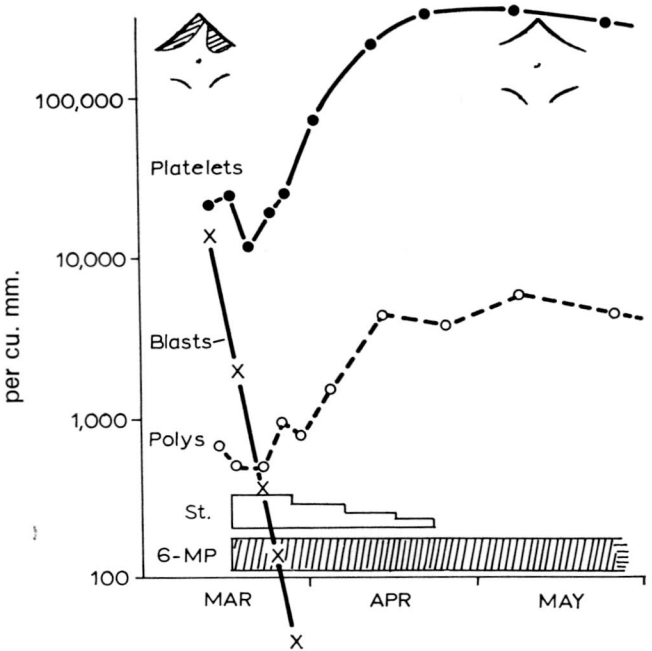

FIG. 4.1. Sequence of peripheral blood changes and regression of hepatosplenomegaly during remission induction.

rods in Myeloblasts or Monoblasts, and P.A.S.-Positive 'blocks' or
'bars' in Lymphoblasts.

Criteria for *complete remission*, similar to those above, as well as for
partial remission and for *no response to therapy* have been defined by
Bisel (1956) and have subsequently been used in the numerous clinical
trials conducted by the Acute Leukaemia Group B (ALGB) and
National Cancer Institute (Bethesda) groups in the U.S.A. Similar
symptomatic, clinical, peripheral blood and bone marrow criteria for
complete remission, partial remission or relapse have been defined by
other groups (National Criteria Committee, 1964; Vietti *et al.*, 1965;
Leiken *et al.*, 1968). In general, persistence of any abnormality attributable to leukaemic infiltration, or the presence of more than 5%
of blast cells in the marrow, precludes complete remission status;
whereas manifestations of chemotherapeutic toxicity such as buccal
ulceration, moderate degrees of marrow hypoplasia or megaloblastic
erythropoiesis do not.

From Table I it is seen that Vincristine (VCR), Steroids (PRED),
Daunorubicin (DAUNO) and Asparaginase (ASP) are the four most

TABLE I

REMISSION INDUCTION IN UNTREATED CHILDHOOD ALL
DRUGS USED SINGLY OR IN COMBINATION

Treatment	No. of patients in study	%CR*
Single drugs		
PRED ⎱	337	63%
VCR ⎰ Inducers	103	57%
DAUNO	25	64%
ASP	21	67%
ARA-C	51	30%
6-MP	43	27%
MTX	48	22%
CYCLO	50	14%
Two drugs		
PRED + VCR	121	86%
PRED + DAUNO	8	87%
PRED + 6-MP	154	82%
PRED + MTX	80	80%
PRED + CYTOX	58	76%
6-MP + MTX	39	43%
Three drugs		
PRED + VCR + DAUNO	33	97%
	11	100%
Four drugs		
PRED + VCR + 6-MP + MTX (POMP)	35	94%

* Complete marrow remission

TABLE II

DURATION OF FIRST REMISSION WITH CONTINUOUS MAINTENANCE THERAPY

Maintenance Drug	Drugs used for remission induction	No. of patients in study	Median complete remission
PRED	PRED	16	11 weeks
ASP	ASP	8	11 weeks
VCR	VCR	37	9 weeks
DAUNO	DAUNO	28	7 weeks
MTX (bi-weekly)	VCR + PRED	22	55 weeks
6-MP	PRED	28	33 weeks
6-MP + MTX	VCR + PRED	37	30 weeks
ARA-C	ARA-C	51	19 weeks
CYCLO	PRED + CYCLO	34	17 weeks

efficient drugs for remission induction in childhood acute lymphoblastic leukaemia (ALL). For this reason, they are referred to as *inducer drugs*. They are relatively ineffective when used alone for purposes of maintaining established remissions compared to drugs such as 6-Mercaptopurine (6-MP) or Methotrexate (MTX) (Table II).

It can also be seen from Table I that combinations of drugs are more effective than single drugs. The % remissions obtained with any two drugs is very close to, and may slightly exceed, the % expected from the independent action of each drug separately. The anti-leukaemic effects of two or more drugs are therefore at least additive, and possibly synergistic, with respect to remission induction (ALGB, 1965b; Zubrod, 1965). Combinations of two or more inducer drugs are therefore particularly effective. The most widely used remission induction schedule employs VCR plus Prednisone or Prednisolone (PRED) in the following doses:

VCR $1\cdot5$–$2\cdot0$ mg/m²/week I.V.
PRED   40 mg/m²/day in divided oral doses.

Complete remissions in untreated ALL are obtained in 84% to 96% by the use of these two drugs (ALGB, 1965 and 1969). The remission rate for patients in their first relapse is 82% and in the second relapse 63% (Hardisty *et al.*, 1969). It is undoubtedly the initial treatment of choice in ALL. Holland (1968) has shown that there is a sigmoid time-remission relationship with 70% of patients achieving remission in 28 days, but with 20% reaching this state in under 20 days and another 20% taking up to 40 days for remission to occur. A three-fold increase in steroid dose, to 120 mg/m², did not increase the speed of remission nor the final % of remissions in this study; but the subsequent duration of remissions maintained by antimetabolites was slightly longer with the higher steroid dose, which may indicate that a greater leukaemic 'cell kill' was obtained with the higher dose (Holland, quoted by Henderson, 1969).

An advantage of using VCR plus steroids is that neither drug is particularly toxic to the normal myeloid or megakaryocyte series in the marrow. At the initial stage of the disease when there is neutropenia and thrombocytopenia with few remaining normal marrow cells it is preferable to avoid further marrow depression. ASP is another drug which produces minimal marrow depression (Oettgen *et al.*, 1967; Hill *et al.*, 1969). Used in combination with VCR, steroids or both, it might further improve the % of remission in ALL over and above the already high rate obtained with VCR plus steroids alone.

Another example of the use of two inducer drugs is the combination of DAUNO plus PRED (Holton *et al.*, 1969). DAUNO was given at a dose of 25 mg/m² for 3 days followed by a 4 day rest. Two thirds of children at an advanced stage of ALL achieved remission, but marrow depression was more marked than with VCR and PRED.

Triple combination therapy using the 3 inducer drugs DAUNO, VCR and PRED has been used by Mathé *et al.* (1967) with apparently 100% complete remission rate. Since DAUNO has marked marrow toxicity these remissions are obtained at the cost of greater marrow depression, requiring nursing in pathogen-free rooms and availability of platelet transfusions. With this reservation it is, however, a very effective remission induction schedule that can be useful in ALL failing to respond to VCR plus steroids alone, and in acute myeloid leukaemia (AML). The doses are as follows:

VCR	$1 \cdot 5$ mg/m^2 Day 1 only.
DAUNO	20 mg/m^2 Days 1 and 2 only.
PRED	100 mg/m^2 orally, daily.

The whole course is repeated at weekly intervals until a complete remission is obtained. An E.C.G. is performed before each course to exclude cumulative cardiac toxicity. For the same reason the total DAUNO dose should be kept below 25 mg/Kg (Tan *et al.*, 1967).

After several relapses the above schedules may fail to achieve a further remission. High doses of I.V. MTX, 3 mg/Kg, at fortnightly intervals, either alone (Perrin *et al.*, 1963) or together with daily oral PRED (Brubaker *et al.*, 1968) are then worth trying, even in patients who have relapsed on continuous smaller doses of MTX. Fortnightly I.V. MTX (3–6 mg/Kg) can also be used for maintenance therapy (Nagao *et al.*, 1970).

The newer drugs Cytosine Arabinoside (ARA-C) and ASP used either separately (ALGB, 1968; Hill *et al.*, 1969), sequentially (McElwain and Hardisty, 1969) or simultaneously may also obtain a remission in a significant proportion of patients at this stage of the disease. Promazine is frequently needed to control the nausea and vomiting caused by ARA-C.

Once a complete remission is obtained by any schedule the steroids are gradually 'tailed off' over a period of 7–10 days and maintenance therapy is begun.

REMISSION MAINTENANCE CHEMOTHERAPY

This phase of management only begins after a patient has reached a state of complete clinical and haematological remission with A1 marrow status. In numerous clinical trials it has been shown that children failing to achieve a complete remission from the induction therapy have an unsatisfactory course in terms of subsequent remission duration. It is therefore better to continue with the induction schedule, or augment it with other inducer drugs, in an attempt to obtain a complete remission before commencing maintenance chemotherapy.

The concept of specifically evaluating the ability of a drug to *maintain* an established remission, rather than to *induce* a remission *de novo*, arose from a trial conducted by the Acute Leukaemia Group B (1963). After PRED induction (40 mg/m²) patients achieving a remission were randomly allocated to 6-MP maintenance (3 mg/Kg/day) or placebo, and the steroids discontinued. The median remission duration was 33 weeks on 6-MP and 9 weeks on placebo. It was clear from this trial that 6-MP could prolong remissions in many patients in whom it would fail to induce a remission. Although it could induce complete remission in only 27% of children with ALL it could substantially prolong the remission in at least 80%. The recognition that a given drug could have widely different activities if tested for remission maintenance on the one hand or remission induction on the other, has led to numerous clinical trials from which the relative value of different drugs for purposes of maintenance therapy can be judged (Table II). For strict comparison between different drugs an identical remission induction schedule should have been employed since the subsequent length of remission could be critically related to the degree of leukaemic cell kill. As indicated in the table, differing induction schedules have been used in some trials. However, it is clear from a comparison of Tables I and II that the inducer drugs are uniformly poor when used for remission maintenance, the best drugs for this latter purpose being 6-MP, MTX, CYCLO and ARA-C.

Until recently it was assumed that daily oral dosage was the optimal form of administration for the first three of these maintenance drugs. The usual dosages were:

6-MP	2·5–3·0 mg/Kg	or 65–90 mg/m².
MTX	0·1–0·125 mg/kg	or 3·0–3·3 mg/m².
CYCLO	3–5 mg/Kg	or 75–100 mg/m².

These doses are in fact the highest that can be tolerated clinically with chronic administration. Combination of 6-MP plus MTX at these daily oral doses greatly increases the marrow toxicity but does not increase the median duration of remission over that of 6-MP alone (ALGB, 1965).

Among the newer drugs only ARA-C is of any value for maintenance therapy. It is given once per week at a dose of 40–80 mg/m² subcutaneously.

With daily oral administration 6-MP appears superior to the other two drugs, the median duration of complete remission being 8 months compared to 3–4 months for MTX or Cyclophosphamide (CYCLO), (Table II). In one trial, however, CYCLO and 6-MP both gave similar remission durations of $3\frac{1}{2}$–4 months, but the induction regimes were not identical (Fernbach *et al.*, 1966). Median total survival in patients given these drugs in a sequential manner, with induction of second and third remissions with steroids and/or VCR and a change of maintenance drug after each relapse, approximates to the sum of the median duration of remission on each of the three drugs. In a report by Saunders *et al.* (1967a) using the 5 drugs PRED, VCR, 6-MP, MTX and CYCLO in this way, the median survival was 17 months. The first remission on 6-MP lasted approximately 6 months and subsequent remissions on MTX and CYCLO were progressively shorter.

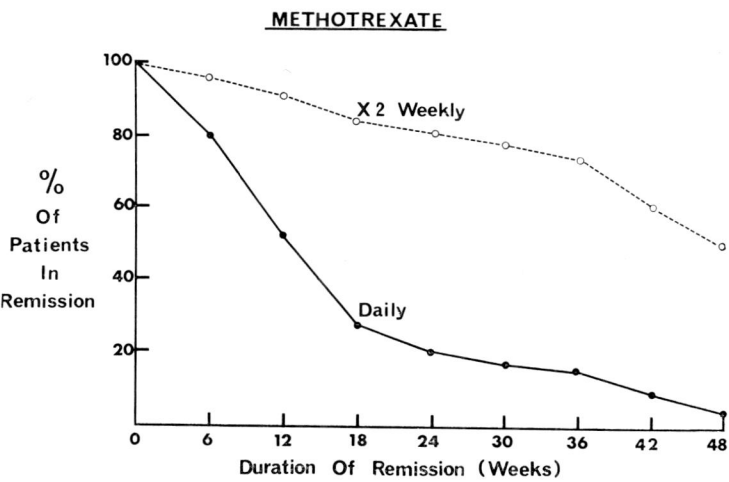

FIG. 4.2. Comparison of duration of drug-maintained remission using either a twice-weekly high-dose of methotrexate or a low daily dose.

A five-fold increase in duration of remission maintenance by MTX is achieved when this drug is given in a high dose twice weekly (20–30 mg/m²) instead of in a small dose daily (3 mg/m²) (Fig. 4.2.) Both dosages are the highest that can be tolerated when given at bi-weekly or daily intervals respectively for prolonged periods. The superiority of the twice-weekly regime was clearly shown in a trial by the ALGB (1965a) with random allocation to the two groups following remission induction to A1 marrow status with VCR plus PRED. In the first such trial the twice-weekly MTX was given intramuscularly but a subsequent trial by the same group showed that twice-weekly oral MTX at the same dose gave a similar prolongation of remission (ALGB, 1969). The improved results were therefore schedule-dependent, not route-dependent. It should be noted that a higher total weekly dose (40–60 mg/m²) can be

tolerated when the drug is given twice-weekly than when it is given daily
(7×3 mg/m^2 = 21 mg/m^2), yet the clinical toxicity (buccal ulceration
and marrow depression) is not significantly greater at the higher weekly
dose providing renal function is normal (Selawry and Holland, 1966).
Severe systemic MTX toxicity is encountered with even quite small
doses of this drug in the presence of renal impairment, and this should
be assessed before using high doses.

It is possible that the greater anti-leukaemic effect of the twice-weekly
schedule is simply related to the higher total weekly dose of drug or to
higher peak blood levels (see later). However the twice-weekly schedule
was tried in human leukaemia as a direct extension of animal studies by
Goldin et al. (1956). Using the L1210 transplantable leukaemia in
mice as a model, it was found that the effectiveness of MTX in controlling the rate of multiplication of small numbers of innoculated L1210
cells was markedly schedule-dependant, the twice-weekly high dose
regime being greatly superior to the equitoxic daily low dose regime.
This difference was not found when large numbers of tumour cells were
present. In order to parallel the experimental conditions used by Goldin
it was necessary in the clinical trial to reduce the number of residual
leukaemic cells present at diagnosis before commencing the MTX
therapy. This was achieved by using VCR plus PRED for induction. It
was a good example of an improved clinical schedule resulting from
experimental work in an animal model system and has focused attention
on the possible importance of time-scheduling of administration of
other drugs. In the case of 6-MP and CYCLO, intermittent high dosage
does not appear to result in a similar advantage as regards remission
maintenance (Pierce et al., 1966; Chevalier and Glidewell, 1967).

Another way in which an improved mode of drug administration for
maintenance of remissions has been achieved is by their 'cyclic' use.
This was pioneered by Zuelzer (1964) and Brubaker et al. (1963).
It involves changing from one drug to another at predetermined intervals
while the patient is still in remission, rather than changing only after a
relapse has occurred on each drug in turn (termed 'sequential' maintenance therapy). The underlying concept of cyclic therapy is that the
acquisition of drug resistance by residual leukaemic cells may be
forestalled by a change of maintenance drug while still in remission.

The results of Zuelzer and Brubaker were impressive at the time
with median first remissions of 48 and 60 weeks respectively. The
superiority of their results over those of others at that period may have
been partly due to their care in haematological surveillance and management of complications. Recent controlled trials have failed to show
improvement in survival (Colebatch, 1968) or total period of 'control
of the disease' (Krivit et al., 1968) using drugs cyclically rather than
sequentially, but both trials can be criticized on the grounds that

they employed inducer drugs, i.e. VCR and PRED, for extended periods of maintenance therapy, a role for which these drugs are known to be relatively ineffective (Table II). When the cyclic rotation is restricted to maintenance drugs following initial remission induction it is possible to evaluate the length of first remission on cyclic therapy. Using conventional drug doses of 6-MP for 10 weeks, followed by MTX for 6 weeks and CYCLO for 6 weeks, then repeating the cycle, a median first remission of 14–15 months was obtained (Willoughby and Laurie, 1968). This was clearly in excess of the remission duration obtainable by any single drug (Table I). It was apparent, however, that overall survival was not increased by the cyclic use of drugs. The median survival in this series was 19 months; a figure closely comparable to that of 17 months reported by Saunders et al. (1967a) who used the same 5 drugs sequentially. The advantage of cyclic therapy is that longer first remissions are obtained, but subsequent remissions are unfortunately short. This suggests that acquired resistance to all three maintenance drugs has developed during their cyclic use. It is undoubtedly better to give MTX twice-weekly rather than daily, as described above, when this drug is incorporated in cyclic therapy.

'Reinduction Therapy', namely the use of short courses of inducer drugs at prescribed intervals while still in remission, was introduced in 1967 by Jacquillat et al. in an attempt to further extend the duration of first remissions. Maintenance therapy with 6-MP and MTX was interrupted at 6 monthly intervals for a period of 2–3 weeks during which the following therapy was given:

PRED   100 mg/m² for 7 days orally.
VCR   1 mg/m² I.V. on Day 1.
           2 mg/m² I.V. on Day 7.

After the second dose of VCR the maintenance therapy is restarted and the steroids tailed off over 10 days. Later modifications included an intrathecal injection of MTX at a dose of 10 mg/m² and shorter intervals between reinduction courses. The length of first remissions in these protocols was impressive, the median duration being in excess of 26 months with very few relapses within the first year of therapy.

The efficacy of reinduction therapy during remission has subsequently been confirmed in controlled trials. Chevalier and Glidewell (1967) compared remission maintenance (in relapsed patients) with 6-MP alone, 90 mg/m²/day, and the same schedule with the addition of monthly reinduction courses of VCR 2 mg/m² plus PRED 40 mg/m² for 7 days. Without reinduction the median length of remission was 16 weeks; with reinduction it was prolonged to 33 weeks. Similarly Holland and Glidewell (1968) have shown that the addition of two VCR plus PRED reinduction courses during an 8-month intensive

MTX schedule increases both the total length of remission and the subsequent period of unmaintained remission, suggesting that the reinduction courses contributed to a greater leukaemic cell kill.

Apart from the statistical evidence that reinduction prolongs remissions it has been observed on occasions that a small number of leukaemic blast cells are present in the marrow just before a routine reinduction course and that these have gone following the course; the marrow remaining in complete remission while on the same maintenance therapy for a year or more thereafter.

The therapeutic advantages of cyclic therapy, twice-weekly MTX and reinduction therapy can be combined. After modifying the cyclic maintenance schedule described by Willoughby and Laurie so as to use twice-weekly MTX, instead of daily, and introducing reinduction at 5–6 month intervals the length of first remissions has exceeded 3 years in 25% of the patients and exceeded 5 years in 10%. Such a scheme could be recommended for paediatric units wishing to employ the most effective palliative therapy for their cases, with a good chance of long first remissions, but without the facilities necessary for intensive therapy (see below).

A somewhat more ambitious composite scheme named 'Total Therapy', requiring a considerable degree of clinical organization but not undue supportive facilities, has been described by George *et al.* (1968). It employs VCR and PRED induction followed by 1 week of high-dose I.V. 'consolidation' therapy (see below) followed in turn by continuous 6-MP maintenance therapy upon which are superimposed weekly I.V. injections of VCR, MTX and CYCLO. An 87% remission rate followed by a median first remission of 78 weeks, and median survival of 135 weeks, was obtained. When this maintenance therapy was preceded by Cranial Radiotherapy (2,400 R) plus intrathecal MTX, for the purpose of eradicating meningeal foci of leukaemic cells, impressive extension of the duration of the first remission was obtained, with two-thirds of the patients still in remission at 30 months (Aur *et al.*, 1971). Later modifications of these schedules have substituted weekly oral MTX and CYCLO, in place of parenteral, without loss of efficacy (Pinkel, 1970). The combined results from the "Total Therapy" schedules show a 17% 5-year leukaemia-free remission rate.

It is not certain that continuous maintenance therapy remains beneficial beyond a certain length of time. In one trial the minority of patients who remained in remission for over $2\frac{1}{2}$ years showed no difference in subsequent relapse rate in the group remaining on chemotherapy compared to a group left on no therapy (Krivit *et al.*, 1970). Also a number of the 132 5-year survivors collected by Burchenal (1966) were continuing in remission without treatment. The 7 5-year survivors reported by Aur *et al.* (1971) had been off chemotherapy for 2 to $3\frac{1}{2}$

years. Determination of the optimum duration of continuous therapy is worthy of investigation by a clinical trial.

INTENSIVE CHEMOTHERAPY

Unlike the palliative aims of maintenance therapy, the hope of intensive chemotherapy is eradication of the disease in at least a proportion of patients. The therapy is primarily intended to be 'Cytoreductive', viz. to reduce the residual leukaemic cells to the smallest possible number. Until such time as dependable eradicative chemotherapy is devised, the relative efficacy of different intensive schedules must be judged by a new parameter not yet considered, viz. the number of residual leukaemic cells present at the end of the therapy. This is of course different from either % rate of remission induction or duration of maintained remission discussed above. In fact it is quite possible that, just as certain drugs and schedules are better for remission induction and others for remission maintenance, so the main activity of yet other drugs or schedules could be 'cytoreductive', achieving a high 'fractional leukaemic cell kill' at a time when the patient is already in a state of apparent clinical remission. One such drug is probably BCNU 1, 3-bis-(2-Chloroethyl)-1-Nitrosourea, NSC 409962 which incidentally has seldom been used for remission induction and is quite unsuitable for maintenance remission because of delayed marrow toxicity.

The concept of possible eradication of the cellular phase of the disease undoubtedly sprung from the work of Skipper et al. (1964, 1967, 1968). A large body of experimental work using the transplantable mouse leukaemia L1210 system has shown that:

1. A single injected leukaemic cell is capable of causing fatal leukaemia. This occurs at an average time of 19 days in the mouse, dependent upon the logarithmic growth of the tumour cells, involving 30 doubling divisions, each occupying 13 hours, so as to reach the number of approx. $1 \cdot 5 \times 10^9$ cells present in the mouse at death.

2. A logarithmic increase in the number of inoculated (or residual) leukaemic cells results in an arithmetically proportionate shortening of the survival time (Fig. 3).

3. A given dose of a particular drug causes a constant proportionate cell kill (fractional cell kill) e.g. 99% whatever the number of leukaemic cells present in the body at the time it is given.

4. In general intermittent high doses of drugs achieve a greater leukaemic cell kill than do equitoxic chronically administered low doses.

5. In the case of drugs such as ARA-C, which are active only against cells in the DNA synthesis (S) phase, so called *cycle-active drugs*, the timing of administration so as to 'catch' as many as possible of the

leukaemic cells in the sensitive S phase is crucial to achieving a high kill (Fig. 5).

6. By employing these principles it is possible to eradicate all L1210 leukaemic cells and to achieve cure in the mouse.

The average child of 6 years at the time of diagnosis or relapse has approx. 1 Kg of leukaemic tissue in the body. This corresponds to approx. 10^{12} leukaemic blast cells (Frei and Freireich, 1965). It would take 41 doubling cell divisions to achieve this number (with none of the progeny entering a resting phase). Estimates of the effective cell doubling-time (not the cell-cycle time) in human acute leukaemia vary between 4 and 6 days. This means that it would take between 164 and 246 days ($5\frac{1}{2}$ to 8 months) for a single leukaemic cell to multiply to the number needed to produce a clinically detectable relapse *assuming that there was no restraining influence from chemotherapy or host resistance affecting cell multiplication or survival.*

During unmaintained remissions following intensive therapy the first of the conditions certainly apply. Calculations have therefore been made relating the observed duration of unmaintained remission to the calculated (and hypothetical) number of residual leukaemic cells following various forms of chemotherapy (Johnson *et al.*, 1966) (Fig. 3). There are undoubted inaccuracies in such calculations but the measurement of unmaintained remission is valuable for comparing the efficacy of different intensive chemotherapy schedules since (1) this is the *only* method of approaching an estimate of the number of residual cells at present available, (2) it is an *absolute* measurement, which can hardly be compromised by variations in local patient care or remission criteria, and (3) even if the calculations of the number of residual cells are fallacious it is nevertheless a measurement which shows how near or far a given form of therapy approaches permanent cure, and permits the rating of different intensive schedules in terms of their approach to cellular eradication of the disease (Table IV).

Support for the concept that relapses following conventional therapy are caused by regrowth from residual surviving cells of the original line, in spite of an intervening period of apparent complete remission, has come from several sources. Reisman *et al.* (1964) have demonstrated that the leukaemic cells at relapse possess the same cytogenetic abnormalities as were present in the original cell lines at diagnosis for any given patient. During remission the cytogenetic analysis of marrow cells is normal, since the marrow is then repopulated by normal haemopoietic cells, and the leukaemic cells are too few to find in chromosome analyses (as well as possibly being in a resting, non-dividing, phase).

By taking multiple biopsies of marrow, liver, kidney and testes and by examining concentrates of C.S.F. and peripheral blood, Mathé *et al.* (1966) demonstrated residual foci of leukaemic cells in 12 out of

31 patients fulfilling the normal criteria for complete remission (see above). Similarly Nies *et al.* (1965) have found histological evidence of leukaemic foci in 10 out of 15 patients dying while in remission. Del Vecchio *et al.* (1965) found leukaemic cells in C.S.F. concentrates from 68% of patients with ALL and 47% of patients with Acute Myeloblastic Leukaemia (AML). It is therefore entirely reasonable to assume that these various residual foci are the source of the tumour cells which repopulate the marrow at times of relapse. Intensive therapy is directed towards the elimination of these unseen foci throughout the body at a time when the patient is apparently in complete remission.

There remains the lurking suspicion, however, that eradication of all identifiable leukaemic cells—the 'cellular phase of the disease'—may not be enough. If a virus plays any part in the initiation of the disease or if there is some intrinsic instability of cellular multiplication, such an underlying leukaemogenic predisposition could persist after all leukaemic blast cells had been eliminated. Neither is it known whether the earliest leukaemic blast cells are produced by unidentified leukaemic stem cells which might be resistant to chemotherapeutic attack, particularly if in a dormant state for long periods. These possibilities are relevant to the small number of patients who relapse after unmaintained remission considerably in excess of 8 months following intensive therapy (Freireich *et al.*, 1968). Alternative explanations are that intensive therapy permanently affects the rate of division of the residual leukaemic cells, preferentially destroying the more rapidly dividing cells thereby selecting out the slower lines (Holland, 1967), or that a host reaction, i.e. immunological, has been partially effective in restraining leukaemic cell growth during the unmaintained period off anti-leukaemic, and immuno-suppressant, drugs (see below).

INTENSIVE CHEMOTHERAPY DRUG SCHEDULES

All intensive therapy schedules employ short, usually 5-day, courses of drugs given at the highest tolerated doses followed by recovery periods, usually approx. 9 days, off drug therapy. In some *combination* chemotherapy schedules up to 5 drugs are used simultaneously; in others single drugs are used at even higher doses than can safely be used in combination. In some schedules employing cycle active drugs i.e. ARA-C or MTX, infusions over a number of hours or at 8-hourly intervals over a period of 48 hours have been used. In most schemes the intensive therapy is not started until a complete remission with a normal marrow has been achieved by the use of the relatively non-toxic combination of VCR + Steroids. When intensive therapy is used in this way while the patient is in remission it is sometimes referred to as 'Consolidation Therapy'.

There are practical advantages in delaying the more toxic therapy until the marrow is in remission referred to above. Moreover it is then easier to know whether any resulting neutropenia or thrombocytopenia is due to the disease, when it will get progressively worse, or to the therapy, when it will spontaneously recover. There are also theoretical advantages. Rall and Homan (1967) have pointed out that a therapeutic advantage is achieved at a time when the marrow is fully repopulated with normal haemopoietic cells, viz. at that time many of the normal stem cells will be in a dormant state and will not be susceptible to the toxic effects of cycle active anti-leukaemic drugs. By contrast at a time when the marrow is heavily infiltrated by leukaemic cells it is known that many of these are in a non-dividing state (Mauer and Fisher, 1966) while the normal haemopoietic cells are presumably acting under stress. Here the situation would be reversed.

When the marrow is in complete remission it has been found possible to administer the following doses of anti-leukaemic drugs over short courses of up to 5 days, with 9-day rest periods between courses, without undue marrow toxicity or other side effects:

6-MP	1,000 mg/m²/day for 5 days I.V.
MTX	15 mg/m²/day for 5 days I.V.
DAUNO	20 mg/m²/day for 5 days I.V.
ARA-C	100 mg/m²/day for 5 days I.V.
PRED	1,000 mg/m²/day for 5 days I.V.
BCNU	100 mg/m²/day for 3 days I.V.
CYCLO	600 mg/m²/day for 1 day I.V.

The rationale behind this type of drug administration is to achieve the highest possible peak blood levels. In the case of cycle-active drugs there is also some advantage in the 5-day course as the separate blood peaks are likely to 'catch' different cohorts of leukaemic cells as they pass through their sensitive S phase during the 4–6 day doubling time (Fig. 5). More prolonged courses than those indicated above cannot be pursued without rest periods because the cumulative toxicity would be too great.

The degree of leukaemic cell kill or 'cytoreductive effect' from these high-dose courses cannot be determined directly since they are given when the blood and marrow are already in complete remission. An indirect assessment can be made, however, from the median length of unmaintained remission following such courses as described above (Fig. 3). There is a scatter of remission durations on either side of the median result, probably because of case to case variation in the sensitivity of the leukaemic cells to the drug in question, or in the rate of multiplication of the residual cells. Median values are used so as to

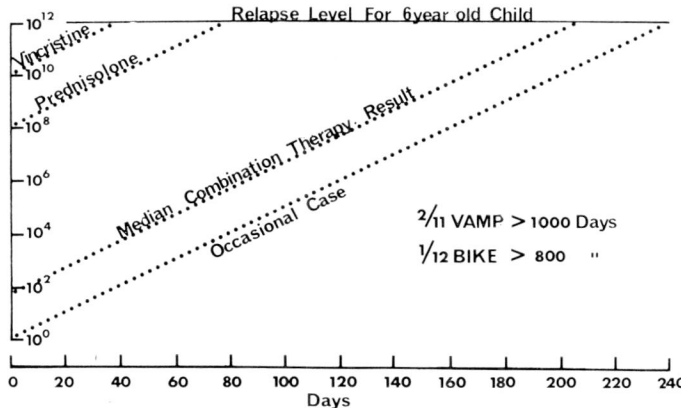

FIG. 4.3. Conceptual relationship between cytoreductive effect of chemotherapy (on a logarithmic scale) and subsequent duration of unmaintained remission. Dotted lines indicate pattern of leukaemic cell regrowth (after SKIPPER).

avoid being misled by fortuitously long or fortuitously short remissions from these causes in certain individual patients.

Table IV shows the results obtained by Holland (1968) in a controlled trial. Also shown is the hypothetical number of residual leukaemic cells corresponding to these median remissions, calculated for the 6-day doubling time as described above. It is clear that a significant cytoreductive effect was achieved by the 6-MP and MTX courses given in this way. The sequence of 6-MP, MTX and CYCLO given as one course each had a greater effect than the single drugs, and was further improved by repeating the whole 3-drug course (BIKE). The addition of 3 doses of BCNU at the end of the 3-drug sequence produced the best cytoreductive effect of all the schedules used by Holland.

It is of importance that it has been established that high-dose courses such as these cause a significant reduction in leukaemic cells well beyond that at the time of complete remission achieved by VCR + PRED alone. From the occasional unmaintained remissions in excess of 1 or 2 years, it is apparent that a small proportion of patients benefit greatly from this type of treatment. But with drugs given *singly at one time* this approach fails in the majority of patients, perhaps because the chance of being highly sensitive to each of the several drugs administered in sequence is small. Lost ground due to regrowth of leukaemic cells can occur during a course of drug to which the patient is fortuitously resistant. It is probably for this reason that *combination chemotherapy*, viz. the administration of multiple anti-leukaemic drugs simultaneously, offers a better hope of very marked reduction of the leukaemic cell population in the human disease. With 4 or 5-drug combinations it is unlikely that the leukaemic cells will be intrinsically resistant to all or even most of the drugs, and no ground will be lost on this account.

HIGH-DOSE COMBINATION CHEMOTHERAPY

The ideal form of combination therapy would employ drugs which had totally dissimilar toxic effects upon the normal tissues of the body, so that these toxic effects were not additive, yet had a common cytocidal effect upon the leukaemic cells (Rall, 1968). Table III lists and grades the major toxic effects of anti-leukaemic drugs and it can be seen that

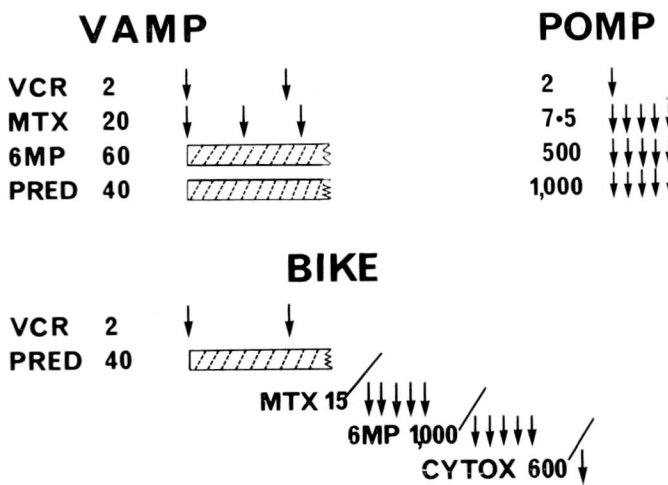

FIG. 4.4. Intensive chemotherapy schedules. ARROWS indicate I.V. administration employing five-day courses in POMP (combination) and BIKE (sequential). VCR doses spaced at weekly intervals. Horizontal blocks indicate daily oral administration. Numerals give dose of drug in mg. per M^2 surface area.

combinations of steroids plus VCR plus an antimetabolite such as 6-MP or MTX largely fulfil this requirement; as does the remission induction scheme of DAUNO, VCR plus steroids, used by Mathé. In fact some of the combination schedules do employ more than one drug with marrow depressing side effects, e.g. 6-MP + MTX in VAMP and POMP, but even this can be tolerated in the majority of patients when given in a short course (Fig. 4).

There is also the hope that combination chemotherapy might achieve a synergistic leukaemocidal effect, i.e. that the leukaemic cell kill might

TABLE III

MAJOR TOXIC EFFECTS OF ANTILEUKAEMIC DRUGS

	Marrow depression	Mucositis esp. buccal	Immuno-suppression	Hepatic toxicity	G.I. toxicity	CNS toxicity	Cardiac toxicity	Other
PRED	−	+	++	+	+	+	−	Obesity, Hypertension, Diabetic acidosis, Fluid retention
VCR	+	−	+	−	+	++	−	Myopathy, Alopecia
ASP	−	−	+	+	+	+	−	Hypoproteinaemia, Allergy
DAUNO	+++	++	+++	−	−	−	+	Alopecia
6-MP	++	+	++	+	+	−	−	
MTX	−+	+	+	+	+	?(I.T.)	−	
CYCLO	+	−	+	−	−	−	−	Alopecia, Cystitis
ARA-C	++	−	+	−	+	−	−	
BCNU	++	−	−	+	−	−	−	

exceed that attributable to the individual drugs (Zubrod, 1965). Although synergism has been shown in animal tumours it has not yet been proved to occur in the human disease.

The first 4-drug combination schedule to be devised was named VAMP. It employed VCR, Amethopterin (Methotrexate), 6-MP and PRED in the dosage and manner shown in Fig. 4. It proved relatively toxic, 11 out of 17 patients completing the course. The median unmaintained remission was 140 days, similar to the BIKE schedule employing high-dose drugs sequentially rather than in combination. There were two long unmaintained remissions of 2 and 4 years with VAMP however, compared to 1 for BIKE (in which 12 out of 15 patients completed the course).

POMP employed the same 4 drugs (the initials standing for PRED, Oncovin (VCR), MTX and Purinethol (6-MP)), but at higher doses given in shorter courses intravenously (Fig. 4).

VCR	2 mg/m² Day 1 only.
PRED	1,000 mg/m² Days 1 to 5 inclusive.
6-MP	500 mg/m² Days 1 to 5 inclusive.
MTX	7·5 mg/m² Days 1 to 5 inclusive.

When 6-MP and MTX are given simultaneously the doses are half those tolerated when given separately as by Holland (1968). In monitoring the possible toxic effects of such therapy liver function (SGPT), diabetic acidosis and hypertension must be considered as well as marrow toxicity and immunosuppression.

POMP may be used for remission induction, when complete remission is achieved in 84% of patients after a median of only two 5-day courses, or for 'consolidation' of an established remission with the objective of cytoreduction (Freireich et al., 1968). After a total of 14 such consolidation courses, 12 being given as 5-day courses once per month, a median unmaintained remission of 240 days (or 8 months) was obtained indicating an exceedingly small number of residual leukaemic cells left in many patients at the end of the course (Henderson, 1967) (Table IV). POMP is therefore superior to VAMP in this respect, as well as being less toxic. The routine of spending 5 days (4 nights) in hospital per fortnight is better tolerated by children than the uninterrupted periods of 6–7 weeks necessary for certain other intensive therapy schedules.

The long term survival of patients initially treated by POMP is better than that recorded after other forms of therapy, giving a median duration of 3 years (Henderson and Samaha, 1969), but total eradication of the disease has not yet been achieved by this form of chemotherapy alone.

TABLE IV

UNMAINTAINED REMISSION DURATION FOLLOWING CHEMOTHERAPY

Initial induction therapy to remission	Consolidation chemotherapy	Subsequent unmaintained remission (median)	Calculated residual leukaemic cells at end of chemotherapy
VCR + PRED	None	9 weeks	10^9
Ditto	5-day 6-MP × 3	13 weeks*	10^7
Ditto	5-day MTX × 3	16 weeks	10^6
Ditto	5-day 6-MP, 5-day MTX, 1-day CYCLO	16 weeks	10^6
Ditto	Ditto × 2 (BIKE)	20 weeks*	10^5
Ditto	Ditto × 1, followed by 3-day BCNU	23 weeks*	10^4
Ditto + 6-MP + MTX	VCR, PRED, 6-MP, MTX in combination (POMP)	34 weeks	10^1

* 1 patient remained in remission for over 1 year.

Nevertheless the high degree of leukaemic cell kill achieved by POMP, may make this an ideal form of chemotherapy for use prior to immunotherapy (*vide infra*).

Combinations of ASP, which is non-toxic to the marrow, with ARA-C and DAUNO are also being explored and might prove useful as adjuvants to POMP for purposes of achieving more profound degrees of leukaemia cell reduction.

CONTINUOUS INFUSION TECHNIQUES

Djerassi first explored the possibility that continuous infusions of MTX might exert a significant anti-leukaemic effect even although the leukaemic cells were resistant to conventional doses of TMX (Djerassi *et al.*, 1967a).

Schedule A employed 18-hour infusions of 36 mg/m², following a rapid 'priming' dose of 12 mg/m². The 18-hour infusions were repeated at daily intervals for up to 3 days. Marked toxicity was encountered including severe buccal ulceration, gastro-intestinal symptoms, hepatic damage, skin rashes and bone marrow depression. Platelet transfusions were necessary at 2–3 day intervals so as to maintain the platelet count above 50,000/cu mm.

All 10 patients treated with this schedule achieved a complete, although short-lived, remission in spite of the fact that 7 were resistant to conventional doses of the drug. In this trial it was remarkable that the therapy was largely conducted on an out-patient basis with overnight admissions for the 18-hour infusions and platelet transfusions in the Out-patient Department. The high toxicity of Schedule A however precludes its widespread use.

Schedule B employed a higher dose, 180 mg/m², given over a shorter period, 4-hours, on 2 successive days. 60% of the dose was given by rapid infusion as a priming dose. It was hoped that a similar degree of drug entry into partially resistant cells could be achieved by increasing the 'drug gradient' but for a shorter time, compared to Schedule A, since clinical toxicity appears to be dependant more upon the duration of infusion than to the total dose. When given to a patient already in remission (i.e. as consolidation therapy) Schedule B was not seriously toxic, producing only mild intestinal upset and transient buccal ulceration plus short-lived elevation of the SGPT. Platelet transfusions were seldom necessary. It has subsequently been used at approx. 28-day intervals, with a single I.V. dose of CYCLO 1,000 mg/m² on Day 14, for purposes of maintenance therapy with all 15 patients surviving over 26 months (Djerassi *et al.*, 1967b).

One theoretical interest in this approach is that sustained blood levels will 'catch' a higher proportion of the randomly-dividing leukaemic cells in their sensitive DNA-synthesis phase than twice-weekly doses which do not persist in the blood for more than 4–6 hours. On the other hand the apparent benefit from 4-hour infusions at a much higher dose and given at monthly intervals suggests that a high drug gradient may saturate even resting cells and perhaps impair their subsequent division. Similar 4-hour infusions of ARA-C on successive days have proved efficacious in AML (*vide infra*). This is another cycle-active drug that is rapidly destroyed in the body, by oxidation to Uracil Arabinoside, and sustained blood levels could be much more damaging to the randomly dividing population of leukaemic cells.

Another way of achieving the same effect with cycle-active drugs is to give a number of shortly spaced injections within the period of 1 or 2 cell cycle intervals (Skipper *et al.*, 1967). In human acute leukaemia the cell cycle is around 60 hours among the dividing population of blast cells, and the DNA-synthesis period approx. 20 hours (Fig. 5) (Saunders *et al.*, 1967b; Killman, 1968). A recent M.R.C. protocol for ALL used MTX intensive consolidation therapy in this way, employing 8 doses of 40 mg/m² given as rapid I.V. injections at 8-hour intervals over a period of 48 hours, i.e. 120 mg/m²/Day. Mathé has used similar schedules and has shown that 75 mg/m²/8 hours or even 150 mg/m²/8 hours can be tolerated, the latter dose on occasions

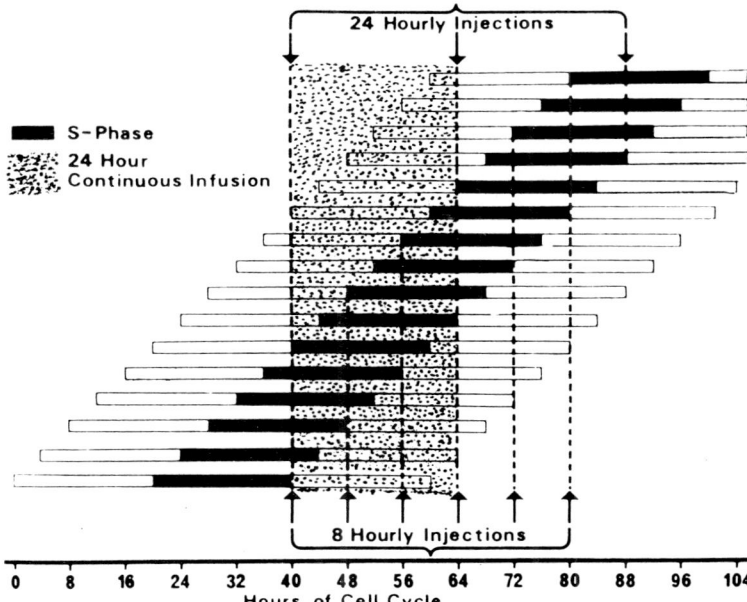

FIG. 4.5. Diagramatic representation of a whole population of randomly dividing leukaemic cells. Drug-Sensitive, DNA-Synthetic S-phases of cells indicated in black. Six 8-hourly injections "catch" the whole population, as do three 24-hourly injections. A single 24-hour infusion (shaded area) fails to "catch" many cells in the drug-sensitive phase.

achieving a remission when the lower dose failed (Mathé, 1969b). Cytosine arabinoside has also been given at 8-hourly intervals over 48 hours (Bodey et al., 1969). Fig. 5 shows that it is less likely that any leukaemic cells will escape being 'hit' in the sensitive S-phase with the 8-hour schedules compared to the daily schedules. The latter, however, may 'catch' more of the more slowly dividing resting cells.

It has been shown by Berenbaum (1964) that Folinic Acid given after MTX can diminish its toxic effects without blocking its immuno-suppressive activity. Folinic acid is the product of the reaction inhibited by MTX. There is probably a close analogy between immunosuppressive and anti-leukaemic activity and it is presumed that the administration of folinic acid (Calcium Leucovorin, Lederle) after high doses of MTX will not significantly reverse the anti-leukaemic effects while sparing the patient serious subsequent toxicity. Folinic acid at a dose of 24 mg/m^2/8 hours for 4 days was given immediately following the MTX in the M.R.C. protocol and a higher dose by Mathé (1969). This principle of 'Folinic Acid Salvage' has also been used in the treatment of solid tumours.

IMMUNOTHERAPY

There is accumulating evidence that cancer cells, including those of acute leukaemia, possess neo-antigens foreign to the host (Klein, 1966; Doré et al., 1967) and that under certain circumstances an immunological reaction is mounted against these antigens which is effective in controlling the tumour growth. Such a reaction normally fails partly because of antigen excess (i.e. 10^{12} cells or 1 Kg of leukaemic tissue in the active stage of the disease) and partly because most of the antineoplastic drugs are also immunosuppressive.

Immunotherapy may be active or passive. Passive immunotherapy is at present impracticable because appropriate immune serum is unavailable and because of the danger from certain antibodies which actually enhance tumour growth. Active immunotherapy may be specific, i.e. using irradiated leukaemic cells, or non-specific using an adjuvant such as B.C.G. which enhances production of a number of different antibodies by the reticulo-endothelial system (see Hamilton Fairley, G., 1969a, for discussion and Chapter 6).

In experiments with transplantable animal tumours it has been known for some time that immunisation of the recipient *before* transplantation could prevent subsequent tumour growth following transplantation. A recent experiment by Mathé (1968) broke new ground in that it showed that immunological stimulation of the recipient immediately *after* transplantation of small numbers of L1210 leukaemic cells in mice prevented the subsequent growth of these cells in about 20% of animals (Fig. 6). Of particular interest in this experiment was the fact that this 'immunotherapy' was effective only if the number of injected L1210 cells was less then 10^5. If more than that number were present immunotherapy failed. Since the lethal number of leukaemic cells in the mouse is approx. 10^9 this would mean that a 4-log reduction or 99·99% cytoreductive cell kill would be necessary before immunotherapy could control the disease in a mouse with the active disease. The experiment was also of interest in that both specific (irradiated L1210 cells) and non-specific (B.C.G.) were effective.

The implication is therefore that immunotherapy might be able to control the disease in a proportion of patients if the number of leukaemic cells could be reduced (? to 10^5 cells) by preceding chemotherapy which would then be stopped at the time immunotherapy was begun. Intensive chemotherapy is more likely to achieve an adequate cell kill than conventional chemotherapy (Table IV). At present this hypothesis is being investigated by clinical trials embodying the above principles which are being conducted both in this country, France and the U.S.A.

At time of writing the results of these controlled trials are not yet available. However, suggestive evidence of a beneficial effect of im-

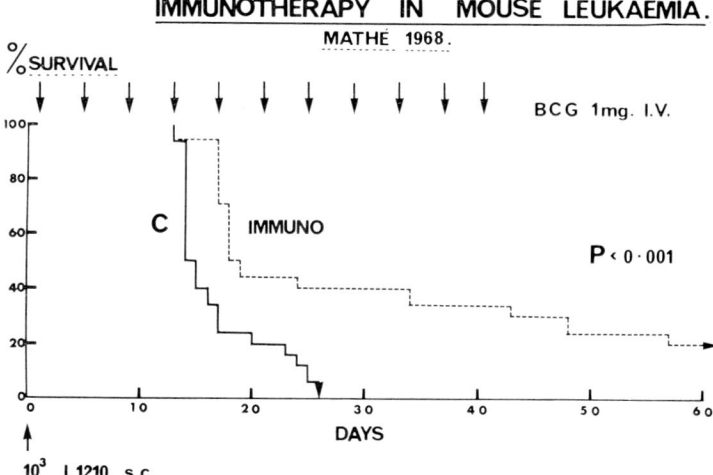

FIG. 4.6. Two groups of mice inoculated with 10^3 L1210 leukaemic cells. All of control group perished by 27 days. 20% of group receiving B.C.G. every fourth day survived indefinitely.

munotherapy in human ALL comes from a report by Mathé et al. (1969). Patients who were still in remission after completing one of three protracted and moderately intensive chemotherapy schedules employing most of the available antileukaemic drugs were randomly allocated to unmaintained or immunotherapy-maintained groups and all chemotherapy was stopped. All 10 patients in the unmaintained group had relapsed by 130 days (median approx. 70 days). Of the 20 patients in the immunotherapy group, 7 were still in remission 325–1,150 days after stopping chemotherapy at the time of the last report (Mathé, 1969a), including 6 for more than a year, 4 for more than 2 years and 1 for more than 3 years. Nine of the immunotherapy group had relapsed by 100 days and it was suggested that an inadequate leukaemic cell kill had been achieved by the preceding chemotherapy in these particular patients, by analogy with the L1210 experiment.

Five patients in the immunotherapy group received weekly subcutaneous injections of irradiated pooled leukaemic lymphoblasts, 8 received B.C.G. given by cutaneous scarification at 4-day intervals and later weekly, while 7 patients received both. There was no obvious difference in the effect of these different forms of immunotherapy. A current M.R.C. trial is employing weekly B.C.G. given by means of a 20 point Heaf gun (Lancet 1971), Guyer and Crowther from the Royal Marsden Hospital in London have recently reported on the use of I.M. Pertussis Vaccine following intensive consolidation chemotherapy (1969). Their results were inconclusive although it appeared possible that the vaccine

delayed the onset of relapse. The longest remission in their immunotherapy group of 8 patients was 455 days off chemotherapy.

The value of immunotherapy in this disease remains *sub judice* at
present. Much more work on both the optimum form of preceding
chemotherapy and optimum form of immunotherapy will be needed.

EXTRAMEDULLARY LEUKAEMIC MANIFESTATIONS

With the increasing length of survival among children with leukaemia
focal recurrence of leukaemic growth including meningeal involvement,
testicular or ovarian tumours, skin, bone and eye involvement are being
seen more frequently.* The peripheral blood and bone marrow are in a
state of remission in approx. 50% of children at the time when these
extramedullary leukaemic manifestations arise (Hardisty and Norman,
1967).

The majority of antileukaemic drugs do not cross the blood-brain
barrier in adequate concentrations to control the proliferation of
leukaemic cells (Rall and Zubrod, 1962) although these cells can
often be detected by concentration techniques even at the onset of the
disease (Del Vechio *et al.*, 1963). Similar drug-permeability barriers
may exist in relation to the other tissues mentioned. Corticosteroids are
an exception among the commonly used drugs. ASP may also exert an
inhibitory effect on meningeal leukaemia, not by virtue of crossing the
blood, but by means of lowering the ASP content of the extracellular
fluid. The nitroso-urea alkylating agent BCNU is a drug which was
specifically synthesized with the object of penetrating the blood-brain
barrier by virtue of its small molecular size and lipid-soluble characteristics (Skipper, 1965). As with other alkylating agents it is probably
active against both resting and dividing cells. It has not been used for
treating active meningeal leukaemia, since other highly effective treatment is available, but has largely been reserved as the final drug in
intensive chemotherapy schedules which aim at eradication of the
disease; the object being to destroy resting leukaemic cells both inside
and outside the C.N.S. Although of proven efficacy in animal experiments using intracerebral inoculation of leukaemic cells, controlled
clinical trials of its use in preventing the recurrence of meningeal
leukaemia are only just beginning.

The standard treatment of meningeal leukaemia is intrathecal MTX
0·25 mg–0·5 mg/Kg or 8·0–12 mg/m² two or three times per week until
the cells in the C.S.F. are less than 10/cu mm. This will achieve remission
of the meningeal disease in close to 100% of patients (Hardisty and
Norman, 1967), within 2–3 weeks. Alternatively the MTX doses can be
given at weekly intervals with similar efficacy but less chance of systemic

* In a recent series of 37 patients 29 developed CNS leukaemia (Aur *et. al.*, 1971).

toxicity. Folinic acid, 3 mg b.d. I.M., can be given to counteract systemic toxicity if it occurs.

The good rate of response, even when the systemic disease has become resistant to MTX, can be attributed to the high drug concentration in the C.S.F., more than 1,000 times that ever achieved in the plasma.

Radiotherapy is also effective if extended to the whole cerebrospinal axis, rather than the cranium only, at a tumour dose of 1,000 rad (Sullivan *et al.*, 1969), but the frequency of alopecia and marrow depression and the somewhat shorter durations of meningeal remissions after radiotherapy make intrathecal MTX the treatment of choice. MTX plus Radiotherapy at this dosage does not have any advantage over MTX alone in the average case. Radiotherapy is of value, however, when there is evidence of deep focal brain involvement. This is sometimes seen coincident with or following meningeal leukaemia and fails to respond to I.T. MTX.

The length of remission following conventional treatment of meningeal leukaemia is unsatisfactory, with a median duration of between 3 and 5 months in most recent studies. Selawry and Odom (1968) have investigated the rate of decline in numbers of leukaemic cells in the C.S.F. following I.T. MTX. From the calculated total number of cells in the subarachnoid space and the rate of cell kill they concluded that 8 or more additional doses of I.T. MTX after apparent normality of the C.S.F. had been achieved might succeed in eradicating the meningeal involvement. This would be a considerable therapeutic advance since many of these patients with recurrent meningeal leukaemia are otherwise in complete remission.

In an elegant trial by Sullivan and Haggard (1970), it was shown that continued 8-weekly doses of I.T. MTX, 12 mg/m², given after initial meningeal remission had been obtained, prolonged the remission to a median of 70 weeks, compared to 17 weeks in patients given no subsequent I.T. therapy. BCNU at a dose of 100 mg/m² I.V. given at 8-week intervals failed to prolong the meningeal remission. This must be the only clinical trial of BCNU in human meningeal leukaemia so far reported.

ARA-C in a dose of 5–70 mg/m² may be given I.T. at weekly or twice-weekly intervals in cases failing to respond to MTX. The median duration of meningeal remission after this drug alone is only 28 days, compared to over 3 months after MTX (Wang and Pratt, 1970).

The interesting concept that residual leukaemic cells in this privileged meningeal environment might be a significant source of the cells responsible for later systemic relapses has been investigated (ALGB, 1965). Monthly prophylactic I.T. MTX was given to one of two groups of patients on cyclic maintenance therapy. Although meningeal leukaemia was prevented in the group receiving prophylactic I.T. MTX there was no difference in the length of the systemic remissions in the two groups, apparently making it unlikely that meningeal leukaemic cells were responsible for systemic relapse. The possible value of prophylactic I.T. MTX in preventing meningeal involvement was, however, evident. More recently this procedure has been incorporated into the Reinduction Therapy Protocol of Jacquillat et al. (1967) and into an M.R.C. intensive therapy protocol. Its clinical benefit remains unknown at the present time. Prophylactic Cobalt[60] irradiation of the C.N.S., total dose 1,200 r, does not significantly reduce the incidence of meningeal leukaemia (George et al., 1968), but the higher dose of 2,400r combined with I.T. MTX both reduces the incidence of Meningeal Leukaemia and prolongs the length of systemic remission (Aur et al., 1971). This observation reopens the question of the role of meningeal cells as a source of later systemic relapse.

Other extramedullary sites of leukaemic relapse include testicular or ovarian lymphoblastic tumours, usually occurring in patients who are otherwise in complete remission for above average durations. Such tumours respond to either corticosteroids or local radiotherapy, but the benefit from radiotherapy is more likely to be permanent. Surgical excision is unnecessary. Although clinically unilateral the leukaemic involvement is bilateral histologically and should be treated as such. Localized skin infiltration, periosteal involvement and retinal involvement are occasionally encountered in patients otherwise in remission, (Fig. 7). Local radiotherapy has proved completely effective for skin and bone manifestations. High systemic steroid dosage can be effective in the retinal disease.

SUPPORTIVE THERAPY

Unfortunately marrow depression and immunosuppression can be caused both by the disease and by its treatment. During remission induction patients are therefore doubly susceptible to the complications of infection and haemorrhage, which together constitute the major causes of death in acute leukaemia (Hersh et al., 1965).

Haemorrhage is almost invariably due to thrombocytopenia and can be satisfactorily controlled or prevented by platelet transfusions. The only exceptions to this are when there is concomitant septicaemia which causes continuing intravascular consumption of platelets (Cohen and Gardiner, 1967), or in Promyelocytic leukaemia when a coagulation defect associated with excessive fibrinolysis may occur.

Platelet transfusions are indicated when there is purpura, bruising or haemorrhage associated with a platelet count below 20,000/cu mm. They can also be used to anticipate bleeding when the platelet count is low or

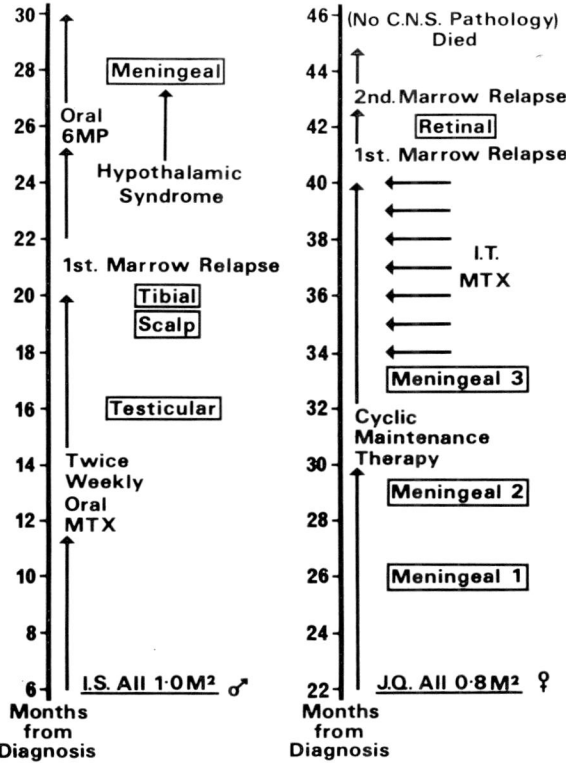

FIG. 4.7. Two patients with prolonged control of systemic ALL by maintenance chemotherapy but developing a series of extramedullary leukaemic manifestations, i.e. testicular, scalp, tibial, meningeal and retinal tumour deposits.

falling and the chemotherapy that is planned, i.e. DAUNO, ARA-C or high doses of MTX, is certain to lower the platelet count further. Practical policy in this situation is to administer the chemotherapy through the same drip that has just been used for the platelet infusion.

Fresh platelet-rich plasma is obtained from donor blood collected into Fenwall ACD double bags by centrifuging at 1,000 r.p.m. (350 g) at 10°C for 20 min (Klein *et al.*, 1967) and separating the platelet-rich plasma from the red cells by using the closed transfer system for which the bags are designed. Two units of platelet-rich plasma (i.e. the platelets from 2 pints of blood) can be given over 30 minutes to a child of 2–5 years, and 3 units to older children. In the presence of blood loss this dose could be repeated the next day, otherwise at 2–3 day intervals or twice-weekly until the danger from thrombocytopenia is past. I.V. Frusemide 5–10 mg can be given at the time of the infusion to lessen the danger of pulmonary oedema. Platelet concentrates have been used to obviate the problems of circulatory overload but unless a more acid anticoagulant than ordinary ACD is used considerable loss of functional platelets occurs due to clumping and subsequent difficulties of resuspension. I have been impressed by the efficacy of platelet-rich plasma in achieving haemostasis and an elevated platelet count compared to platelet concentrates. Blood of the same ABO group as the recipient is used since there is evidence that ABO incompatible platelets have a lower recovery *in vivo*. Special platelet-giving sets (Fenwall) must be used but siliconed scalp-vein needles (Abbot "Butterfly") (size 21) can be used instead of the larger needles originally thought necessary. A rapid infusion of platelet-rich plasma, followed if necessary by a slow infusion of the packed red cells, appears to be more effective than the slow infusion of the equivalent volume of whole blood, by analogy with the use of fresh frozen plasma in haemophilia. A good response is shown in Fig. 8.

In future the organization of platelet transfusion may be greatly simplified if satisfactory methods of preserving viable platelets in a concentrated form become available e.g. in Dimethyl Sulphoxide (Djerassi and Roger, 1965).

It is most important to avoid all I.M. injections while patients are thrombocytopenic and also to apply prolonged pressure over venepuncture sites so as to preserve the veins for future use and to avoid haematomata.

Infection during the active phase of acute leukaemia is common and is the most frequent cause of death (Hersh *et al.*, 1965). The incidence is related to the circulating granulocyte count (Bodey *et al.*, 1966).

Granulocyte count	*Incidence of infection (% Patient/days)*
100/cu mm	53%
100–500/cu mm	36%
500–1,000/cu mm	20%
1,000/cu mm	10%

Schneider *et al.* (1969) found that the granulocytes were less than 500/cu mm in 31 out of 40 such patients with infection. Defective granulocyte function or ability to leave the vascular compartment also occurs in acute leukaemia and may contribute to the liability to infection (Spivak *et al.*, 1969).

The organisms responsible for these infections are now less frequently staphylococcal or streptococcal, but more commonly 'opportunist' organisms of endogenous origin including *Pseudomonas*, coliforms, *Proteus*, *Klebsiella*, fungi, cytomegalovirus, *Pneumocystis carinii*, herpes simplex virus and *Toxoplasma* (Frei *et al.*, 1966; Cangir

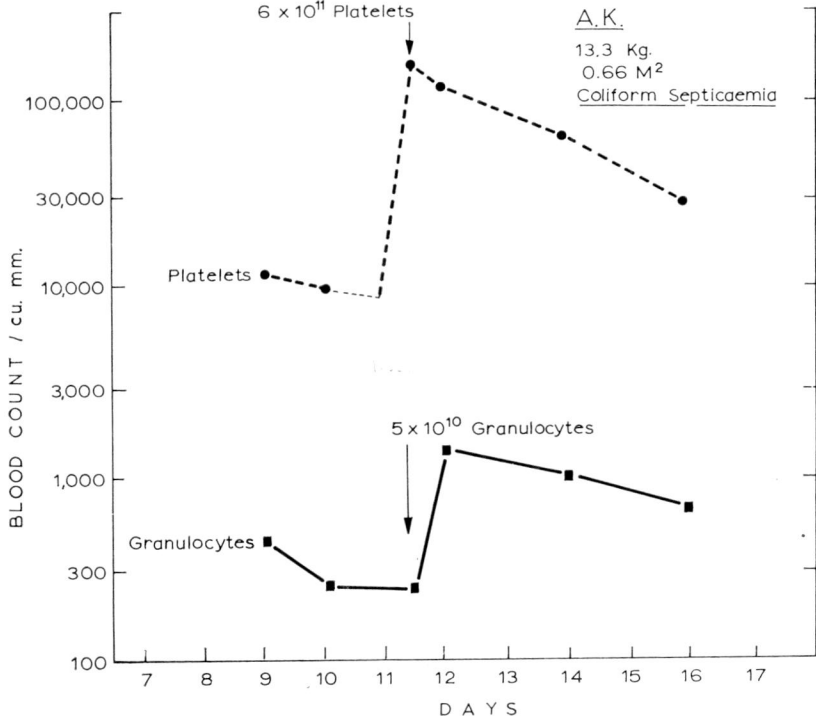

Fig. 4.8. Rise in circulating platelets and granulocytes as a result of platelet and granulocyte transfusion in a leukaemic patient with pancytopenia and coliform septicaemia, who subsequently recovered. The donor was a patient with Chronic Granulocytic Leukaemia having a white count of 260,000/cu.mm. and a platelet count of 689,000/cu.mm. Approximately 200 mls. of his leucocyte-rich plasma was given.

and Sullivan, 1966; Abell and Holland, 1969; ALGB, 1969). Common types and sites of the infections include septicaemia, pneumonia, osteomyelitis, cutaneous, buccal and intestinal.

Prophylactic systemic antibiotics are thought to do more harm than good. Nursing the patient in a sterile environment either by means of a plastic patient isolator (Schartz and Perry, 1966) or a laminar air flow unit (Bodey *et al.*, 1969), together with stringent attempts to reduce both the skin and gut flora, lower the incidence of serious infection to less than a third of the expected incidence (Levitan and Perry, 1967). Schneider *et al.* (1969) found infection in 80% of acute leukaemia patients nursed in a conventional ward but only 33% in leukaemic patients nursed in pathogen-free rooms, the latter group being selected for isolation because of their more severe marrow aplasia. Some of the practical problems associated with patient isolation are discussed by James *et al.* (1967) and Robertson *et al.* (1968). Reduction of gut flora may be more valuable than physical isolation or air filtration (Preisler *et al.*, 1970).

The following policy of patient protection has been found of value at the Royal Hospital for Sick Children in Glasgow:

At granulocyte levels below 1,000/cu mm a 'Neutropenia Regime' is instituted for patients being nursed in an open ward:

1. 0·1% Hibitane mouth washes q.d.s., p.c.
2. Naseptin cream to anterior nares t.d.s.
3. Daily phisohex baths.
4. Use chewing gum instead of toothbrush.

If the granulocytes fall below 500/cu mm the patient should in addition be reverse barrier nursed in a separate room. If it is necessary to continue administration of marrow depressing drugs such as DAUNO or ARA-C at a time when the granulocytes are less than 500/cu mm it is safer to attempt a totally sterile environment using a plastic isolator system such as that manufactured by Vickers Ltd. (Fig. 9). In addition removal of pathogenic gut flora is attempted by the use of oral:

Neomycin	0·5 G b.d.
Amphotericin B (tab)	100 mg b.d.
Amphotericin B lozenges	10 mg t.d.s. (to suck)
Enpac (Lactobacillus Acidophillus)	t.d.s.

A gut sterilizing régime using oral Gentamicin, Vancomycin and Nystatin combined with cooked, but not totally sterile, food has proved both bacteriologically and clinically effective in neutropenic patients (Preisler *et al.*, 1970).

Great attention must be paid to sterility in performing all venepunctures and intravenous infusions for which scalp vein needles are preferred (Darrell and Garrod, 1969).

The availability of platelet transfusions and protection from endogenous or exogenous infections as described above permits one to 'press on' with planned antileukaemic therapy in the face of thrombocytopenia and neutropenia, rather than having to interrupt therapy as in the past. The chance of obtaining a remission, followed by full regeneration of normal marrow elements, is thereby enhanced.

If a severe infection develops in the presence of neutropenia high-dose bactericidal antibiotic therapy should be instituted without delay rather than awaiting the results of blood and other cultures. Gentamycin plus Cloxacillin or Cephaloridine are useful initial drugs to use. Gram negative septicaemia presents the greatest immediate hazard.

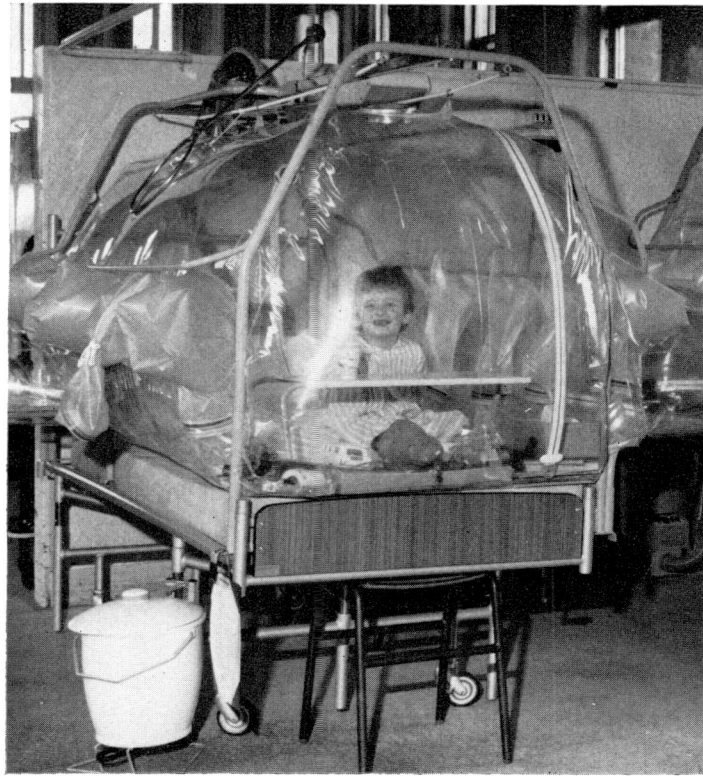

FIG. 4.9. A child being nursed in a sterile environment achieved by the use of a plastic isolator inflated by filtered air under pressure. Isolator system supplied by Vickers Ltd.

Granulocyte transfusions also have a place in the treatment of the severely neutropenic patient with septicaemia. The procedure involves plasmaphoresis of one or more patients with Chronic Granulocytic Leukaemia having white cell counts in excess of 100,000/cu mm. The procedure is similar to that for platelet transfusion but the red cells are separated either at 1G or at 200 r.p.m. for 10 min (Freireich *et al.*, 1967). Dramatic defervescence of fever follows upon the use of granulocyte transfusion more often than an actual rise in circulating granulocytes. A correction of neutropenia and thrombocytopenia can sometimes also be achieved (Fig. 8). More recently a continuous flow centrifuge has been developed (Buckner *et al.*, 1969). With this type of apparatus adequate numbers of leucocytes can be obtained from normal donors. A possible hazard with all leucocyte transfusions is a graft versus host reaction, but this is rare in practice.

The most commonly seen infection in patients on steroid therapy is oral thrush. This responds rapidly to Amphotericin B Lozenges, 10 mg t.d.s. It is thought that liability to fungus infection is dependent upon impaired lymphocyte function, which is particularly likely during systemic steroid therapy. Generalized moniliasis has been seen in a patient given an unusually protracted course of steroids. Varicella can result in a generalized fatal infection, and measles in fatal giant-cell pneumonia in patients on any of the immunosuppressant antileukaemic drugs, including MTX or 6-MP in conventional maintenance doses. Chemotherapy has to be withheld in susceptible contacts.

The relationship between immunological impairment and liability to infection is less certain in acute leukaemia than in chronic leukaemia. The antibody response to challenge with a number of antigens is very nearly normal (Silver *et al.*, 1960) but transient depression of immunoglobulin G is found during relapse (Kiran and Gross, 1969) and intensive chemotherapy (McKelvey and Carbone, 1965). There is no correlation between the level of immunoglobulins and the development of infection. It must be remembered that blood or platelet-rich plasma transfusion will contribute significant amounts of normal immunoglobulins.

Supportive therapy also includes the prevention and correction of dehydration and of hyperuricaemic acidosis following chemotherapeutic destruction of leukaemic cells where the initial tumour mass is large or blast cell count high (over 50,000/cu mm). Allopurinol in divided daily dosage (8 mg/Kg/day) and alkalinisation of the urine with a high urinary output are instituted in such patients (Holland and Holland, 1968). The dose of 6-MP must be reduced to approx. 25 % if Allopurinol is being given since it inhibits Xanthine Oxidase, which participates in the breakdown of 6-MP as well as of other purines.

MYELOBLASTIC, MYELOMONOCYTIC AND CHRONIC GRANULOCYTIC LEUKAEMIA

Fortunately 70 % of cases of childhood leukaemia are of the lymphoblastic variety since this is the type most responsive to currently available chemotherapy. Approximately 15 % of childhood leukaemia is, however, of the myeloblastic variety. The remaining 15 % is made up of mixed forms of acute leukaemia such as myelomonocytic and erythroleukaemia together with the rare Chronic Granulocytic Leukaemia of Childhood.

The same principles of chemotherapy apply to all the acute forms of leukaemia but the chance of an easily obtained or long maintained remission is considerably less in AML, although probably better than in adults with AML.

Complete remissions lasting 3–6 months or more have been obtained in 5 out of 8 patients by the use of VCR plus PRED plus 6-MP in conventional doses, but a total of 6–8 weekly doses of VCR were needed compared to 3–4 for ALL.

DAUNO alone (Bornstein et al., 1969) in combination with VCR plus steroids as used by Mathé or in combination with ARA-C (Crowther et al., 1970) can achieve remissions in a proportion of adult cases and these schedules are equally applicable to children. Bernard et al. (1968) reported 50% complete remission rate in childhood AML using DAUNO alone at a dose of 60 mg/m²/day for 5 days.

ARA-C appears to be one of the most active drugs in myeloblastic leukaemia. Henderson et al. (1968) reported a 78% remission rate by the use of 4-hourly infusions of this drug at a dose of 75–100 mg/m²/day, given for 4 successive days, followed by a similar period for recovery from toxicity. It has also been used in combination with Thioguanine (similar to 6-MP) in adults achieving a complete remission in 15 out of 36 patients with an additional 4 achieving good partial remissions (Gee et al., 1969). ARA-C has also been successfully used in combination with VCR and steroids for remission induction in acute myeloblastic leukaemia (Burke et al., 1968).

POMP achieves a remission in 70% of childhood AML (Henderson, 1968).

The combination of DAUNO, ARA-C plus 6-MP and steroids is currently being investigated as a form of intensive chemotherapy for myeloblastic leukaemia. The value of ASP in this type of leukaemia is less well established than in ALL (Hill et al., 1969).

CHRONIC MYELOID LEUKAEMIA

Chronic Myelocytic Leukaemia is rare in childhood but can occur in two forms. A 'juvenile' type is found in younger children and is characterized by thrombycytopenia, a high level of foetal haemoglobin and an absence of the Philadelphia chromosome; while an 'adult' type is found in older children and is identical in all its features with the disease in adults, including the presence of a Philadelphia chromosome and very low leucocyte alkaline phosphatase level (Reisman and Trujillo, 1963; Hardisty et al., 1964).

The subdivision of the two types is of more than academic interest since the response to chemotherapy is different. The juvenile type responds best to continuous oral 6-MP at conventional doses; the adult type best to Busulphan (0·05 to 0·1 mg/Kg/day).

In both types massive splenomegaly may be present, causing both hypersplenism and local discomfort. Carefully graded doses of local irradiation, while temporarily stopping the Busulphan, can be of great benefit in this repect in the adult type.

The chemotherapy merely controls the leukaemic process without ever attaining a complete remission as in acute leukaemia. The median survival is 9 months in the juvenile and 2 years 9 months in the adult form (Hardisty *et al.*, 1964).

GROWING POINTS IN LEUKAEMIA
MANAGEMENT

Particular areas of current research that may lead to improved management of this disease in the future include finer methods for determining small numbers of residual leukaemic cells during apparent remission, cytokinetically orientated time schedules of antileukaemic drug therapy and selection of such drugs on the basis of *in vitro* sensitivity tests performed on the patient's leukaemic cells.

While small numbers of leukaemic blast cells can be identified in white cell concentrates from peripheral blood of patients in apparent remission (Mathé *et al.*, 1966), or in a preleukaemic phase of the disease (Willoughby and Whitelaw, 1964), this technique is tedious. The elegant approach of Godwin *et al.* (1968) showed that the *in vivo* injection of tritiated Thymidine in normal individuals gave rise to a peak in circulating leukocyte radioactivity at approximately 5 days, due to the emergence of labelled polymorphs. In patients with active acute leukaemia 'early' peaks of blood radioactivity at 24 to 48 hours occurred due to labelled blast cells. Most patients in complete remission gave normal curves but others with impending relapse or with extramedullary leukaemic foci showed 'early' peaks even although conventional examination of the peripheral blood and marrow was normal. These early peaks were undoubtedly due to small numbers of circulating leukaemic blast cells undetectable by normal means.

A subsequent paper by the same group (Zimmerman *et al.*, 1968) showed that incubation of peripheral venous blood with tritiated Thymidine allows one to distinguish between groups of normal individuals, leukaemic patients in a state of complete remission with no leukaemic cells in their marrow, and those in a state of apparent remission but with up to 5% leukaemic cells in their marrow. It appears that tritiated Thymidine uptake *in vitro* is a much more sensitive index of the presence of small numbers of circulating blast cells than conventional morphological criteria. By the application of such techniques it may be possible to monitor the levels of the residual unseen leukaemic cells at different stages of the disease, including the period following intensive cytoreductive therapy.

Reference has already been made to the 'cycle active' drugs that only damaged cells in their DNA synthesis phase and to drug schedules designed to 'catch' as many cells in this phase as possible. It is only recently that direct experiments have been made to determine the precise cytokinetic effects of the commonly used antileukaemic drugs upon the blast cells in human acute leukaemia. These are important since there must be reservations in the uncritical application of data derived from the L1210 mouse leukaemia, where all the cells are in cyclic DNA synthesis, to the human disease where the majority of leukaemic cells are in a resting phase (Foadi et al., 1968).

Lampkin et al. (1969a) demonstrated by serial marrow cytokinetic studies in children that corticosteroids caused direct lysis of the blast cells and suppressed their entry into DNA synthesis. VCR arrested the cells in mitosis. ARA-C inhibited DNA synthesis and thereafter produced a partial synchronization of the cell cycle of the survivors. Subsequently this group have exploited the possibilities of this synchronization by administering VCR 72 hrs later at a time when many more of the blast cells were in the sensitive phase of their cell cycle. There was also apparent clinical benefit in this timing (Lampkin et al., 1969b). An increased proportion of 'resting' leukaemic blast cells may also be brought into the sensitive S-phase by extracorporeal irradiation (Bullimore et al., 1969). This type of study is still in its infancy but could have far-reaching consequences in the design of improved anti-leukaemic drug schedules in the future.

The possibility of selecting the drugs to which a leukaemic cell line is most sensitive or alternatively of excluding those to which it is resistant now appears feasible for a number of agents. ASP, corticosteroids, VCR and ARA-C inhibit RNA synthesis in vitro in leukaemic cells from patients sensitive to these drugs (Oettgen et al., 1967; Cline and Rosenbaum, 1968); DAUNO plus VCR impairs cell viability in vitro in patients achieving a complete remission on this combination of drugs (Laurie and Willoughby, 1969); in vitro MTX uptake (Kessel et al., 1968), 6-MP and ARA-C phosphorylation (Kessel et al., 1969; Kessel and Hall, 1969) are also hopeful indices of clinical responsiveness. The application of these techniques could transform 'blind' chemotherapy in the individual patient to 'tailor-made' chemotherapy.

REFERENCES

ABELL, C., & HOLLAND, P. (1969). Acute toxoplasmosis complicating leukemia. Am. J. Dis. Child., 118, 782.

ALGB* (1963). The effect of 6-mercaptopurine on the duration of steroid-induced remission in acute leukemia: a model for evaluation of other potentially useful therapy. Blood, 21, 699.

* Acute Leukaemia Group B.

ALGB (1965a). New treatment schedule with improved survival in childhood leukemia. Intermittent parenteral vs. daily oral administration of methotrexate for maintenance of induced remission. *J. Am. med. Ass.*, **194**, 75.

ALGB (1965b). The effectiveness of combinations of antileukaemic agents in inducing and maintaining remissions in children with acute leukemia. *Blood*, **26**, 642.

ALGB (1968). Arabinosyl cytosine: a useful agent in the treatment of acute leukemia in adults. *Blood*, **32**, 507.

ALGB (1969). Acute lymphocytic leukemia in children. Maintenance therapy with methotrexate administered intermittently. *J. Am. med. Ass.*, **207**, 923.

AUR, R. J. A., SIMONE, J., HUSTU, H. O., WALTERS, T., BORELLA, L., PRATT, C., & PINKEL, D. (1971). Central Nervous System Therapy and Combination Chemotherapy of Childhood Lymphocytic Leukemia. *Blood*, **37**, 272.

BERENBAUM, M. C. (1964). Prolongation of homograft survival by methotrexate with protection against toxicity by folinic acid. *Lancet*, **ii**, 1363.

BERNARD, J., BOIRON, M., JACQUILLAT, C., & WEIL, M. (1968). Rubidomycin in 400 patients with leukemia and other malignancies. Abstracts of the simultaneous sessions, XIIth Congress, International Society of Hematology, 1968, p. 5.

BISEL, H. F. (1956). Criteria for the evaluation of the response to treatment in acute leukemia. *Blood*, **ii**, 676.

BODEY, G. P., BUCKLEY, M., SATHE, Y. S., & FREIREICH, E. J. (1966). Quantitative relationships between circulating leukocytes and infection in patients with acute leukemia. *Ann. intern. Med.*, **64**, 328.

BODEY, G. P., FREIREICH, E. J., & FREI, E. (1969). Studies of patients in a laminar air flow unit. *Cancer*, **24**, 972.

BORNSTEIN, R. S., THEOLOGIDES, A., & KENNEDY, B. J. (1969). Daunorubicine in acute myelogenous leukemia in adults. *J. Am. med. Ass.*, **207**, 1301.

BRUBAKER, C. A., WHELLER, H. E., SONLEY, M. J., WILLIAMS, K. O., & HAMMOND, D. (1963). Cyclic chemotherapy for acute leukemia in children. *Blood*, **22**, 820.

BRUBAKER, C. A., GILCHRIST, G. S., HAMMOND, D., HYMAN, C. B., SHORE, N. A., & WILLIAMS, K. O. (1968). Induction of remission in acute leukemia with prednisone and intravenous methotrexate. *J. Pediat.*, **73**, 624.

BUCKNER, D., GRAW, R. G., EISEL, R. J., HENDERSON, E. S., & PERRY, S. (1969). Leukapheresis by continuous flow centrifugation in patients with chronic myelocytic leukemia. *Blood*, **33**, 353.

BULLIMORE, J. A., CHAN, B. W. B., & HAYHOE, F. G. J. (1969). Changes in leukaemic marrow blast cells following ECIB. Abstracts of Papers at International Symposium of Extracorporeal Irradiation of the Blood. Rehovoth, Israel. *Br. J. Haemat.*, **17**, 407.

BURCHENAL, J. H. (1966). Results of treatment of acute leukaemia. Proceedings of the XIth Congress of the International Society of Haematology. Plenary Sessions, p. 69.

BURKE, P. J., LENHARD, R. E., & OWENS, A. H. (1968). Therapy for acute leukemia in adults with cytosine arabinoside, vincristine and prednisone. *Cancer Chemother. Rep.*, **52**, 305.

CANGIR, A., & SULLIVAN, M. P. (1966). The occurrence of cytomegalovirus infections in childhood leukemia. Report of three cases. *J. Am. med. Ass.*, **195**, 616.

CHEVALIER, L., & GLIDEWELL, O. (1967). Schedule of 6-mercapto-purine and effect of inducer drugs in prolongation of remission maintenance in acute leukemia. *Proc. Am. Ass. Cancer Res.*, **8**, 10.

CLINE, M. J., & ROSENBAUM, E. (1968). Prediction of *in vivo* cytotoxicity of chemotherapeutic agents by their *in vitro* effect on leukocytes from patients with acute leukemia. *Cancer Res.*, **28**, 2516.

COHEN, P., & GARDINER, F. H. (1966). Thrombocytopenia as a laboratory sign and complication of gram-negative bacteremic infection. *Arch. intern. Med.*, **117**, 113.

CROWTHER, D., BATEMAN, C. J. T., VARTAN, C. P., WHITEHOUSE, J. M. A., MALPAS, J. S., HAMILTON FAIRLEY, G., & BODLEY SCOTT, R. (1970). Combination Chemotherapy using l-Asparaginase, Daunorubicin and Cytosine Arabinoside in Adults with Acute Myelogenous Leukaemia. *Br. Med. J.*, **4**, 513.

COLEBATCH, J. H. (1968). Cyclic drug regimen for acute childhood leukaemia. *Lancet*, **i**, 313.

DARRELL, J. H., & GARROD, L. P. (1969). Secondary septicaemia from intravenous cannulae. *Br. med. J.*, **2**, 481.

DEL VECCHIO, P. R., CHU, E. W., MALMGREN, R. A., & FREIREICH, E. J. (1963). Cytology of spinal fluid in leukemia. Abstracts of the American Society of Cytology, Inc., Eleventh Annual Meeting.

DORE, J. F., MOTTA, R., MARHOLEV, L., HRASK, Y., COLAS DE LA NOUE, H., SEMAN, G., DE VASSAL, F., & MATHÉ, G. (1967). Preliminary results of researches for new antigens in human leukaemic cells, and antibody in the serum of leukaemic patients. *Lancet*, **ii**, 1396.

DJERASSI, I., & ROY, A. (1968). A method for preservation of viable platelets: combined effect of sugars and dimethylsulphoxide. *Blood*, **22**, 703.

DJERASSI, I., FARBER, S., ABIR, E., & NEIKIRK, W. (1967a). Continuous infusion of methotrexate in children with acute leukemia. *Cancer*, **20**, 233.

DJERASSI, I., ROYER, G., TREAT, C., & ABIR, E. (1967b). Survival of children with acute lymphatic leukemia—role of methotrexate and intensive supportive management. *Proc. Am. Ass. Cancer Res.*, **8**, 14.

FERNBACH, D. J., GRIFFITH, K. M., HAGGARD, M. E., HOLCOMB, T. M., SUTOW, W. W., VIETTI, T. J., & WINDMILLER, J. (1966). Chemotherapy of acute leukemia in childhood—comparison of cyclophosphamide and mercaptopurine. *New Engl. J. Med.*, **275**, 451.

FOADI, M. D., COOPER, E. H., & HARDISTY, R. M. (1968). Proliferative activity of leukaemic cells at various stages of acute leukaemia of childhood. *Br. J. Haemat.*, **15**, 269.

FREIREICH, E. J., JUDSON, G., & LEVIN, R. H. (1965). Separation and collection of leukocytes. *Cancer Res.*, **25**, 1516.

FREIREICH, E. J., HENDERSON, E. S., KARON, M. R., & FREI, E. (1968). The Treatment of Acute Leukemia Considered with Respect to Cell Population Kinetics. *The Proliferation and Spread of Neoplastic Cells*, p. 441. Baltimore: Williams and Wilkins.

FREI, E., & FREIREICH, E. J. (1965). Progress and Perspectives in the Chemotherapy of Acute Leukemias. *Advances in Chemotherapy*, p. 286. Goldin, A., Hawking, F., and Schnitzer, R. J. (Eds.). New York: Academic Press.

FREI, E., LEVIN, R. H., BODEY, G. P., MORSE, E. E., & FREIREICH, E. J. (1965). The nature and control of infections in patients with acute leukemia. *Cancer Res.*, **25**, 1511.

GEE, T. S., KOU-PING YU, & CLARKSON, B. D. (1969). Treatment of adult acute leukemia with arabinosylcytosine and thioguanine. *Cancer*, **23**, 1019.

GEORGE, P., HERNANDEZ, K., HUSTU, O., BORELLA, L., HOLTON, C., & PINKEL, D. (1968). A study of 'total therapy' of acute lymphocytic leukemia in children. *J. Pediat.*, **72**, 319.

GODWIN, H. A., ZIMMERMAN, T. S., & PERRY, S. (1968). Peripheral leukocyte kinetic studies of acute leukemia in relapse and remission and chronic myelocytic leukemia in blastic crisis. *Blood*, **31**, 686.

GOLDIN, A., VENDITTI, J. M., HUMPHREYS, S. R., & MANTEL, N. (1956). Modification of treatment schedules in the management of advanced mouse leukemia with amethopterin. *J. natn. Cancer Inst.*, **17**, 203.

GUYER, R. J., & CROWTHER, D. (1969). Active immunotherapy in treatment of acute leukaemia. *Br. med. J.*, **4**, 406.

HAMILTON FAIRLEY, G. (1969). Immunity to malignant disease in man. *Br. med. J.*, **2**, 467.

HARDISTY, R. M., SPEED, D. E., & TILL, M. (1964). Granulocytic leukaemia in childhood. *Br. J. Haemat.*, **10**, 551.

HARDISTY, R. M., & NORMAN, P. M. (1967). Meningeal leukaemia. *Archs. Dis. Childh.*, **42**, 441.

HARDISTY, R. M., McELWAIN, T. J., & DARBY, C. W. (1969). Vincristine and prednisone for the induction of remissions in acute childhood leukaemia. *Br. med. J.*, **2**, 662.

HENDERSON, E. S. (1967). Combination chemotherapy of acute lymphocytic leukaemia of childhood. *Cancer Res.*, **27**, 2570.

HENDERSON, E. S. (1968). Treatment of acute leukemia. Editorial, *Ann. intern. Med.*, **69**, 628.

HENDERSON, E. S., SERPICK, A., LEVENTHAL, B., & HENRY, P. (1968). Cytosine arabinoside infusions in adult and childhood acute myelocytic leukemia. *Proc. Am. Ass. Cancer Res.*, **9**, 29.

HENDERSON, E. S., & SAMAHA, R. J. (1969). Evidence that drugs in multiple combinations have materially advanced the treatment of human malignancies. *Cancer Res.*, **29**, 2272.

HERSH, F. M., BODEY, G. P., NIES, B. A., & FREIREICH, E. J. (1965). Causes of death in acute leukemia. *J. Am. med. Ass.*, **193**, 105.

HILL, J. M., LOEB, E., MacLELLAN, A., KHAN, A., ROBERTS, J., SHIELDS, W. F., & HILL, N. O. (1969). Response to highly purified l-Asparaginase during therapy of acute leukemia. *Cancer Res.*, **29**, 1574.

HOLLAND, J. F. (1967). Intensive High-Dose Treatment of Children in Complete Remission of Acute Lymphocytic Leukemia. *Treatment of Burkitt's Tumour*. U.I.C.C. Monograph series, Vol. 8, p. 163. Burchenal, J. H., and Burkitt, D. P. (Eds.). Heidelberg: Springer-Verlag.

HOLLAND, J. F. (1968). Progress in the Treatment of Acute Leukemia, 1966. *Perspectives in Leukemia*, p. 218. Dameshek, W. (Ed.). New York: Grune and Stratton.

HOLLAND, J. F., & GLIDEWELL, O. (1968). Induction, consolidation, intensification, reinduction, and maintenance chemotherapy of acute lymphocytic leukemia. Abstracts of the simultaneous sessions, XIIth Congress, Int. Soc. Hemat., p. 9.

HOLLAND, J. F., quoted by Henderson, E. S. (1969). Treatment of Acute Leukemia, in Seminars in Hematology, Vol. 6, No. 3, p. 285.

HOLLAND, P., & HOLLAND, N. H. (1968). Prevention and management of acute hyperuricemia in childhood leukemia. *J. Pediat.*, **72**, 358.

HOLTON, C. P., VIETTI, T. T., NORA, A. H., DONALDSON, M. H., STUCKEY, W. J., WATKINS, W. L., & LANE, D. M. (1969). Clinical study of daunomycin and prednisone for induction of remission in children with advanced leukemia. *New Engl. J. Med.*, **280**, 171.

JACQUILLAT, C., BOIRON, M., WEIL, M., NAJEAN, Y., & BERNARD, J. (1967). Traitement actuel des leucémies aiguës lymphoblastiques; effets de la méthode de 'réinduction'. *Marseille méd.*, **104**, 1.

JAMES, K. W., HAMESON, B., KAY, H. E. M., LYNCH, J., & NGAN, H. Some practical aspects of intensive cytotoxic therapy. *Lancet*, **i**, 1045.

JOHNSON, R. E., ZELEN, M., & FREIREICH, E. J. (1966). Evaluation of human acute leukemia data using a murine leukemia model system. *Cancer*, **19**, 481.

KESSEL, D., HALL, T. C., & ROBERTS, DE W. (1968). Modes of uptake of methotrexate by normal and leukemic human leukocytes *in vitro* and their relation to drug response. *Cancer Res.*, **28**, 564.

KESSEL, D., HALL, T. C., & ROSENTHAL, D. (1969a). Uptake and phosphorylation of cytosine arabinoside by normal and leukemic human blood cells *in vitro*. *Cancer Res.*, **29**, 459.

KESSEL, D., & HALL, T. C. (1969b). Retention of 6-mercaptopurine by intact cells as an index of drug response in human and murine leukemias. *Cancer Res.*, **29**, 2116.

KILLMANN, S. A. (1968). The Kinetics of Leukemic Blast Cells in Man. *Cell Kinetics in Human Leukemia*, p. 54. *Series Haematologica, Vol. I, 3*. Copenhagen: Munksgaard.

KIRAN, D., & GROSS, S. (1969). The G-immunoglobulins in acute leukemia in children. Hematologic and immunologic relationships. *Blood*, **33**, 198.

KLEIN, G. (1966). Tumour antigens. *A. Rev. Microbiol.*, **20**, 223.

KLEIN, E., FARBER, S., & DJERASSI, I. (1965). Control and prevention of hemorrhage: platelet separation. *Cancer Res.*, **25**, 1504.

KRIVIT, W., BRUBAKER, C., THATCHER, L. G., PIERCE, M., PERRIN, E., & HARTMANN, J. R. (1968). Maintenance therapy in acute Leukemia of childhood. Comparison of cyclic vs. sequential methods. *Cancer*, **21**, 352.

KRIVIT, W., GILCHRIST, G., & BEATTY, E. C. (1970). The need for chemotherapy after prolonged complete remission in acute leukemia in children. *J. Pediat.*, **76**, 138.

LAMPKIN, B. C., NAGAO, T., & MAUER, A. M. (1969a). Drug effect in acute leukemia. *J. clin. Invest.*, **48**, 1124.

LAMPKIN, B. C., NAGAO, T., & MAUER, A. M. (1969b). Synchronization of the mitotic cycle in acute leukemia. *Nature, Lond.*, **222**, 1274.

Lancet (1971). Medical Research Council Trial of treatment of Leukemia in children (in press).

LAURIE, H. C., & WILLOUGHBY, M. L. N. (1969). *In-vitro* prediction of clinical response to chemotherapy in childhood leukaemia. I. Combination of daunorubicin, vincristine and prednisolone. *Br. J. Haemat.*, **17**, 251.

LEIKEN, S. L., BRUBAKER, C. A., HARTMAN, J., MURPHY, M. L., WOLFF, H. A., & PERRIN, E. (1968). Varying prednisone dosage in remission induction of previously untreated childhood leukemia. *Cancer*, **21**, 346.

LEVITAN, A. A., & PERRY, S. (1967). Infectious complications of chemotherapy in a protected environment. *New Engl. J. Med.*, **276**, 881.

MATHÉ, G., SCHWARZENBERG, L., MERY, A. M., CATTAN, A., SCHNEIDER, M., AMIEL, J. L., SCHLUMBERGER, J. R., POISSON, J., & WAJCNER, G. (1966). Extensive histological and cytological survey of patients with acute leukaemia in 'complete remission'. *Br. med. J.*, **i**, 640.

MATHÉ, G., HAYAT, M., SCHWARZENBERG, L., AMIEL, J. L., SCHNEIDER, M., CATTAN, A., SCHLUMBERGER, J. R., & HASMIN, C. (1967). Acute lymphoblastic leukemia treated with a combination of prednisone, vincristine and rubidomycin. *Lancet*, **ii**, 380.

MATHÉ, G. (1968). Immunothérapie active de la leucémie L1210, appliquée après la greffe tumorale. *Revue fr. Étud. clin. biol.*, **13**, 881.

MATHÉ, G. (1969a). Approaches to the immunological treatment of cancer in man. *Br. med. J.*, **4**, 7.

MATHÉ, G. (1969b). Therapeutic Strategy in Acute Leukaemia: Chemotherapy and Immunotherapy. Fifth Annual Guest Lecture. Leukaemia Research Fund. London: Queen Anne Press.

MATHÉ, G., AMIEL, J. L., SCHWARZENBERG, L., SCHNEIDER, M., CATTAN, A., SCHLUMBERGER, J. R., HAYAT, M., & DE VASSAL, P. (1969). Active immunotherapy for acute lymphoblastic leukaemia. Lancet, i, 697.

MAUER, A. M., & FISHER, V. (1966). Characteristics of cell proliferation in four patients with untreated acute leukemia. Blood, 28, 428.

McELWAIN, T. J., & HARDISTY, R. M. (1969). Remission induction with cytosine arabinoside and L-asparaginase in acute lymphoblastic leukaemia. Br. med. J., 4, 596.

McKELVEY, E. M., & CARBONE, P. P. (1965). Serum immune globulin concentrations in acute leukemia during intensive chemotherapy. Cancer, 18, 1292.

NAGAO, T., LAMPKIN, B. C., & MAUER, A. M. (1970). Maintenance therapy in acute childhood leukemia. J. Pediat., 76, 134.

NATIONAL CRITERIA COMMITTEE (1964). Criteria for evaluating chemotherapy in acute leukemia. Cancer Chemother. Rep., 42, 27.

NIES, B. A., BODEY, G. P., THOMAS, L. B., BRECHER, G., & FREIREICH, E. J. (1965). The persistence of extramedullary leukemic infiltrates during bone marrow remission of acute leukemia. Blood, 26, 133.

OETTGEN, H. F., OLD, L. J., BOYSE, E. A., CAMPBELL, H. A., PHILLIPS, F., CLARKSON, S., TALLAL, B. D., LEEPER, R. D., SCHWARTZ, M. K., & KIM, J. H. (1967). Inhibition of leukemia in man by l-asparaginase. Cancer Res., 27, 2619.

PERRIN, J. C. S., MAUER, A. M., & STERLING, T. D. (1963). Intravenous methotrexate therapy in the treatment of acute leukemias. Pediatrics, 31, 833.

PIERCE, M., SHORE, N., SITARZ, A., MURPHY, M. L., LOUIS, J., & SEVERO, N. (1966). Cyclophosphamide therapy in acute leukemia of childhood: co-operative study conducted by members of Children's Cancer Co-operative Group A. Cancer, 19, 1551.

PINKEL, D. (1970). Personal communication.

PREISLER, H. D., GOLDSTEIN, I. M., & HENDERSON, E. S. (1970). Gastrointestinal "sterilization" in the treatment of patients with acute leukemia. Cancer, 26, 1076.

RALL, D. P., & ZUBROD, C. G. (1962). Mechanisms of drug absorption and excretion. A. Rev. Pharmac., 2, 109.

RALL, D. P., & HOMAN, E. R. (1967). Possible approaches to selective toxicity: new concepts in cancer chemotherapy. Cancer Chemother. Rep., 51, 247.

RALL, D. P. (1968). Selective aspects of chemotherapy in acute leukemia and Burkitt's tumour. Cancer, 21, 4.

REISMAN, L. E., & TRUTILLO, J. M. (1963). Chronic granulocytic leukemia of childhood. J. Pediat., 62, 710.

REISMAN, L. E., MITANI, M., & ZUELZER, W. W. (1964). I. Evidence for the origin of leukemic stem lines from anenploid mutants. New Engl. J. Med., 270, 590.

ROBERTSON, A. C., LYNCH, J., KAY, H. E. M., JAMESON, B., GUYER, R. J., & EVANS, I. L. (1968). Design and use of plastic tents for isolation of patients prone to infection. Lancet, ii, 1376.

SAUNDERS, E. F., KAUDER, E., & MAUER, A. M. (1967a). Sequential therapy of acute leukemia in childhood. J. Pediat., 70, 632.

SAUNDERS, E. F., LAMPKIN, B. C., & MAUER, A. M. (1967b). Variation of proliferative activity in leukemic cell populations of patients with acute leukemia. J. clin. Invest., 46, 1356.

SCHNEIDER, M., SCHWARTZERBERG, L., AMIEL, J. L., CATTAN, A., SCHLUMBERGER, J. R., HAYAT, M., DE VASSAL, F., JASMIN, C., ROSENFELD, C., & MATHÉ, G. (1969). Pathogen-free isolation unit—three years' experience. Br. med. J., 1, 836.

SCHWARTZ, S. A., & PERRY, S. M. (1966). Patient protection in cancer chemotherapy. *J. Am. med. Ass.*, **197**, 623.
SELAWRY, O. S., & HOLLAND, J. F. (1966). Methotrexate in leukemia intramuscularly. Letter to *J. Am. med. Ass.*, **196**, 460.
SELAWRY, O. S., & ODOM, S. (1968). On eradication of leukemic meningopathy. *Proc. Am. Ass. Cancer Res.*, **9**, 62.
SKIPPER, H. E., SCHABEL, F. M., & WILCOX, W. S. (1964). On the criteria and kinetics associated with 'curability' of experimental leukemias. *Cancer Chemother. Rep.*, **35**, 1.
SKIPPER, H. E. (1965). Summary of informal discussion on pharmacology protected areas. *Cancer Res.*, **25**, 1578.
SKIPPER, H. E., SCHABEL, F. M., & WILCOX, W. S. (1967). Scheduling of arabinosylcytosine to take advantage of its S-phase specificity against leukemia cells. *Cancer Chemother. Rep.*, **51**, 125.
SKIPPER, H. E. (1968). Cellular Kinetics Associated with 'Curability' of Experimental Leukemias. *Perspectives in Leukemia*, p. 187. Dameshek, W. (Ed.). New York: Grune and Stratton.
SPIVAK, J, L., BRUBAKER, L. H., & PERRY, S. (1969). Intravascular granulocyte kinetics in acute leukemia. *Blood*, **34**, 582.
SILVER, R. T., UTZ, J., FREI, E., KOLE, R., KASSEL, R., & SZWED, C. (1960). Antibody response in patients with acute leukemia. *J. Lab. clin. Med.*, **56**, 634.
SULLIVAN, M. P., & HAGGARD, M. E. (1970). Comparison of the prolongation of Remission in Meningeal Leukemia with Maintenance Intrathecal Methotrexate and Intravenous BCNU. *Proc. Am. Ass. Cancer Res.*, **11**, 77.
SULLIVAN, M. P., VIETTI, T. J., FERNISACH, D. J., GRIFFITH, K. M., HADDY, T. B., & WATKINS, W. L. (1969). Clinical investigations in the treatment of meningeal leukemia: radiation therapy regimens vs. conventional intrathecal methotrexate. *Blood*, **34**, 301.
TAN, C., TASAKA, H., KOU-PING YU, MURPHY, M. L., & KARNOFSKY, D. A. (1967). Daunomycin, an antitumour antibiotic, in the treatment of neoplastic disease. *Cancer*, **20**, 333.
VIETTI, T. J., SULLIVAN, M. P., BERRY, D. H., HADDY, T. B., HAGGARD, M. E., & BLATTNER, R. J. (1965). The response of acute childhood leukemia to an initial and a second course of prednisone. *J. Pediat.*, **66**, 18.
WANG, J. J., & PRATT, C. B. (1970). Intrathecal Arabinosyl Cytosine in Meningeal Leukemia. *Cancer*, **25**, 531.
WILLOUGHBY, M. L. N., & WHITELAW, J. W. (1964). The Diagnosis of Preleukaemia. Abstracts of Simultaneous Sessions. Xth Congress of the International Society of Haematology. A: 33, Stockholm.
WILLOUGHBY, M. L. N., & LAURIE, H. C. (1968). Cyclic chemotherapy in childhood acute leukaemia. *Archs Dis. Childh.*, **43**, 187.
ZIMMERMANN, T. S., GODWIN, H. A., ZELEN, M., & PERRY, S. (1968). The remission and relapse status of acute leukemia as studied by the *in-vitro* uptake of tritiated thymidine by peripheral blood leucocytes. *Blood*, **32**, 292.
ZUBROD, C. G. (1965). Combinations of drugs in the treatment of acute leukaemia. *Proc. R. Soc. Med.*, **58**, 987.
ZUELZER, W. W. (1964). Implications of long-term survival in acute stem cell leukemia of childhood treated with composite cyclic therapy. *Blood*, **24**, 477.

5 Burkitt's Lymphoma

PETER CLIFFORD

The association of lymphocytic lymphomatous jaw, visceral and osseous tumours in African children was first described by Burkitt (1958), Burkitt and Davies (1961), and Burkitt and O'Conor (1961). This clinical syndrome was initially termed the 'Lymphoma of African Children' or the 'African Lymphoma', but as other tumours of the reticuloendothelial system also occur in African children, the eponym 'Burkitt's Tumour or Lymphoma' was adopted to describe a poorly differentiated lymphocytic lymphoma with a particular clinical presentation, commonly seen in certain areas of Africa and New Guinea.

Epidemiological studies by Burkitt (1961, 1962) indicated that the tumour distribution in Africa was dependent on temperature and humidity. This 'Lymphoma Belt' extending across tropical Africa 15° north and south of the Equator and down the East Coast of the continent was found to exclude areas where the annual rainfall was 20 inches or less, or where the mean temperature fell below 60°F at any time during the year. In the countries of Equatorial Africa, temperature relates directly to altitude and cases occurred very rarely in areas over 5,000 feet.

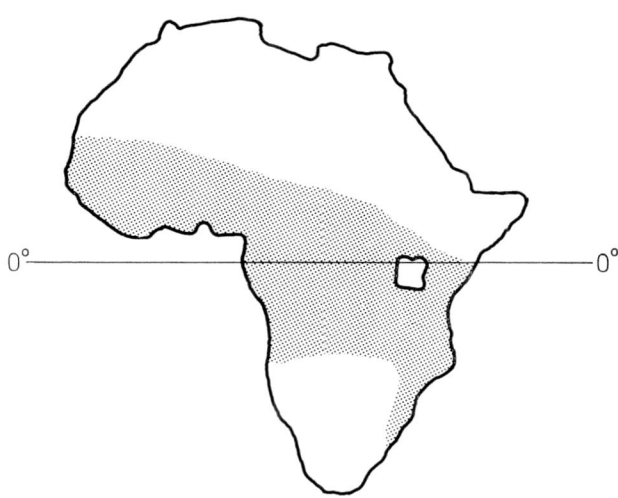

FIG. 5.1. African 'Lymphoma Belt'.

For every 5° north or south of the Equator the 60°F isotherm falls 1,000 feet so that the altitude up to which cases occur falls as distance from the Equator increases. This suggested to Burkitt and Davies (1961) that the tumour might be virus induced. The development of the yellow fever and dengue viruses is temperature dependent and Haddow (1961, 1963) in a bioclimatic study of the distribution of Burkitt's lymphoma noted the similarity to the distribution of yellow fever cases and antibodies. Haddow suggested that the 60°F limitation may relate to the minimal temperature at which the oncogenic virus could develop within the vector as in areas with an annual rainfall of 20 inches or less, most of the mosquitoes belong to species which depend on drought resistant eggs for survival. During periods of drought the adult mosquitoes die out completely, which would cause a break in the transmission of any oncogenic viruses these arthropods might carry.

Subsequent to the recognition of this tumour as a clinical syndrome in Africa, cases were reported from other areas of the world, and Wright (1967) and Burkitt (1970a) have reviewed the world-wide distribution. The disease may be endemic in New Guinea (ten Seldam et al., 1966) and is recognized with increasing frequency in parts of Brazil and Malaysia. Isolated case reports have appeared from many European countries and over 20 cases have been recorded from the United States of America.

VIRUSES AND BURKITT'S LYMPHOMA

The close parallel between the geographical distribution of Burkitt's lymphoma and other well-known arthropod borne viral diseases in Africa stimulated the search for a causal virus. The recognition of a small number of isolated cases in Europe and North America in areas where the temperature/humidity conditions of the African lymphoma belt and its associated arthropods did not prevail, suggested that these sporadic cases might be due to vertical virus transmission. In tropical Africa the high incidence of this tumour, higher than the combined incidence of all other childhood tumours, might be due to free horizontal transmission by an arthropod (Gross, 1961), or to a hyperviraemia following direct blood stream infection by a haemophagous vector. Alternatively the tumour may not be associated with a specific virus but arise as the result of some factor in a patient's external or internal environment or genetic composition rendering oncogenic a ubiquitous and perhaps normally simple virus or viruses.

Though a number of viruses have been isolated either directly or from cultures of tumour lymphoblasts (Bell, 1967), only two are considered at present to have possible aetiological significance.

REOVIRUS

Bell *et al.* (1964) isolated a double strand RNA reovirus from Burkitt tumour culture fluids inoculated into indicator cells. Since then reovirus type 3 has been recovered from 27 out of 85 Burkitt lymphoma biopsies and neutralizing antibodies were present in the serum of 73% of 72 Burkitt lymphoma patients as compared with 18% of controls (Bell, 1970). Infection with all three types of reoviruses occurs frequently throughout the world in men and animals. Infection with reovirus 3 is usually spread via the respiratory tract or by faecal oral routes. Under certain circumstances this virus can be transmitted by mosquitoes. Clinical disease arising from infection with this virus is confined almost entirely to children with an age incidence similar to that of Burkitt's lymphoma. But a direct relationship between reovirus 3 and Burkitt's lymphoma has not yet been established (Levy *et al.*, 1968; Harris, 1970).

EPSTEIN-BARR VIRUS

Epstein *et al.* (1964) identified an intracellular DNA herpes type virus now known as the Epstein-Barr virus (EBV) in an established strain of cultured Burkitt's lymphoma cells. The particles observed were smaller than herpes simplex and probably belong to the varicella-cytomegalovirus sub-group. The virus has not been seen in fresh tumour biopsy cells but has been observed in culture lines established from patients in Uganda, Kenya, Nigeria, New Guinea and the United States (Epstein and Achong, 1970). Henle and Henle (1966) and Henle *et al.* (1968) have related infection with this virus to infectious mononucleosis. Infection with EBV revealed by the presence of antibodies, usually in low titres, is world-wide. Infection is most widely spread and occurs at an earlier age in populations of low socio-economic levels. In East Africa 82% of children in the 1–5, and 94% in the 6–10 year age groups have low titres ($\leqslant 1 : 10$) of specific anti-EBV antibodies (Diehl *et al.*, 1969). High anti-EBV antibody titres ($\geqslant 1 : 160$) have to date only been found regularly associated with infectious mononucleosis, Burkitt's lymphoma and nasopharyngeal carcinoma, irrespective of the patient's race or country of origin (Henle and Henle, 1969).

There is now a vast amount of circumstantial evidence which suggests that EBV plays a causative role in Burkitt's lymphoma and perhaps in anaplastic carcinoma of the nasopharynx (de Schryver *et al.*, 1969; de Thé *et al.*, 1970). Herpes type viruses possibly antigenetically related to EBV have been shown to cause Marek's lymphomatous syndrome of chickens (Churchill *et al.*, 1967, 1969) and probably Lucke's renal carcinoma of leopard frogs (Fawcett, 1956).

By adapting the indirect membrane immunofluorescence technique (Möller, 1961) for use with sera and tumour cells from patients with Burkitt's lymphoma, Klein *et al.* (1966, 1967a, b, c) demonstrated a humoral factor directed against tumour associated antigens expressed on the Burkitt tumour cell membrane. The presence of these neo-antigens is determined by infection with EBV (Klein *et al.*, 1968a, b). Most patients with Burkitt's lymphoma have high titres of antibodies directed against these viral neo-antigens which are not present on the patient's normal cells (Klein, E. *et al.*, 1967). Using an indirect immunofluorescence test on acetone fixed smears of cells from EBV carrying cell lines, Henle and Henle (1966, 1967) and Henle *et al.* (1969) identified antibodies directed against intracellular EBV determined antigens. The membrane reactive antibodies are 7SIgG immunoglobulins (Smith *et al.*, 1967, Klein *et al.*, 1967b) and by isolating these from a highly reactive Burkitt reference serum and coupling the active fractions with fluorescein isothiocyanate (Goldstein *et al.*, 1969), a more specific direct membrane immunofluorescence test was possible.

Using this test the anti-EBV titre of sera is now assessed as the ability to block the reaction of a standard fluorescent reference serum with cells from various Burkitt tissue culture lines. The results are expressed as a *blocking index*. This method though less sensitive than the indirect technique is more specific detecting fewer irrelevant and misleading antibody/antigen reactions (Klein *et al.*, 1969a). Blocking experiments have shown that there are at least two antibody complexes directed against membrane antigens and that these are distinct from antibodies formed against the intracellular antigens (Pearson *et al.*, 1969; Klein, 1970; Svedmyr *et al.*, 1970; Gunvén *et al.*, 1970). These antibodies are specifically directed against the three EBV determined antigen complexes identified to date (Klein *et al.*, 1970, 1971; Henle *et al.*, 1970, 1971). In these tests high antibody titres were in general confined to sera from patients with infectious mononucleosis, Burkitt's lymphoma and anaplastic carcinoma of the post-nasal space when tested against Burkitt lymphoma biopsy cells or more usually EBV carrying Burkitt tumour cell lines.

Complement fixation tests have also demonstrated antibodies in the sera of Burkitt lymphoma patients directed against antigens in disintegrated cultured Burkitt tumour cell (Armstrong *et al.*, 1966; McCormack *et al.*, 1969) and a precipitating antibody has been found in the sera of Burkitt lymphoma patients reactive against an antigen isolated from EBV carrying Burkitt lymphoma cells (Old *et al.*, 1966; Oettgen *et al.*, 1967).

It is impossible at present to decide whether EBV plays a causative role or is merely a passenger virus in Burkitt's lymphoma and nasopharyngeal carcinoma. This can only be done by a prospective serological study in children and young adults in areas of high tumour incidence, so that antibody patterns can be determined preceding and subsequent to tumour development. It could then be assessed if tumour development was associated with recurrent EBV infections or with high antibody levels reflecting an extensive viral carrier state (Henle and Henle, 1969). Alternatively it might be found that tumours develop in those whose primary EBV infection has been delayed until a time when the reticuloendothelial system has been 'primed' by the hyperplasia associated with repeated malarial or other parasitic infections (Dalldorf *et al.*, 1964; Burkitt, 1969; Kafuko and Burkitt, 1970). Such a situation might apply in New Guinea as well as in East Africa where Burkitt's tumour is endemic in areas where malaria is holo-endemic; also in countries such as Brazil and Malaysia where the disease is relatively common but which are also malarial. Stewart (1970) has suggested that clinical presentation of the tumour may relate to malarial infections in infancy.

OTHER FACTORS OF POSSIBLE AETIOLOGICAL SIGNIFICANCE

The high incidence of this disease in tropical Africa and New Guinea suggests that a particular environment or genetic factors may be of importance.

1. *Proximity to domestic animals and fowls.* African children in the 'lymphoma belt' live in very primitive dwellings, often in close proximity to domestic animals. Sheep, goats and hens often share the same hut as humans, and cattle are usually kept in a 'boma' or enclosure near the hut (Figs. 2 and 3). Fowl leukaemia and bovine leukosis are transmissible viral diseases and though very little is known about malignant disease in African domestic stock, the proximity of these animals to poorly nourished children may be significant.

2. *Malnutrition.* The highest incidences of Burkitt's lymphoma occur in populations living at a very low socio-economic level and liable to suffer from malnutrition (Clifford *et al.*, 1967). There is a vast interface between malnutrition and medicine in the tropics. Ramalingswami (1969) has reviewed the effects of kwashiorkor and protein-calorie malnutrition in young growing children in the tropics. The resulting syndrome includes retardation of the body's biochemical enzyme systems, impairment of cell division, differentiation and organ growth. The reactive capacity of the body is severely restricted. Alleyne and Young (1966) have shown that protein-calorie malnutrition results in adreno-cortical hyperfunction. The high plasma levels of 11-hydroxycortico-steroids may be of fundamental importance in many of the biochemical disturbances of kwashiorkor and will depress the body's immunological surveillance system. Thus the anergy associated with malnutrition may

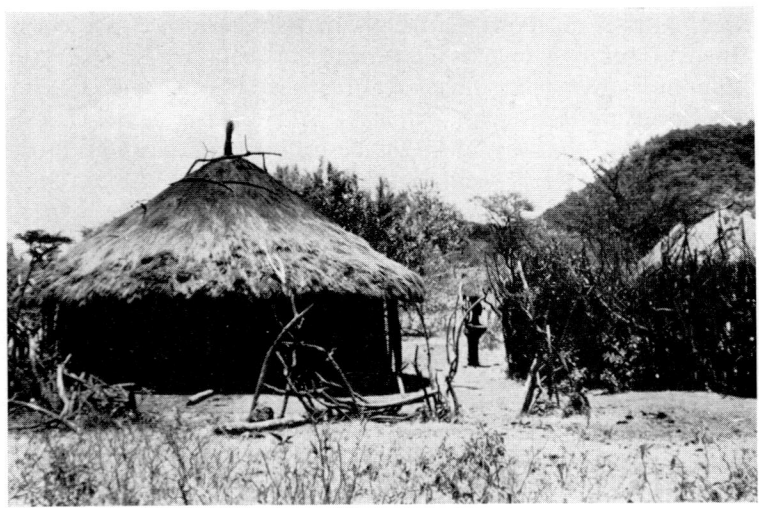

Fig. 5.2. The home of a patient with Burkitt's lymphoma; the walls of the hut are made of mud and wattle and the roof of grass thatch. At night fowl and young goats and sheep occupy the hut along with the family.

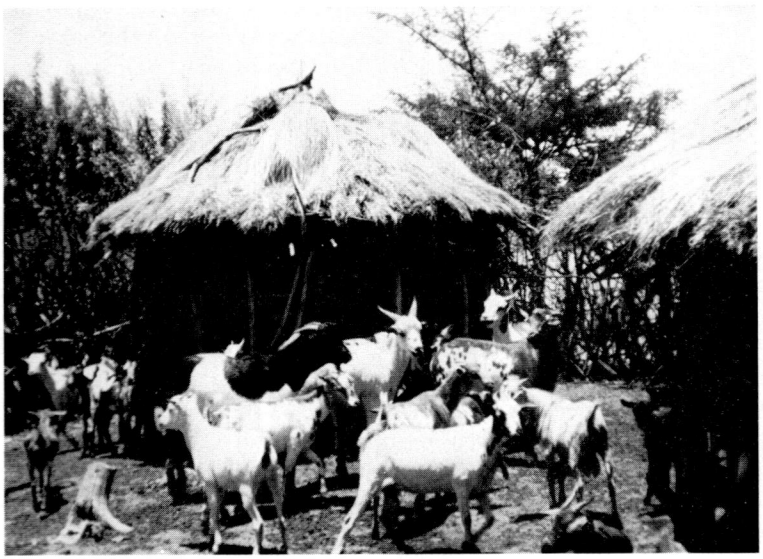

Fig. 5.3. Domestic stock in the compound of a Burkitt's lymphoma patient's homestead.

be a factor in altering the usual non-malignant response to EBV infection.

3. *Herbs and Food.* Little is known about African herbal medicines but herbs are used in the treatment of fever, headache, dysmenorrhoea and constipation, as abortifacients and to ease childbirth. Flora as well as fauna are influenced by temperature and humidity and in Africa many wild plants are used as food or as food additives. Phytomitogens may be widely distributed in wild and cultivated plants. Farnes *et al.* (1964) and Chessin *et al.* (1966) have described the mitogenic activity of extracts of the roots of *Phytolacca Americana* which grows throughout tropical Africa, and the mitogenic property of the broad bean (*Vicia faba*) has been noted by Nowell (1960). Hashem and Kabarity (1966) tested various legumes and vegetable seeds and found that extracts of lentils (*Lens esculenta*), broad beans, fenugreek (*Trigoonella faenum gracum*) and the common bean (*Phaseolus vulgaris*) contained strong mitogenic agents. *Phaseolus vulgaris* is frequently used as a food-stuff in tropical Africa, and children are often fed bean milk as a substitute for animal milk. These beans are a rich source of phytohaemagglutinin, a substance widely used as a stimulant of leucocyte mitosis and growth. Normal cells so stimulated retain their normal chromosome pattern. Initially it may seem absurd to associate beans with malignancy but it is reasonable to consider that the association of such a stimulus with other factors may result in malignancy (Pulvertaft, 1964).

4. *Genetic factors.* The clustering of cases in particular areas (Pike *et al.*, 1967) suggests a genetic susceptibility to this disease similar to that postulated by Lilly *et al.* (1964) for viral murine leukaemogenesis. These authors found a close relationship between the susceptibility to develop viral leukaemia and a histocompatibility factor associated with a single gene or a group of closely linked genes. Ellman *et al.* (1970) have suggested that immunological responsiveness to an oncogenic virus in man may be linked to the gene coding for histocompatibility surface antigens. But factual information is scant for the situation in humans and nothing definite can be said until the results of analysis of the isoantigens responsible for tissue incompatibility in humans are known.

5. *Transplacental and Arthropod Transmission.* Burnett (1969) has suggested that Burkitt's lymphoma may arise as a graft versus host reaction, the graft originating from maternal immunocytes following a leak through the placental barrier. Green *et al.* (1960) had previously suggested that Hodgkin's disease might arise as a maternal-to-foetal lymphocyte chimoera, and Turner *et al.* (1966) have provided cytogenic evidence concerning the possibility of the transplacental transfer of leucocytes in pregnant women. A recent observation (Manolov *et al.*, 1970) lends support to Burnett's suggestions. It was found that whereas the chromosomes of normal tissues of 3 male children with Burkitt's

lymphoma were of a male karyotype, those of the tumours were female.

It has also been suggested that tumour cells might be transmitted by mosquitoes. Scanlon *et al.* (1965) showed that a homotransplanted melanoma could grow and kill the recipient, and Banfield *et al.* (1966) demonstrated the capacity of female *Aedes Aegypti* mosquitoes to transmit reticulum cell sarcoma in a colony of Syrian hamsters. It was estimated that tumour cells were transmitted by 1–2% of mosquitoes, the rate of transmission was 5–10% and the tumour cells were found to be viable for 8 hours after ingestion by the mosquitoes. Recently Fialkow *et al.* (1971) have used isozyme typing to compare fresh normal and tumour material with tumour cell culture lines from 13 patients. Cultured tumour cells from 5 were genetically foreign to their host and may have been introduced by blood transfusions or through the bite of a haemophagous vector to an immunologically incompentent host.

INCIDENCE

Burkitt's lymphoma accounts for over 50% of all malignant tumours of childhood in tropical Africa (Burkitt, 1970b). In Ibadan in Nigeria it accounts for 70% of all neoplasms of childhood with an incidence estimated as 15 cases per 100,000 children between the ages of 5 and 9 years (Edington and Maclean, 1964).

Age and Sex. No cases have been reported under 1 year of age. The highest incidence occurs in both sexes between the ages of 4 and 7, and between 8 and 16 years the incidence falls steeply. Rare cases have been reported over the age of 20 years; the majority have been pregnant women in whom the disease has presented as a breast tumour. The majority of patients with jaw tumours present under 8 years of age.

The male to female ratio is approximately 2 : 1 irrespective of the site of the presenting tumour. Jaw tumours occur most frequently in males but the incidence of abdominal tumours, (including ovarian) is equal in both sexes.

CLINICAL FEATURES

The first description of this syndrome related to tumours of the jaws (multiple in 40% of cases) but it is now recognized that patients may present with retroperitoneal, ovarian or long bone tumours and the jaws may not be affected. Growths of the jaw are more obvious (Fig. 4) than retroperitoneal tumours but the incidence of intrarenal and para-pancreatic tumours is much higher (Fig. 5). Spinal paresis is another frequent presentation which may or may not be associated with a clinically obvious tumour. Burkitt and O'Conor (1961), Burkitt (1964, 1970b) have fully described the clinical presentations of this tumour

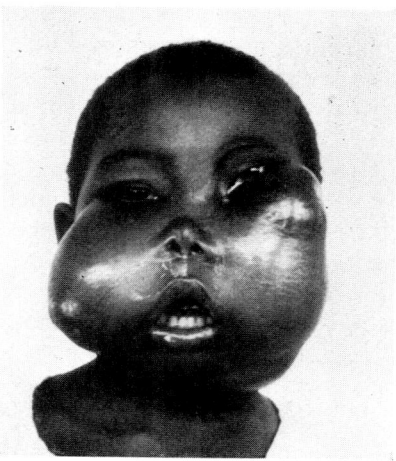

Fig. 5.4. Burkitt's lymphoma involving four jaw quadrants and left orbit and submandibular area in an 8-year-old female child (Kenya Cancer Council Number (K.C.C. No.) 816).

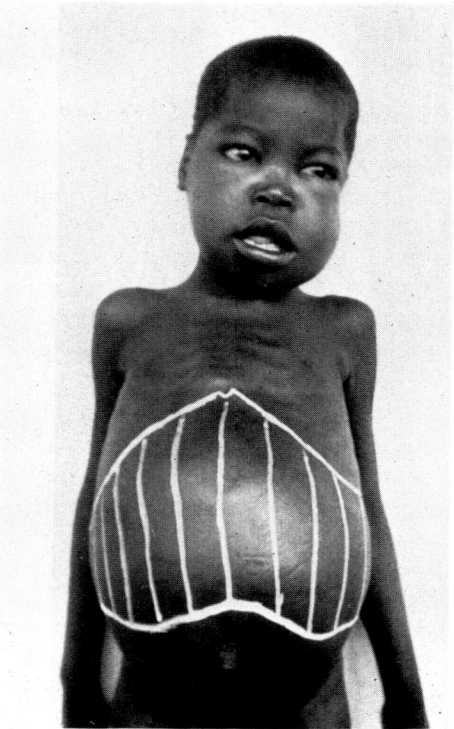

Fig. 5.5. Burkitt's lymphoma of abdomen and left mandible in a 7-year-old boy (K.C.C. 896). The kidneys, suprarenals, retroperitoneal tissues, root of the mesentery and liver were involved by one large tumour mass,

syndrome and O'Connor (1961) and Wright (1970) have recorded sites of tumour involvement in post-mortem series.

An estimation of the extent of the disease is important as this may relate to the immunological status of the patient and the form and response to treatment. This necessitates a careful clinical examination, radiological examination of any suspected tumour areas and should always include chest, kidneys, ureters and bladder. Tumour cells may be evident in the C.S.F., bone marrow and peripheral blood. The entire clinical status of the patient must be reviewed at regular intervals as this may alter even while the patient is under treatment. A staging classification is used to denote the extent of tumour spread in the body (Clifford, 1970a).

Stage I   Disease limited to one anatomical area.

Stage II (a) Disease limited to two contiguous areas.
           (b) Disease occurring in two or more non-adjacent areas, but on the same side of the diaphragm.

Stage III (a) Disease involving structures on both sides of the diaphragm.
           (b) Tumour cell involvement of the bone marrow or in the blood stream.

Stage IV Disease involving the central nervous system.

The majority of patients are in Stage III (a) or (b) when first seen. Involvement of the pleura, lung parenchyma, mediastinum or heart is not common and will be obvious on routine chest radiographs (Figs. 6 and 7). Tomography is helpful in assessing the extent and site of any cardiac involvement (Fig. 8). Pleural and pericardial effusions may be massive (Fig. 9), and the entire endothelial linings of these cavities may be infiltrated by tumour cells which can be recovered from the effusions.

The kidneys are involved in over 90% of patients with Stage III Burkitt's lymphoma, usually by multiple small tumours in the cortex and medulla of both kidneys. These multiple small tumours may grow and coalesce and eventually destroy the renal parenchyma. Intravenous pyelography (I.V.P.) may indicate enlargement or irregularity of the renal outline of one or both kidneys with serration and distortion of the renal calyces and pelvis (Figs. 10, 11, 12 and 13). Most patients with Burkitt's lymphoma have high plasma levels of membrane reactive antibodies and these initially small intra-renal tumours may represent antibody/antigen emboli formed with circulating tumour cells which have been trapped in the renal arterioles. Tumour cells can be identified in properly prepared 'buffy coat' preparations from peripheral blood in about 10% of patients (C. Hershko, *pers. comm.* 1970).

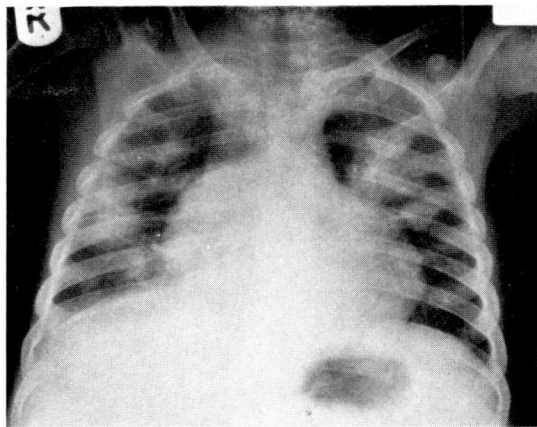

FIG. 5.6. Burkitt's lymphoma of the heart and lungs (K.C.C. 1140, vide Figs. 12, 20, 21). The heart shadow is enlarged and globular with an irregular left margin. Tumour opacities are evident in the left upper and right middle lobes of the lungs.

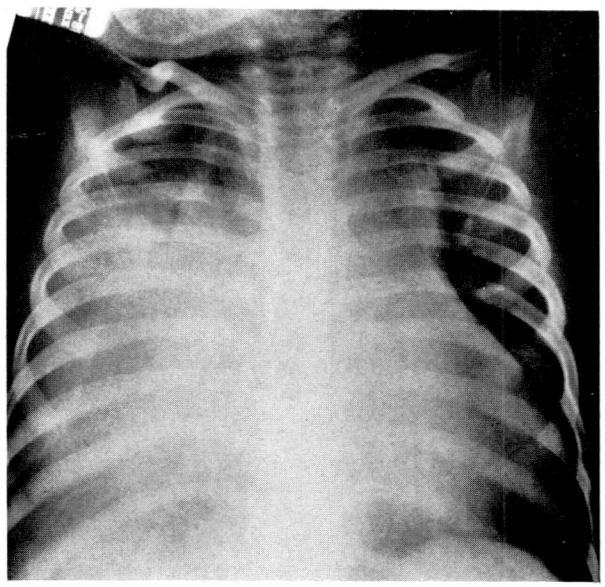

FIG. 5.7. Burkitt's lymphoma of the heart with a large pericardial effusion and collapse of the right middle lobe of the lung (K.C.C. 812, vide Figs. 10, 26, 27). The child was treated 3 years previously and had been discharged from hospital in total tumour regression.

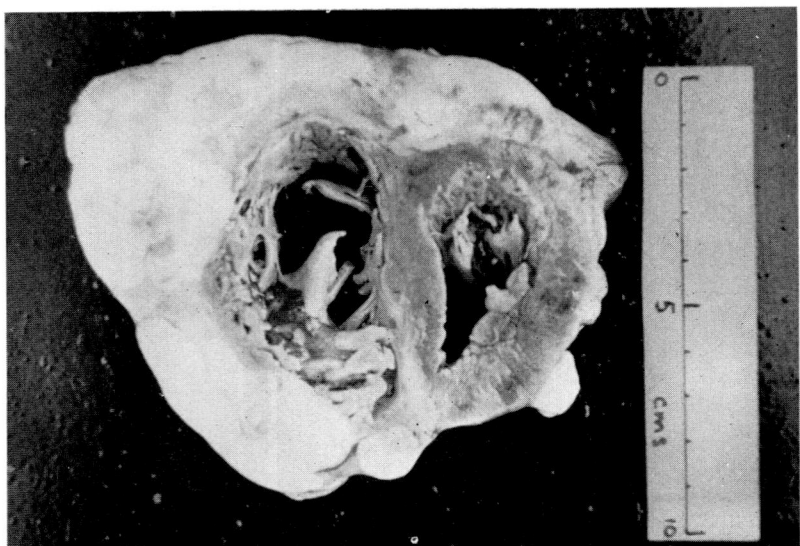

FIG. 5.8. Burkitt tumour of the heart and pericardium which caused the death of a 10-year-old girl (K.C.C. 674). Tumour formation is maximal over the epicardium of the right ventricle. The myocardium was infiltrated and small subendocardial tumours were noted at the bases of the trabeculae carneae, particularly in the right ventricle.

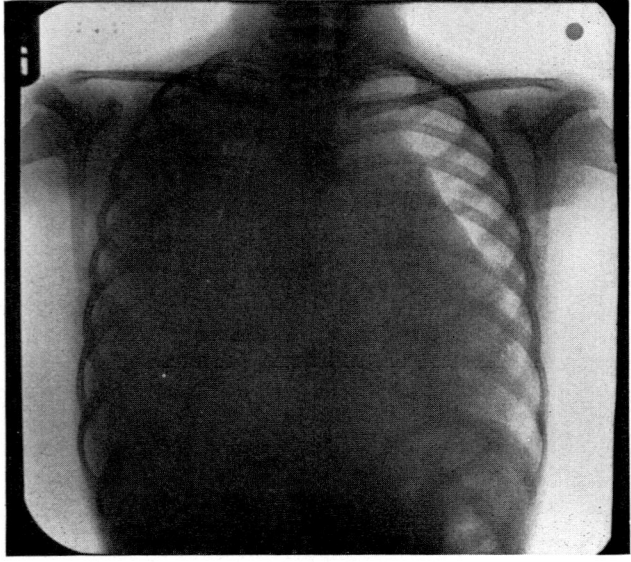

FIG. 5.9. Burkitt's lymphoma of the pleura in a 6-year-old girl (K.C.C. 904). The pleural effusion (550 cc on a single aspiration) contained many Burkitt lymphoma cells. Both ovaries and kidneys were also involved (stage IIIa). Treatment with Orthomerphalan 1·4 mg/Kg $\times$ 6 over $4\frac{1}{2}$ months produced total tumour regression and the girl is now classified as a long-term survivor to day 860.

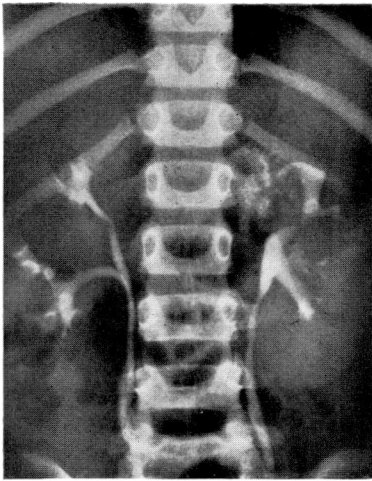

FIG. 5.10. Bilateral renal involvement in a Burkitt's lymphoma. The floccular calcification in the left upper pole represents tumour treated 3 years previously (K.C.C. 812, vide Figs. 7, 26, 27). Calyceal deformity is marked in the left kidney and tumour has separated the right upper and middle calyces.

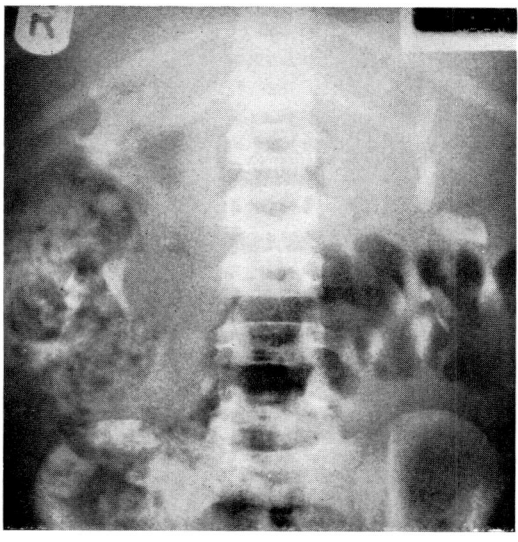

FIG. 5.11. Bilateral renal involvement in Burkitt's lymphoma in an 8-year-old boy (K.C.C. 1170). The I.V.P. shows extension and stretching of both calyceal systems.

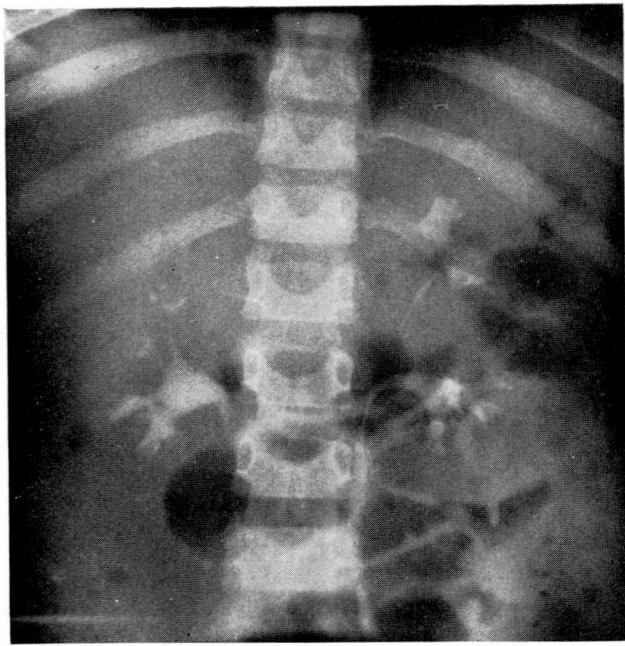

Fig. 5.12. Involvement of the left kidney by Burkitt's lymphoma (K.C.C. 1140, vide Figs. 6, 20, 21). The left renal pelvis is stretched and tumour has separated the calyces.

Ureteric displacement and failure to visualize the outline of the psoas muscle may be the only indication of a retroperitoneal mass (Fig. 14). Tumours of this area, involving the pancreas and surrounding areolar tissue are difficult to detect and define clinically until they have reached a large size. Distortions of the bladder outline may indicate ovarian involvement which otherwise might have escaped notice (Whittaker, 1970).

The evaluation of the effect of treatment on renal tumours is very difficult as residual scarring and fibrosis even in the absence of tumour causes calyceal deformities. Renal needle biopsy is of great value in these cases.

The central nervous system (C.N.S.) is involved in over 60% of patients at some time during the course of the disease, not infrequently after treatment of the systemic lesions has started (Clifford et al., 1967; Clifford, 1970a). Tumour cells may reach the C.N.S. through the blood stream or less frequently by direct extension, for instance following cranial erosion by a large orbito-ethmoidal tumour. Spread from the blood stream may occur through the choroid plexuses, which often

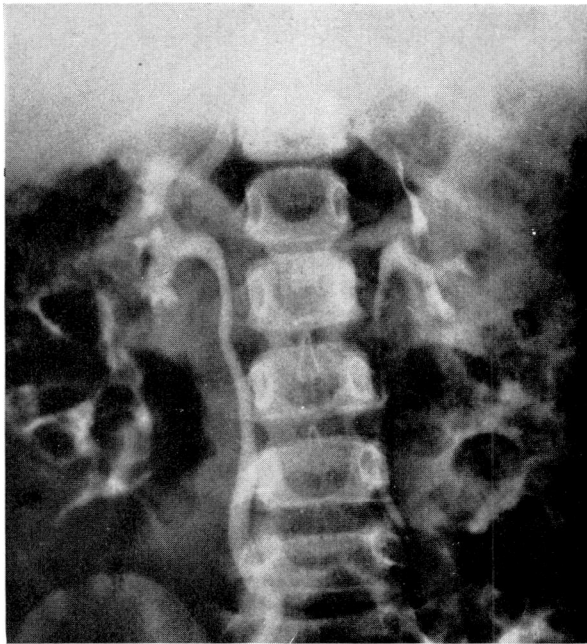

FIG. 5.13. Involvement of the left kidney by Burkitt's lymphoma (K.C.C. 1106, vide Figs. 18, 19). The left upper and mid calyces are in a straight line having been displaced medially by a tumour in the cortex of the upper pole of the kidney. The left ureter may be displaced medially.

show extensive tumour cell infiltration. Retrograde tumour spread may occur along cranial or peripheral nerves traversing large tumours, probably along the peri-neural arterioles and Virchow-Robin spaces. Extension to the spinal theca and cord may follow involvement of the anterior external and internal venous plexuses by retroperitoneal tumour. Wright (1970) has suggested that many cases of paraplegia are due to ischaemia following compression of the anterior spinal and radicular arteries by extradural tumours. Myelography will determine whether the lesion is intra- or extramedullary (Figs. 15 and 16).

This extension of the disease may give rise to a diffuse lymphomatous leptomeningitis, similar to that seen in acute lymphoblastic leukaemia; inflammatory and tumour cells can be identified in the C.N.S. Tumours may develop about the cavernous sinus, the trigeminal ganglion or form plaques on the dura, most frequently on the floor of the mid-cranial fossa. Tumour nodules may grow on the surface of the brain, usually adjacent to the large venous sinuses. Individual cranial nerves may be affected, the 3rd, 4th and 6th being the most frequently involved,

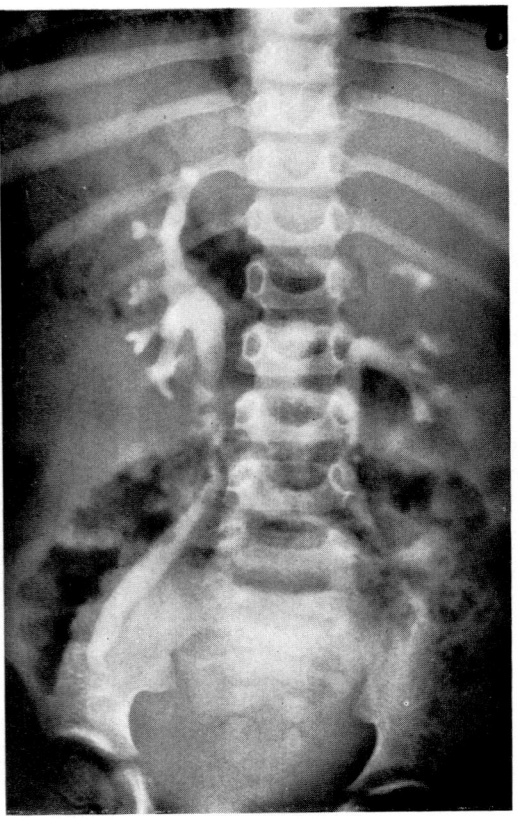

Fɪɢ. 5.14. Involvement of both kidneys by Burkitt's lymphoma in a 4-year-old boy (K.C.C. 1170). The calyceal pattern of both kidneys is enlarged, the left more than the right. The left lower ureter is displaced by retroperitoneal tumour. The bladder is enlarged and the boy could not completely empty the bladder but was not incontinent.

and these lesions may be bilateral. A lymphomatous ependymitis may obstruct the aqueduct leading to an internal hydrocephalus, and this may also occur associated with tumorous infiltration of the floor of the 4th ventricle. Intracerebral tumours do occur but are rare.

Clinically intracranial involvement may present as a focal lesion, i.e. a 3rd, 4th or 6th cranial nerve lesion, or paresis of an arm, or with general signs usually initially manifest by an alteration in behaviour associated with signs of increased intracranial pressure. The lumbar area is that part of the cord most frequently involved, either by intra- or extra-medullary tumours, but multiple small tumours may develop on the cauda equina. Spinal lesions are usually associated with retroperitoneal or retropleural tumours.

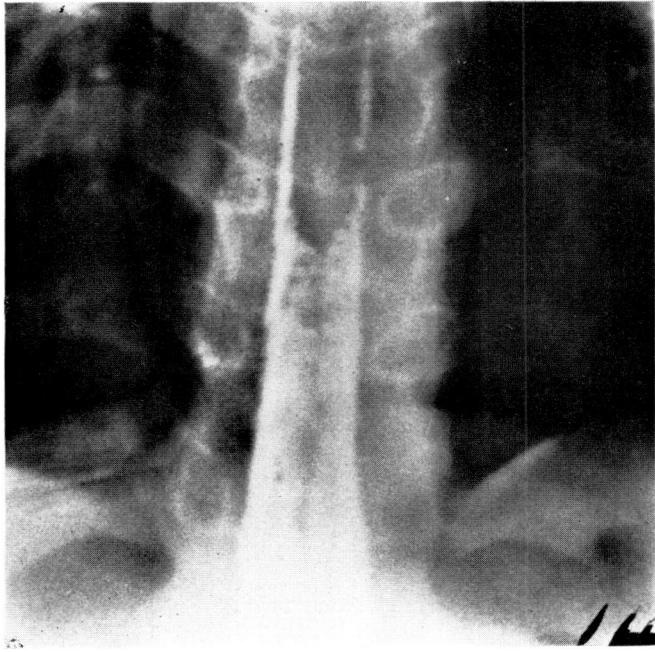

Fig. 5.15. Extramedullary Burkitt's lymphoma in a 10-year-old boy (K.C.C. 1003). At the site of the block, at the L2 L3 level, the myodil column is convex upwards with a filling defect on the left at the level of L2. The boy (disease stage IIIa and b, IV) was treated with chemotherapy and radiotherapy. Post mortem examination confirmed an extramedullary tumour with infiltration of L4, L5 vertebral bodies.

THE ORIGIN OF MULTIPLE BURKITT TUMOURS

The cytogenetic studies of Jacobs *et al.* (1963) and Stewart *et al.* (1965) on 14 patients with Burkitt's lymphoma favoured the hypothesis that this multifocal lymphoma is virally induced. Four of the tumours studied showed a normal karyotype but in all the others numeric or structural variations in the diploid range were noted. One of the No. 2 chromosomes served as a marker chromosome in six of the tumours and in five of these the other No. 2 chromosome was missing. In Burkitt lymphoma cell lines another marker chromosome, one of the small c group, probably a No. 10 has been noted (Rabson *et al.*, 1966, 1970; Miles and O'Neill, 1967; Bishun and Sutton, 1967; Kohn *et al.*, 1967; Toshima *et al.*, 1967; and Tomkins, 1968). These studies suggest that a specific causal virus commonly produces similar chromosome changes in lymphoid cells of different human hosts and that these changes may be associated with malignant transformation. As Jacobs *et al.* (1963) found normal karyotypes in the tumour cells of 4 of the 13 patients

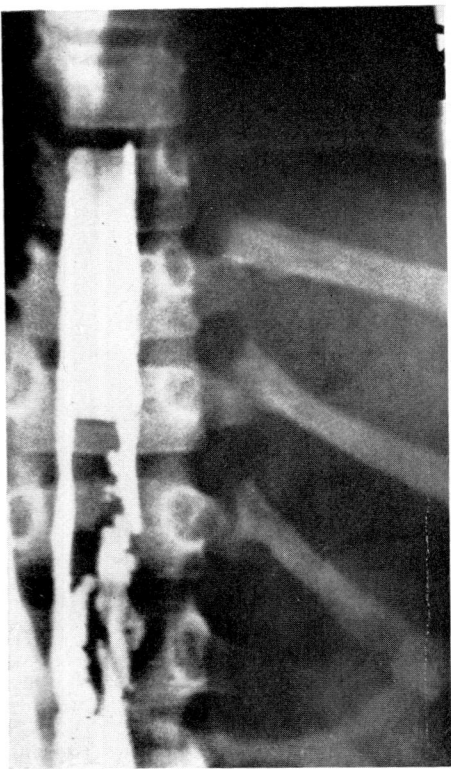

FIG. 5.16. Myelogram in a 7-year-old Burkitt lymphoma patient (K.C.C. 1151, stage IIb, IV). The obstruction at disc space T8-9 indicates that the paresis of both legs was due to an intramedullary tumour.

they studied, visible chromosomal abnormalities are not a *sine qua non* for the development of Burkitt's lymphoma.

Gripenberg *et al.* (1969) did serial cytogenetic studies on a Burkitt lymphoma patient with bilateral maxillary tumours and 'metastases' to the submaxillary and neck glands. The chromosomal stem lines were different on the left and right sides. Both were diploid, the left side representing the normal karyotype, but the right exhibited a number of marker chromosomes. Similar differences were noted in the submaxillary and neck gland tumours. Though the results of cytogenetic studies support the theory of a viral factor in the development of Burkitt's lymphoma, these results do not provide proof relating to a particular virus, nor to the rate and manner of malignant transformation following infection.

The fact that the majority of patients with Burkitt's lymphoma present with multiple tumours has led to speculation as to whether the disease process gives rise to multiple independent tumours or whether these represent a primary tumour and its metastases. In a study designed to try and determine whether Burkitt's lymphoma has a single or multiple cell origin, Fialkow *et al.* (1970) have used a technique which depends on the fact that in females, inactivation of one of the two X chromosomes in each somatic cell occurs early in embryogenesis and all descendants from any one cell have the same active X chromosome. The genes for the A and B types glucose-6-phosphate dehydrogenase (G-6-PD) are X linked and the isoenzymes are electrophoretically distinguishable. Cultures of normal skin fibroblasts from heterozygous females contain both A and B type enzymes but any one cell from these females will give rise to a clone containing only one type of enzyme. Fialkow *et al.* (1970) have reported such a study on 7 female Burkitt lymphoma patients with 12 tumours, who were identified as heterozygous at the G-6-PD locus by identifying both isoenzymes in normal tissue. Only a single enzyme type was found in each of the 12 tumours examined. This is highly suggestive that these multiple tumours had a monoclonal origin, but there are alternative explanations. The original oncogenic agent or process may have involved many cells but the tumours may have developed from a cell clone (either type A or B) which had very marked and strong proliferative advantages so that it outgrew all others. Or lymphocytes of either phenotype A or B may have been for some reason more susceptible to malignant transformation, thus the multiple tumours would represent clones derived from many cells but all of the same phenotype. It would be interesting to see if in the case of patients classified as long-term survivors (Clifford *et al.*, 1967) recurrent tumours were of the same phenotype as the initial tumour. If not, it will be possible to speak of a fresh induction and not a recurrence. Other isoenzyme genetic markers such as the phosphoglucomitase and adenosinedeaminase phenotypes are now used to classify normal and tumour cells (P. Fialkow, *pers. comm.* 1970).

The epidemiological evidence to date suggests that Burkitt's lymphoma arises as a rare manifestation of infection with EB virus. In most African children the virus gives rise to no signs or symptoms and in a few to African Glandular Fever (Diehl *et al.*, 1969). If it is accepted that malignant transformation is a rare event, this may only involve one cell or one cell type, giving rise to a clone or clones from which multiple tumours develop (The Lancet, 1970).

IMMUNOLOGICAL ASPECTS

Serological reactivity. Three different EBV-determined antigen systems have been identified to date using immunofluorescence and absorption techniques:

(a) *Early antigen* (*EA*). This is a soluble intracellular antigen which appears soon after infection of EBV-negative lymphoblastoid cell lines with EBV concentrates (Henle *et al.*, 1970), possibly representing a group of antigens (Henle *et al.*, 1971).

(b) *A membrane antigen complex* (*MA*) found on the outer surface of viable cells in carrier culture (Nadkarni *et al.*, 1969). MA is considered to represent viral envelope components built into the cell membrane (Klein *et al.*, 1969; Pearson *et al.*, 1970; Gunvén *et al.*, 1970; Klein *et al.*, 1970, 1971).

(c) *Viral capsid antigen* (*VCA*) demonstrated in cells containing viral particles (Henle and Henle, 1966; Henle *et al.*, 1969, 1970, 1971).

These antigens, though all EBV-determined, are distinct and are associated with different antibody specificities (Pearson *et al.*, 1969, 1970; Svedmyr *et al.*, 1970). Using a two-colour immunofluorescence technique, Klein *et al.* (1971) have demonstrated that the EBV membrane antigen complexes are distinct from isoantigenic HL-A receptors. Only lines with more than 1% of VCA positive cells show a significant number of MA positive cells which as a general rule are ten times more frequent. EA positive cells can be VCA positive or negative. EA positive, VCA negative cells may be MA positive or negative, but VCA positive cells are always MA positive. The appearance of MA and EA after infection with EBV is independent of viral DNA synthesis, so both are considered as 'early' viral products. VCA represents a 'late' viral product requiring viral DNA and viral capsid protein synthesis (Henle *et al.*, 1969, 1970, 1971; Klein *et al.*, 1970, 1971).

Antibody fractions directed against these antigen complexes are distinct and the strength of each in sera specimens can be estimated using immunofluorescence and absorption techniques. Comparisons of sera from Burkitt's lymphoma patients and various African controls has shown significantly higher anti-MA and VCA titres in the sera of the former. MA and VCA antibody levels were concordant in over 80% of the Burkitt lymphoma patients and in many the discrepancies could be related to the clinical state of the patient. The majority of Burkitt lymphoma patients had high titres of anti-MA and anti-VCA antibodies. The highest anti-VCA titres were found in patients with large tumours prior to treatment, and lower values in those classified as being in long-term remission. This may relate to the presence and absence of the specific antigenic stimulus. Low anti-VCA titres have also been noted in patients with advanced disease, moribund on admission to hospital, and these may have been incapable of responding to antigenic stimulus. Patients with large or recurrent tumours had relatively low anti-MA titres; all of these had high anti-VCA titres. In the majority of patients anti-MA titres rose as tumour bulk was reduced by treatment and it is possible that low anti-MA titres were due to absorption of antibody by a large mass of tumour cells (Henle *et al.* 1969, 1970; Klein *et al.*, 1970). Generally in patients who respond well to chemotherapy anti-MA titres rise as tumour is destroyed. Einhorn *et al.* (1970) have also shown that local irradiation of a Burkitt tumour is followed 6–9 weeks later by a rise in anti-MA titres. This may be due to a reaction following antigen release from the irradiated tumour or alternatively to a reduction in anti-MA absorption. In those patients who go into long-term regression anti-MA titres fall slowly after approximately two years, but a sudden decrease may indicate tumour recurrence (Klein *et al.*, 1969b).

General and cellular immunological reactivity. The cellular immunological reactivity of treated and untreated patients with Burkitt's lymphoma has been investigated by Stjernswärd by *in vivo* and *in vitro* tests. The results related to the clinical stage and tumour burden of the patients and to the response to therapy.

Delayed hypersensitivity. Patients with large Burkitt tumours were found to have a decreased ability to produce a delayed hypersensitivity reaction to 1, 2-dinitrochlorobenzene (D.N.C.B.). Children in maintained remission for more than 6 months showed the same reactivity level as age matched normal controls. An age dependent variation in the delayed hypersensitivity to D.N.C.B. was evident in the control group (Stjernswärd *et al.*, 1968, 1970). Similar results were obtained by Fass *et al.* (1970a) using an autologous tumour extract to test the capacity of Burkitt lymphoma patients before and after treatment to exhibit a delayed hypersensitivity reaction. Negative results were obtained in patients with multiple tumours and in those who responded poorly to subsequent chemotherapy. Positive reactions occurred in those with localized disease and in the patients who maintained tumour regression following treatment.

Mixed lymphocyte—Target cell interaction test (MLTI test). This test depends on the tumour cells containing recognizably foreign antigens. When mixed with autochthonous lymphocytes, the tumour antigens may stimulate the lymphocytes to undergo transformation to pyroninophilic blast cells, synthesize nucleic acid and divide. DNA synthesis in the target tumour cells was inhibited by Mitomycin C, and this was measured in the lymphocytes by adding radioactive tritiated thymidine to the culture. Mitomycin C treated bone marrow target cells were used in parallel control tests. The ability of the patient's lymphocytes to be stimulated was checked by recording the effect of phytohaemagglutinin on DNA synthesis *in vitro*. It was found in this test that only about 19% of patients showed a significant cellular reaction against the tumour cells. Stjernswärd noted that this figure approximates to the percentage of patients in most series who maintain prolonged remission of the disease after chemotherapy. The non-reactivity of the remainder was ascribed as being due to a specific paralysis or tolerance possibly associated with prolonged exposure to a weak antigenic stimulus. Alternatively the non-reactivity of lymphocytes may have been due to other factors associated with the target cells as it was noted that in autochthonous situations tumour cells from previously established tissue culture lines provoked a significantly higher reaction than fresh biopsy cells. The latter may not have functioned optimally as target cells because of *in vitro* antibody coating. The administration of an irradiated autochthonous tumour vaccine altered this non-reactive state in 16 patients tested. Lymphocytes from glands draining the injection area reacted strongly in the M.L.T.I. test and this change may have been due to a minor change in the antigenic structure of the injected tumour cells following irradiation (Stjernswärd *et al.*, 1968, 1970; Stjernswärd and Clifford, 1970). The results of these tests, corresponding closely with the effects of chemotherapy, are highly significant in determining modes of treatment.

TREATMENT

Radiotherapy. A cobalt 60 unit provided by Sweden and operated by personnel from the Radiumhemmet, Stockholm, has been functioning at the Kenyatta National Hospital, Nairobi, since the beginning of 1969. Practically all Burkitt's lymphoma patients admitted during this period were in disease Stage III and IV and so were not ideally suited for treatment with local radiotherapy. A small number of tumours, such as growths of the jaw, brain, spine, abdomen and limbs, have however been selected for this treatment either before or after chemotherapy. Initially the same dose and fractionation as is usual in treating malignant lymphomas was used to treat separate areas. Though immediate tumour regression was obvious in a few cases, in some tumour regrowth occurred before the next daily treatment.

This tumour has not proved to be as sensitive to conventional radiotherapy as initially hoped. By changing the time/dose relationship (by thrice daily superfractionation) better results have been achieved but data on optimal doses and modes of treatment for such areas as the brain and abdomen are not yet available (Norin *et al.*, 1971). The finding by Einhorn *et al.* (1970) that anti-MA antibody titres rise following local radiotherapy may be of significance in the management of patients in disease Stages I and II (J. Einhorn, A. de Schryver, B. Johannson and T. Norin, *pers. comm.* 1969, 1970).

Chemotherapy. Studies on the treatment of Burkitt's lymphoma conducted over the past ten years have indicated that the kinetics of the Burkitt tumour cell, host responses, and the probably related disease stage, as well as the drug used and the manner of administration, are all closely related to the response to treatment.

Studies in freshly biopsied Burkitt tumour cells by Cooper *et al.* (1966, 1968) using cytochemical and autoradiographic methods to record DNA content and synthesis confirmed the high proliferative activity of the cell population without any marked aneuploidy or arrest of the cells in the S period. A potential doubling time of less than 24 hours was found in 41 % of the biopsies and in 89 % this was less than two days. The actual doubling time of a Burkitt tumour is very much slower because, though the cell proliferation rate is high, so is the cell death rate with a mean generation time of 24–36 hours. This is highly pertinent to treatment as different drugs affect different phases of the cell cycle. A Burkitt tumour cell having a mean generation time of 24 hours is illustrated in Fig. 17. The various types of drugs, alkylating

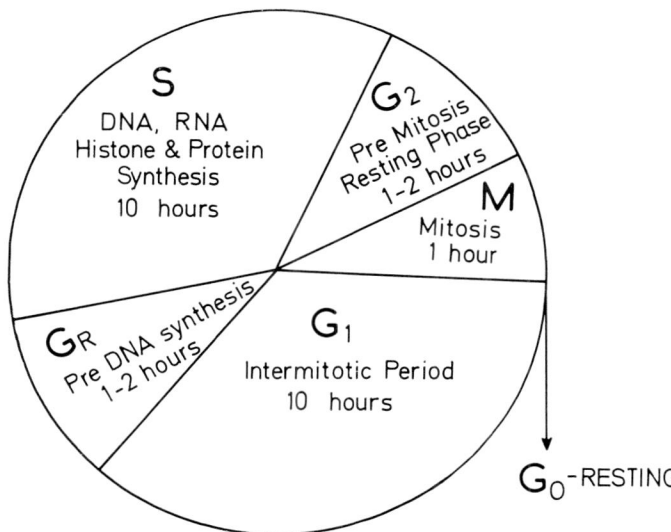

FIG. 5.17. Diagram of a Burkitt lymphoma cell with a 24-hour life cycle.

agents, antimetabolites, antibiotics and steroids selectively effect different parts of this cycle (Connors, 1969a, b; Mueller, 1969; Schabel, 1969). It is considered that normally few if any Burkitt tumour cells enter the G_0 phase. Such 'resting' cells, not synthesizing DNA, are extremely resistant to chemotherapy. The alkylating agents kill tumour cells (and sensitive normal cells) by cross-linking guanine bases of fully formed adjacent DNA strands during the interphase so that cell mitosis is inhibited (Brookes 1964; Connors 1969a) and for tumour cells with a short life span this is equivalent to death.

Bruce (1967) classified chemotherapeutic drugs into three types related, not to chemical composition, but to their effects on the cell cycle. The first type such as HN_2 are *non-specific* and kill normal and malignant cells in all phases of the cell cycle including those at rest. These drugs have a low therapeutic index. The second class are *phase specific* and kill only during a particular phase of the cell cycle. Examples of phase specific drugs are Methotrexate, Cytosine Arabinoside and Vincaleukoblastine. These act during the S phase. The antifolics, antipurines and antimetabolites, by interrupting at some point the formation of nucleotides and DNA synthesis or by incorporation, may lead to the formation of abnormal nucleic acid. It is thought that Vincaleukoblastine effects the formation of protein and enzymes by blocking the synthesis of transfer RNA. The third group are *cycle specific* drugs such as cyclophosphamide, 5-Fluorouracil, BCNU (Bischloroethyl nitrosourea) and Actinomycin-D which kill cells in cycle more effectively than those at rest. The sensitivity of a tumour to drugs of this type depend on the fraction of proliferating cells. Most of these drugs exert their effects during the G_R and S phases. Mitomycin C reacts directly with DNA and prevents its continued synthesis due to the presence of an aziridine group in the Mitomycin C molecular structure (Webb *et al.* 1962). Actinomycin-D interferes with the formation of messenger RNA and so with protein, enzyme, and DNA and RNA synthesis. The mode of action of the steroids is obscure but they may have an effect on protein and RNA synthesis (Connors, 1969a). Theoretically there should be advantages in treating tumours in which the different phases of all cells were synchronized. All cells might be halted at G_R by a reversible inhibitor of DNA synthesis so that the entire tumour entered the S phase at the same time (Mueller, 1969).

The initial attempts to treat Burkitt's lymphoma with chemotherapy were directed to determining the most effective agents and methods of administration. Clifford (1970a) has reviewed the effectiveness of 17 drugs which have been used to date in the treatment of this disease. The alkylating agents Merophan (C.B. 1729, Orthomerphalan), Melphalan (Alkeran, phenylalanine mustard) and Cyclophosphamide (Cytoxan, Endoxan) and the anti-metabolites, Methotrexate (Amethopterin) and Cytosine Arabinoside are the most effective drugs used to date. Experience has shown that in most instances a single large dose of a drug given intravenously is more effective than the same or a larger total dose divided over a number of days (Clifford *et al.*, 1967; Clifford, 1966, 1970a). Initially the significance of disease staging, and in particular the importance of assessing the extent of retroperitoneal and intrarenal disease was not fully appreciated. Intracranial involvement (Stage IV) occurs in over 60% of patients presenting with systemic disease Stage IIIa or b. This may be present on admission or shortly afterwards, but may be evident for the first time two years after the initial presentation, as occurred in a child classified as a long term survivor.

Two drug schedules are at present in use at the Kenyatta National Hospital, Nairobi.

CYTOSINE ARABINOSIDE AND CYTOXAN

The pyramidine neucleoside analogue, Cytosine Arabinoside, is given in doses of 200 mg/m² body surface, as a 12 hour intravenous infusion daily for 4 days. Cytoxan 10 mg/Kg is given intravenously on the completion of each daily infusion. Skipper (1967) has shown that Cytosine Arabinoside is selectively cytotoxic to cells in the DNA synthetic phase or S period of the cell cycle; the drug is non-toxic to non-dividing cells. Most of the anti-DNA effect of Cytoxan occurs in

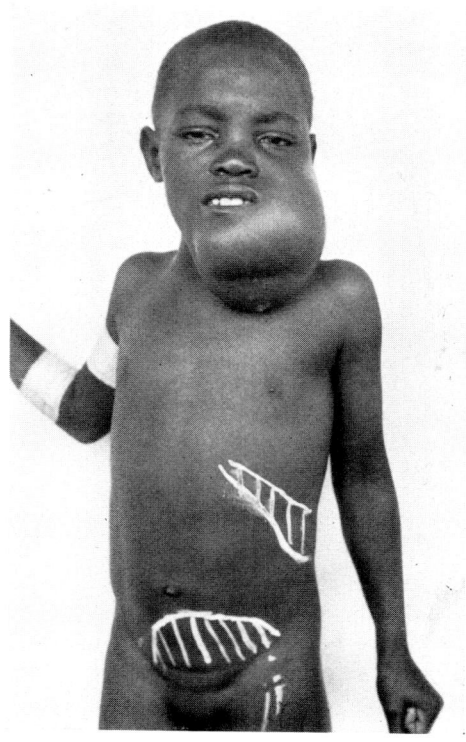

FIG. 5.18. Burkitt's lymphoma in a 7-year-old girl (K.C.C. 1106). The disease involved the left mandible, both ovaries, left kidney (Fig. 13), and bone marrow. The larger ovarian tumour (left) was removed prior to chemotherapy. Three weeks later tumour cells were identified in the C.S.F. (disease stage IIIa and b, IV).

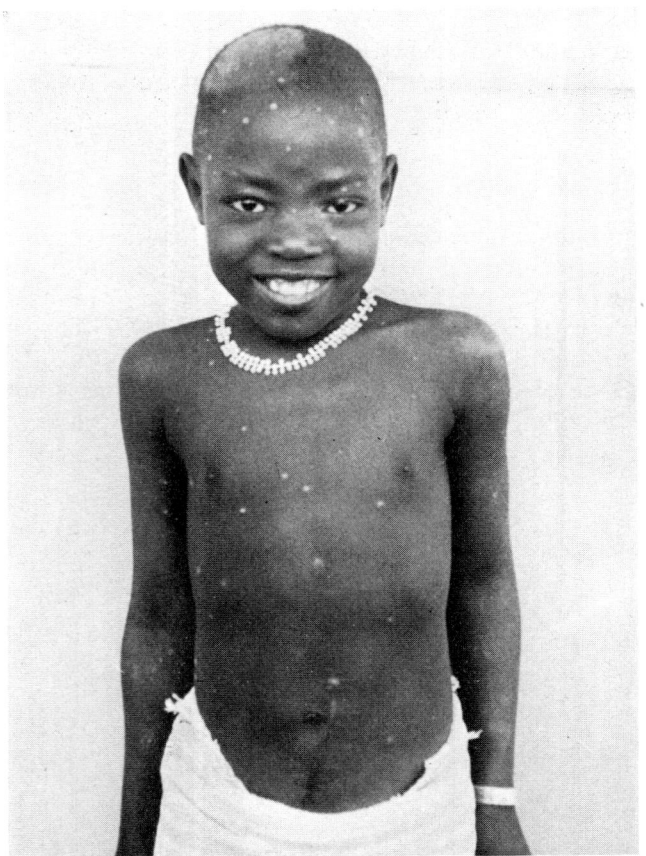

FIG. 5.19. Patient shown in Fig. 18 9 months later. Over a 2-month period she received Merophan 0·8 mg/Kg × 3 concurrently with weekly Methotrexate 10 mg intrathecally. This produced complete regression of the jaw tumour. Subsequently a tumour developed in the left submandibular area and repeat I.V.P. suggested persistent tumour in the left kidney. Following four courses of Cytosine Arabinoside and Cytoxan she is now classified as being in total tumour regression. Her spotted appearance follows an attack of chickenpox.

the first few hours after injection but the drug kills cells in most parts of the cycle. By repeating both drugs each day for 4 days it is hoped that the metabolic inhibitor will have an opportunity of effecting all or most of the tumour cells during an S period, and that tumour cells not affected by Cytosine Arabinoside will be damaged or killed by the alkylating agent (D. Galton, *pers. comm.* 1970). The course is repeated after a fortnight's interval, and most patients are given three or four courses.

   With this therapy haematological toxicity has been minimal. The results of treatment in patients in all disease stages has been very

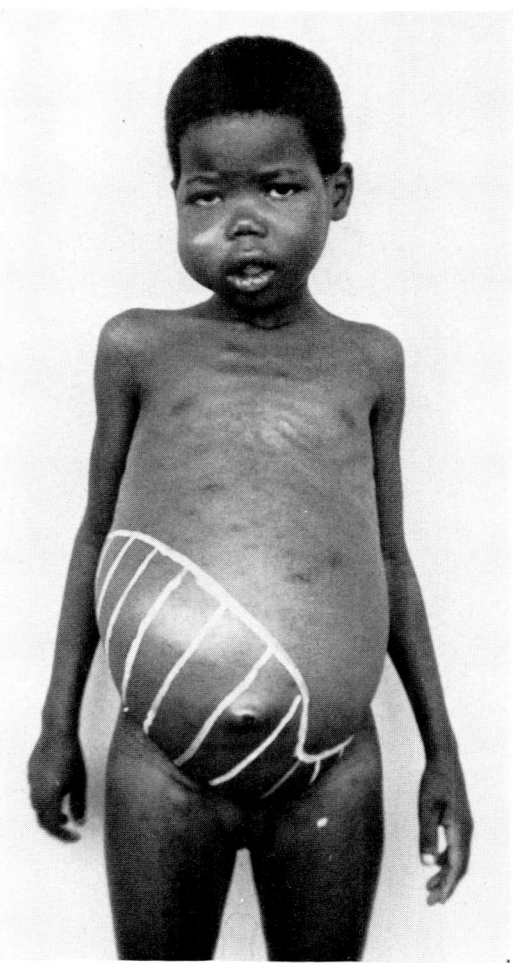

FIG. 5.20. An 8-year-old girl (K.C.C. 1140) with Burkitt's lymphoma of right maxilla, heart, lungs (Fig. 6) and left kidney (Fig. 12). The child had paresis of both legs and incontinence of urine but not of faeces (disease stage IIIa, IV). At laparotomy it was found impossible to remove the larger ovarian tumour (right) which had spread to involve the intestines. Tumour cells were found in the C.S.F.

encouraging and over 60% of patients in Stage III have attained total tumour regression (Figs. 18, 19, 20, 21).

Howard *et al.* (1966) suggested that an appreciable concentration of Cytosine Arabinoside occurred in the C.S.F. after intravenous administration. It may be significant that no patient on this treatment has developed frank C.N.S. involvement through tumour cells have been found in isolated instances in the early weekly C.S.F. examinations.

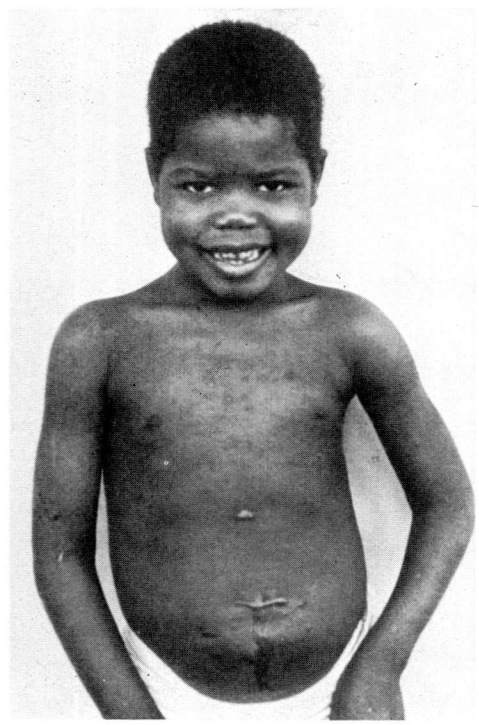

FIG. 5.21. Patient shown in Fig. 20 classified as being in total tumour regression following four courses of Cytosine Arabinoside and Cytoxan. She has full
bladder control and leg movements are normal. She received no specific
intrathecal therapy.

MEROPHAN AND VINCRISTINE SULPHATE

Merophan (C.B. 1729) is one of the most potent and useful alkylating
agents available for treating this lymphoma (Figs. 22, 23, 24, 25, 26, 27).
At present it is used in doses of 0·8 mg/Kg repeated at three weekly
intervals for as long as there is evidence of tumour or until a decision to
change therapy has been made. The nadir of haematological toxicity
occurs 5–7 days later and though the African child can withstand and
recover from relatively large doses of chemotherapeutic agents (Clifford
et al., 1963), this capacity is reduced by repeated chemotherapy. Consequently Vincristine Sulphate 2 mg/m² body surface is given 10 days
after each injection of Orthomerphalan. Burkitt (1966) has reported
good results following the use of Vincristine alone and a dose of 2 mg/m²
is not associated with haematological toxicity.

Zeigler et al. (1970) have reported the effects of single and multiple
doses of Cytoxan at 40 mg/Kg. The remission rates for patients in Stage

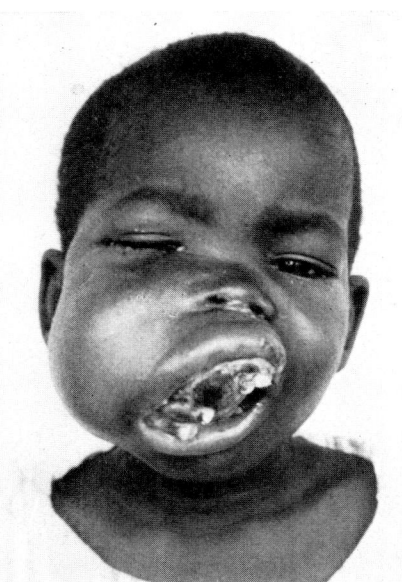

Fig. 5.22. A 4-year-old boy (K.C.C. 959) with Burkitt's lymphoma of right maxilla and both kidneys. Tumour cells were identified in the C.S.F. (disease stage IIIa, IV). The boy was treated with Merophan 0·8 mg/Kg × 6 and intrathecal Methotrexate 10 mg weekly × 10. This led to total tumour regression. He then received ten B.C.G. inoculations at 3-week intervals with a Heaf apparatus.

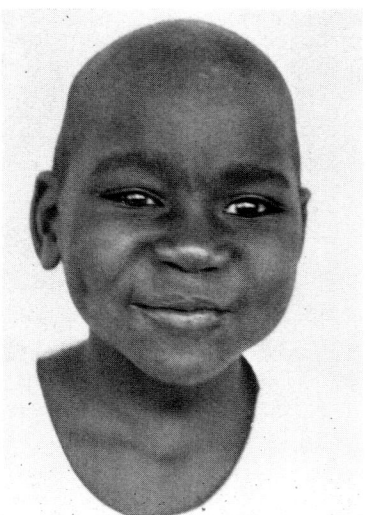

Fig. 5.23. Patient shown in Fig. 22 before discharge. The boy is now classified as a long-term survivor and has remained well without treatment for over 12 months.

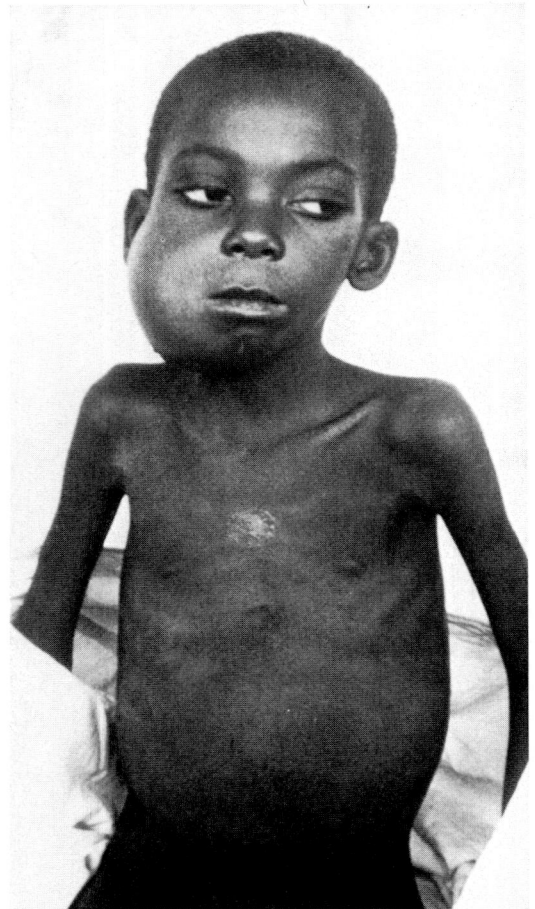

Fig. 5.24. A 7-year-old boy (K.C.C. 801) with Burkitt's lymphoma of the right
mandible, left kidney and para-pancreatic area (disease stage IIIa).

I and II given either one or six treatments with Cytoxan were similar,
but patients in Stage III and IV did better on multiple treatments.
(The staging classification used in their series—Morrow *et al.*, 1967—
differs from that described above.) Patients who relapsed were subsequently treated with cyclic chemotherapy consisting of Vincristine
Sulphate 1·4 mg/m² I.V. on Day 1; Methotrexate 15 mg/m² p.o. Day 1–4;
followed after a 10–14 day interval by Cytosine Arabinoside 250 mg/m²
as a 24 hour I.V. infusion for 3 days. This cycle was repeated twice.

Though over 90% of patients have total or near total regression of
the presenting tumour with initial chemotherapy, the long-term survival in the series reported to date (including all stages) is approximately

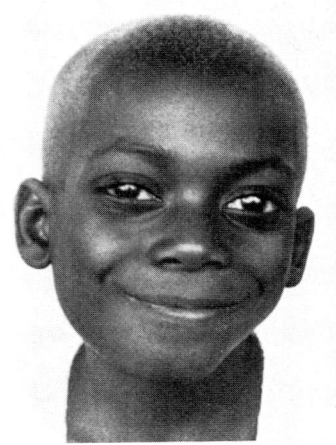

FIG. 5.25. Patient shown in Fig. 24 in total tumour regression following Merophan 1·4 mg/Kg × 3 over 6 weeks. The boy is now classified as a long-term survivor and has remained free of tumour without treatment for 3 years.

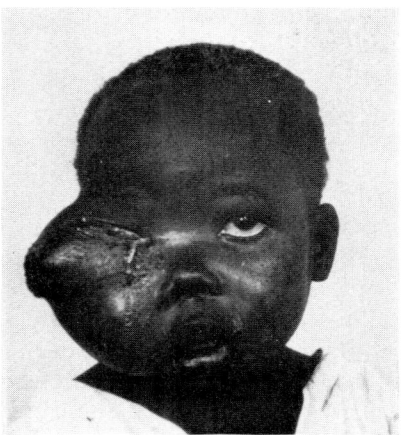

FIG. 5.26. A 4-year-old girl (K.C.C. 812) admitted with Burkitt's lymphoma of the left maxilla and orbit, retroperitoneal area and both kidneys. Treatment with I.T.C.V. × 3 followed by Merophan 1·3 mg/Kg was considered to have produced total tumour regression. Three years from the date of her first admission the child was readmitted in cardiac failure (Fig. 7) and with bilateral renal involvement (Fig. 10).

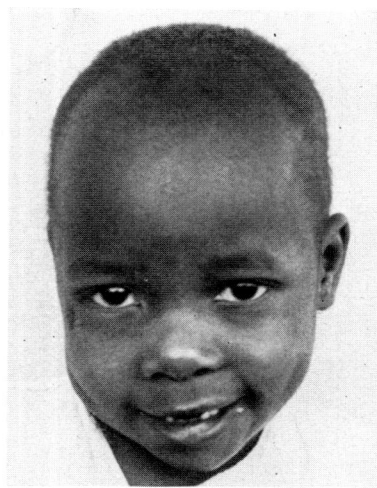

Fig. 5.27. Patient K.C.C. 812 following Merophan 0·8 mg/Kg given alternately with Vincristine Sulphate 2·0 mg/m² × 5. The recurrent tumours of the heart and kidneys now appear to have totally regressed.

20% (Burchenal, 1969). The incidence of patients going into long-term regression is highest in Stage I and falls progressively to Stage IV. This high initial total regression (?) rate with a low incidence of long-term survivors indicates that many patients are incorrectly classified as being free of tumour; the alternative hypothesis is to relate recurrences to new tumour induction. Tumour recurrences have occurred in 4 Burkitt lymphoma patients classified as long-term survivors, in 2 after four years (Clifford et al., 1968), in 1 after three years, and in 1 after two years. In 2 of these patients the recurrence presented as a regrowth of the original tumour. The exact establishment of total tumour regression is perhaps impossible, but the assessment must include in particular a reappraisal of the kidneys and retroperitoneal area. If the kidneys have been involved, as occurs in over 90% of the Kenya Stage III cases, it may be difficult to decide whether the calyceal deformities are solely due to scarring or residual tumour. In these instances renal needle biopsy is extremely useful. Once the patient has been classified as being in total tumour regression immunotherapy is started.

CENTRAL NERVOUS SYSTEM INVOLVEMENT

Once tumour cells have passed the blood/brain barrier, the situation regarding treatment and prognosis alters radically. With the possible exception of Cytosine Arabinoside (Howard *et al.*, 1966; Dixon and Adamson, 1965; Carey and Ellison, 1965) and BCNU[1–3Bis(2-chloroethyl-1-Nitrosourea] (Iriarte *et al.*, 1966; Schambel *et al.*, 1963) none of the drugs used to date in the treatment of systemic tumours attain adequate concentration in the C.S.F. to kill tumour cells. The only drugs at present available which can be administered intrathecally are Methotrexate and Cytosine Arabinoside.

In patients presenting without C.N.S. involvement attempts have been made at prophylaxis by routinely giving all patients on admission intrathecal injections of 10 mg of Methotrexate at weekly intervals for 10–12 weeks. This failed to affect the incidence ($>60\%$ of Stage III patients) of patients developing this complication.

Treatment of C.N.S. extension was initially attempted with Methotrexate 5 mg dissolved in 10 ml distilled water injected intrathecally at weekly intervals. This did reduce the number of tumour cells in the C.S.F. but all patients so treated died with central nervous system involvement. Subsequently the weekly intrathecal dose was increased to 10 mg which was also ineffective and later to 25·0 mg and eventually to 50·0 mg. Nausea and vomiting, headache and neck stiffness were usual after the larger doses but no fatalities occurred which could be ascribed solely to these larger doses. Treatment was repeated two or three times after the C.S.F. became free of tumour cells. Initially Citrovorum 6·0 mg was given i.m. twice daily to patients on intrathecal Methotrexate, but this has been discontinued. As the tumour has spread from areas supplied by the systemic circulation treatment of an intracranial extension is combined with systemic therapy. Methotrexate excreted from the C.S.F. can lead to haematological toxicity and this must be taken into account in deciding the dosage of drugs to be given systemically. The larger doses of Methotrexate, i.e. 50 mg, were only given to patients in whom further systemic treatment was considered unnecessary.

As it is known that the concentration of Methotrexate in the C.S.F. falls rapidly (Rall *et al.*, 1962) smaller doses, i.e. 25 mg, are now given twice weekly with the aim of maintaining adequate drug levels to affect the tumour cells in the C.N.S. during the S phase. Little is known of the kinetics of the Burkitt tumour cell in the C.N.S. and these cells may be biologically different from those in other parts of the body. At present, approximately 25% of patients who have had intracranial involvement are discharged from hospital as possible long-term survivors.

For patients with paraplegia, due either to extra- or intramedullary tumours which may occlude the spinal canal, the drug may be given into the cisterna magna or preferably through an Ommaya assembly into the lateral ventricle (Ommaya, 1963; Clifford, 1970a). This form of administration may have advantages as the drug is then at the source and flows with the C.S.F. Tumour involvement of the ependyma of the choroid plexus and the aqueduct is not uncommon, and a drug solution flowing against the C.S.F. current may never reach these areas. Some of these patients develop hydrocephalus due to tumour obstructing the aqueduct or 4th ventricle. In these cases the ventricles may be aspirated through the assembly and drugs injected into the cisterna magna as well as the ventricles.

Cytosine Arabinoside in doses of 50–100 mg/m² has also been used intrathecally and Zeigler *et al.* (1970) administer 25 mg/m² Methotrexate sequentially with 50 mg/m² Cytosine Arabinoside at 4-day intervals. Treatment is continued for 8 days after the C.S.F. is normal. These drugs cannot be given together as the disparity in the pH of the solutions precipitates the Methotrexate. The absence of tumour cells from the C.S.F. following intrathecal treatment does not however mean that the C.N.S. is free of disease, nor does the persistence of a cranial nerve lesion after prolonged treatment indicate the presence of intracranial tumour. Arteriography and ventriculography are usually of little help. Many aspects of the treatment of this complication are still largely empirical.

IMMUNOTHERAPY

The early studies of Klein *et al.* (1966) have indicated that patients with small and limited tumours and those that responded well to chemotherapy had high titres of a serum fraction(s) specifically directed against antigens on the Burkitt tumour cell. Patients with high titres responded well to chemotherapy and a number became long-term survivors. This suggested a synergism between the strength of the patient's reaction against the tumour and the response to chemotherapy. The report by Burkitt and Kyalwazi (1967) and Ngu *et al.* (1970) of several patients in whom the disease has undergone spontaneous regression also confirms the importance of host defence mechanisms.

Attempts to stimulate host defences against the antigenic tumour cells have been made using specific and non-specific methods (Clifford, 1966, 1967; Clifford *et al.*, 1967; Clifford, 1970a, b).

Specific immunization. An irradiated (9–15,000 r) autochthonous tumour vaccine (I.C.T.V.) prepared from fresh biopsy material was given to 25 Burkitt lymphoma patients weekly for four weeks prior to chemotherapy. Each injection contained 10^{6-7} irradiated tumour cells. Stjernswärd *et al.* (1968, 1970) have described the preparation of the vaccine and *in vitro* studies suggested that lymphocytes from the lymph glands draining the injection area had been specifically sensitized against the tumour cells. Figure 28 indicates that the percentage of Stage I and

LONG TERM SURVIVORS

Synergy of chemotherapy and irradiated tumour cell
vaccine in Burkitts Lymphoma

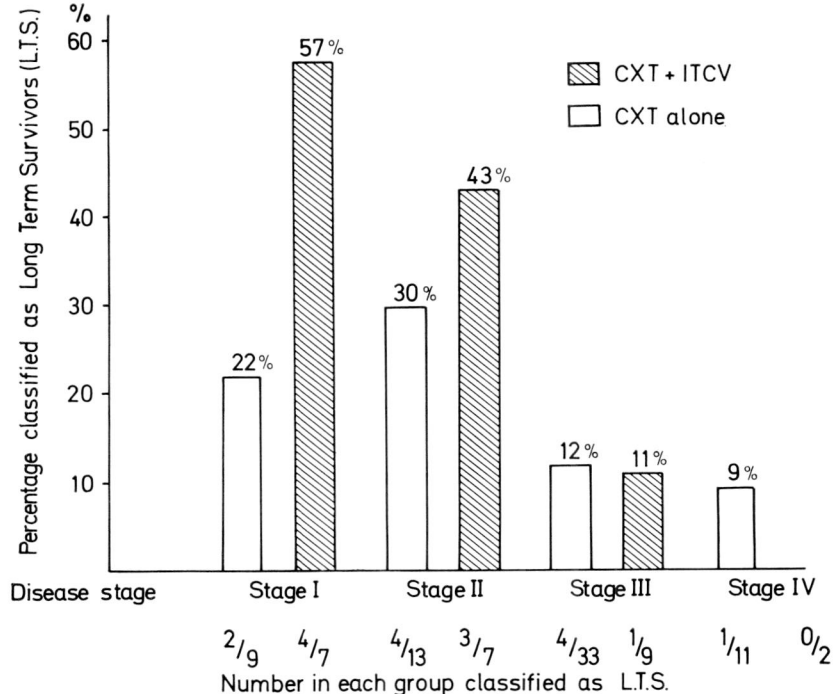

FIG. 5.28.

II patients in prolonged remission was significantly higher in the group that received I.C.T.V. as compared with a group seen in the same time period and who were treated with chemotherapy alone.

In Stages III and IV the differences are not so marked and the forms of chemotherapy used at present probably will give better results. The poor results in Stages III and IV may have been due to paralysis by a large mass of tumour absorbing antibody, though an alternative explanation may be that many of these tumours were protected by a state of self enhancement, the tumour cells being completely coated by IgG.

Non-specific immunisation. BCG, oleic acid, and pertussis-diphtheria-tetanus vaccine ('Trivas' triple antigen, Burroughs Wellcome Co., London) have been used in the hope that an established specific response would be strengthened. Active non-specific immunotherapy is now given to all patients in whom chemotherapy has induced total tumour regression. Glaxo Laboratories' freeze-dried percutaneous B.C.G. vaccine is used once every third week with a Heaf multiple puncture apparatus. It is estimated that on each occasion two firings of a 20 needle apparatus injects approximately one million viable organisms subcutaneously (Burland, 1969). Mathé et al. (1967, 1969) have also demonstrated the value of immunotherapy using irradiated allogenic leukaemic cells and B.C.G. in the treatment of acute lymphoblastic leukaemia.

Passive immunotherapy. Burkitt (1967) and Ngu (1967b) reported temporary tumour regression following the administration of 95–150 c.c.s. of convalescent serum. In both cases tumour regrowth was obvious after two weeks. Clifford et al. (1967) treated 2 patients with serum highly reactive on the indirect membrane immunofluorescence test (Klein et al., 1966, 1967a, b). No effect was noted in one patient, but in the other it was thought that tumour growth was stimulated. Fass et al. (1970b) found no evidence that plasma from patients in remission had an effect on tumour growth and it is now considered that the remissions previously reported were due to other factors (Ngu et al., 1970). In view of the danger of enhancement in treating solid tumours by passive immunization (Kaliss, 1958; Möller, 1965) this form of treatment has been abandoned.

ADVERSE IMMUNOLOGICAL FACTORS

Self enhancement. The results of the serial serological examinations by Klein and Henle suggest a direct relationship between titres of EBV determined antibodies and the response to chemotherapy. High titres of anti-MA antibodies are noted in patients with little or no tumour, these also have low values of anti-VCA antibodies, perhaps because of lack of the stimulating antigen. The presence of high titres of antibodies directed against the early antigen (EA) and VCA indicates a poor prognosis (Gunvén et al., 1970; Henle et al., 1970, 1971). Though in the majority of cases humoral antibody acts against the tumour, there are instances where antibodies provide a protective coating over the tumour cell membrane protecting the antigenic sites from the effects of cytotoxic antibodies. Möller (1965) working with mice recommended splenectomy to break this state of self enhancement but this was ineffective in 4 Burkitt lymphoma patients whose resistance to chemotherapy was thought to be related to marked IgG coating of the tumour cells. Hellström et al. (1969) have shown that in some experimental and human tumours, serum factors may *in vitro* specifically or non-specifically protect tumour cells from the cytotoxic effects of autochthonous lymphocytes.

ANTIGENIC LOSS

A Burkitt tumour may not be composed of biologically uniform tumour cells, and recurrent tumours may represent clones arising from a small number of cells which had an initial or acquired resistance to chemotherapy. Fenyö et al. (1968) have described the outgrowth of an immuno-resistant Maloney lymphoma with decrease concentration of tumour specific surface antigens. Possibly some repeatedly treated but resistant Burkitt tumours may be derived from tumour cells which have undergone antigenic depletion, and are so rendered resistant to cyto-toxic antibodies and (?) chemotherapy (A. Cochrane, 1970).

RESULTS OF TREATMENT

The majority of Burkitt lymphoma patients show a dramatic initial response to treatment with drugs of proven efficacy. In many this response may be marked and in some considered total; but it is known that disease may recur either in the same or a different area after an apparent disease-free interval of as long as four years (Clifford et al., 1968). Because of this the term 'long-term survivor' is preferred to 'cured' in describing those patients who have gone into prolonged total remission. Actuarial calculations by Pike (1966) indicated that patients who remained in total tumour regression for 250 days without treatment could be classified as 'long-term survivors'. In the series of patients reported by Burkitt (1967), Clifford (1966), Clifford et al. (1967), Ngu (1967a) and Morrow (1967) the overall survival rate was approximately 1 in 5; but if patients are classified by disease stage it is strikingly apparent that those in Stage I have a very much better prognosis than those in Stage IV. With the methods of treatment at present in use it can be expected that 80–90% of Stages I and II, 50–60% of Stage III and 20–30% of Stage IV patients will have total tumour regression. Immunotherapy may help many of these to maintain that state, so they become 'longterm survivors'.

ACKNOWLEDGEMENTS

I wish to acknowledge the help and stimulus I have received over the years from Professor George Klein and his associates at the Department of Tumour Biology, Karolinska Institutet, Stockholm. I am very grateful to Professor Sir Alexander Haddow, Dr. David Galton and Professor W. C. Ross of the Chester Beatty Institute for Cancer Research for their advice and encouragement and for supplies of Melphalan and Merophan. Dr. Gordon Zubrod and Dr. Paul Carbone of the National Cancer Institute, Bethesda, have always been very helpful and supplied the Cytosine Arabinoside, Methotrexate and Vincristine Sulphate.

I am also very grateful to my hospital colleagues. Dr. L. R. Whittaker's radiographs are included as Figs. 6–16 and the captions are derived from his reports.

Professor H. Cameron and other members of the Department of Pathology provided cytological, histological and post mortem reports. Dr. V. B. Bhardwaj anaesthetized many of these patients who were often in a poor physical state with large jaw tumours.

My wife, Jayne Clifford, typed the text, arranged the references, and drew Figs. 1, 17 and 28. The Burkitt lymphoma study is supported by a grant from the Cancer Research Campaign.

REFERENCES

ALLEYNE, G. A. O., & YOUNG, V. H. (1966). Adrenal function in malnutrition. *Lancet*, **i**, 911.

ARMSTRONG, D., HENLE, G., & HENLE, W. (1966). Complement fixation tests with cell lines derived from Burkitt's Lymphoma and acute leukemias. *J. Bact.*, **91**, 1257.

BANFIELD, W. G., WOKE, P. A., & MACKAY, C. M. (1966). Mosquito transmission of lymphomas. *Cancer*, **19**, 1333.

BELL, T. M., MASSIE, A., ROSS, M. G. R., & WILLIAMS, M. C. (1964). Isolation of a reovirus from a case of Burkitt's Lymphoma. *Br. med. J.*, **1**, 1212.

BELL, T. M. (1967). Review of the Evidence for a Viral Aetiology of Burkitt's Lymphoma. *Treatment of Burkitt's Lymphoma. U.I.C.C. Monograph Series*, *Vol. 8*, pp. 52–8. Burchenal, J. H., and Burkitt, D. P. (Eds.). Berlin, Heidelberg, New York: Springer-Verlag.

BELL, T. M. (1970). Isolation of Reovirus Type 3. *Burkitt's Lymphoma*, pp. 222–30. Burkitt, D. P., and Wright, D. H. (Eds.). Edinburgh and London: E. and S. Livingstone.

BISHUN, N. P., & SUTTON, R. N. P. (1967). Cytogenetic and other studies on the EB4 line of Burkitt tumour cells. *Br. J. Cancer*, **21**, 675.

BROOKES, P. (1964). Reaction of Alkylating Agents with Nucleic Acids. *Chemotherapy of Cancer*, pp. 32–43. Plattner, A. (Ed.). Amsterdam, London, New York: Elsevier.

BRUCE, W. R. (1967). The Action of Chemotherapeutic Agents at the Cellular Level and the Effect of These Agents on Hematopoietic and Lymphomatous Tissue. *Canadian Cancer Conference, 1966*, I, 53–64. Morgan, J. F., Noble, R. L., Rossiter, R. J., Taylor, R. M., Wallace, A. C., and Whitelaw, D. M. (Eds.). Oxford, London, Edinburgh, New York, Toronto, Paris and Frankfurt: Pergamon Press.

BURCHENAL, J. H. (1969). Success and failure in present chemotherapy and the implications of asparaginase. *Cancer Res.*, **29**, 2262.

BURKITT, D. (1958). Sarcoma involving jaws in African children. *Br. J. Surg.*, **46**, 218.

BURKITT, D. P. (1961). Observations on the geography of malignant lymphoma. *E. Afr. med. J.*, **38**, 511.

BURKITT, D., & DAVIES, J. N. P. (1961). Lymphoma syndrome in Uganda and Tropical Africa. *Med. Press*, **245**, 367.

BURKITT, D., & O'CONOR, G. T. (1961). Malignant lymphoma in African children: a clinical syndrome. *Cancer*, **14**, 258.

BURKITT, D. P. (1962). A tumour safari in East and Central Africa. *Br. J. Cancer*, **16**, 379.

BURKITT, D. (1964). A Lymphoma Syndrome Dependent on Environment. *The Lymphomareticular Tumours in Africa*, pp. 80–93. Roulet, F. C. (Ed.). Basel, New York: Karger.

BURKITT, D. (1966). Observations on response to vincristine sulphate therapy. *Cancer*, **19**, 1131.

BURKITT, D. (1967). Chemotherapy of Jaw Tumours. *Treatment of Burkitt's Tumour*, pp. 94–101. *U.I.C.C. Monograph Series, Vol. 8*. Burchenal, J. H., and Burkitt, D. P. (Eds.). Berlin, Heidelberg, New York: Springer-Verlag.

BURKITT, D. P., & KYALWAZI, S. K. (1967). Spontaneous remission of African lymphoma. *Br. J. Cancer*, **21**, 14.

BURKITT, D. P. (1969). Etiology of Burkitt's Lymphoma: an alternative hypothesis to a vectored virus. *J. natn. Cancer Inst.*, **42**, 19.

BURKITT, D. P. (1970a). Geographical distribution. *Burkitt's Lymphoma*, pp. 186–96. Burkitt, D. P., and Wright, D. H. (Eds.). Edinburgh and London: E. and S. Livingstone.

BURKITT, D. P. (1970b). General features and facial tumours. *Burkitt's Lymphoma*, pp. 6–15. Burkitt, D. P., and Wright, D. H. (Eds.). Edinburgh and London: E. and S. Livingstone.

BURLAND, W. L. (1969). Glaxo Laboratories Ltd. Personal communication.

BURNET, McF. (1969). *Cellular Immunology*, pp. 568–70, 726. Melbourne University Press and Cambridge University Press.

CAREY, R. W., & ELLISON, R. R. (1965). Continuous cytosine arabinoside infusions in patients with neoplastic disease. *Clin. Res.*, **13**, 337.

CHESSIN, L. N., BORJESON, J., WELSH, P. D., DOUGLAS, S. D., & COPPER, H. L. (1966). Studies on human peripheral blood lymphocytes *in vitro*. II. Morphological and biochemical studies on the transformation of lymphocytes by Pokeweed mitogens. *J. exp. Med.*, **124**, 873.

CHURCHILL, A. E., & BIGGS, P. M. (1967). Agent of Marek's disease in tissue culture. *Nature, Lond.*, **215**, 528.

CHURCHILL, A. E., PAYNE, L. E., & CHUBB, R. C. (1969). Immunization against Marek disease using live attenuated virus. *Nature, Lond.*, **221**, 744.

CLIFFORD, P., CLIFT, R. A., & GILLMORE, J. H. (1963). Oral melphalan in advanced malignant disease. *Br. J. Cancer*, **18**, 381.

CLIFFORD, P. (1966). Further studies in the treatment of Burkitt's Lymphoma. *E. Afr. med. J.*, **43**, 179.

CLIFFORD, P. (1967). Observations on the treatment of Burkitt's Lymphoma, Treatment of Burkitt's Tumour, pp. 77–93. *U.I.C.C. Monograph Series, Vol. 8*. Burchenal, J. H., and Burkitt, D. (Eds.). Berlin, Heidelberg, New York: Springer-Verlag.

CLIFFORD, P., SINGH, S., STJERNSWÄRD, J., & KLEIN, G. (1967). Long term survival of patients with Burkitt's Lymphoma: an assessment of treatment and other factors which may relate to survival. *Cancer Res.*, **27**, 2578.

CLIFFORD, P., GRIPENBERG, U., KLEIN, E., FENYO, E. M., & MANOLOV, G. (1968). Treatment of Burkitt's Lymphoma. *Lancet*, **ii**, 517.

CLIFFORD, P. (1970a). The Response to Particular Chemotherapeutic and Other Agents and the Treatment of CNS Involvement. *Burkitt's Lymphoma*, pp. 52–63. Burkitt, D. P., and Wright, D. H. (Eds.). Edinburgh and London: E. and S. Livingstone.

CLIFFORD, P. (1970b). Immunotherapy in the Treatment of Nasopharyngeal Carcinoma and Burkitt's Lymphoma. *Proceedings of the 9th International Congress of Otorhinolaryngology. Mexico City*, pp. 843–51. Gurria, A. B. (Ed.). Amsterdam: Excerpta Medica Foundation.

COCHRANE, A. J. (1970). Personal communication.

Connors, T. A. (1969a). Anti-Cancer Agents. Their Detection by Screening Tests and Their Mechanism of Action. *The Scientific Basis of Cancer Chemotherapy*, pp. 1–17. Mathé, G. (Ed.). London: Heinemann Medical Books. Berlin, Heidelberg, New York: Springer-Verlag.

Connors, T. A. (1969b). The need for additional alkylating agents. *Cancer Res.*, 29, 2443.

Cooper, E. H., Frank, G. L., & Wright, D. H. (1966). Cell proliferation in Burkitt's Tumours. *Eur. J. Cancer*, 2, 377.

Cooper, E. H., Frank, G. L., & Wright, D. H. (1968). Cell Proliferation in Burkitt's Tumours. *Cancer in Africa*, pp. 259–63. Clifford, P., Linsell, C. A., and Timms, G. L. (Eds.). Nairobi: East African Medical Journal/East African Publishing House.

Dalldorf, G., Linsell, C. A., Barnhart, F. E., & Martyn, R. (1964). An epidemiologic approach to the lymphomas of African children and Burkitt's sarcoma of the jaws. *Perspect. Biol. Med.*, 7, 435.

Diehl, V., Taylor, J. R., Parlin, J. A., Henle, G., & Henle, W. (1969). Infectious mononucleosis in East Africa. *E. Afr. med. J.*, 46, 407.

Dixon, R. L., & Adamson, R. H. (1965). Antitumour activity and pharmacologic disposition of cytosine arabinoside (NSC-63878). *Cancer Chemother. Rep.*, 48, 11.

Edington, G. M., & Maclean, C. M. U. (1964). Incidence of Burkitt tumour in Ibadan, Western Nigeria. *Br. med. J.*, i, 264.

Einhorn, J., Klein, G., & Clifford, P. (1970). Increase in antibody titre against the EBV associated membrane antigen complex in Burkitt's Lymphoma and nasopharyngeal carcinoma after local irradiation. *Cancer*, 26, 1013.

Ellman, L., Green, I., & Martin, W. J. (1970). Histocompatability genes, immune responsiveness and leukemia. *Lancet*, i, 1104.

Epstein, M. A., Achong, B. G., & Barr, Y. M. (1964). Virus particles in cultured lymphoblasts from Burkitt's Lymphoma. *Lancet*, i, 702.

Epstein, M. A., & Achong, B. G. (1970). The EB Virus. *Burkitt's Lymphoma*, pp. 231–48. Burkitt, D. P., and Wright, D. H. (Eds.). Edinburgh and London: E. and S. Livingstone.

Fass, L., Herberman, R. B., & Zeigler, J. (1970a). Delayed cutaneous hypersensitivity to Burkitt Lymphoma cells. *New Engl. J. Med.*, 282, 776.

Fass, L., Herberman, R. B., Zeigler, J., & Morrow, R. H. (1970b). Evaluation of the effect of remission plasma on untreated patients with Burkitt's Lymphoma. *J. natn. Cancer Inst.*, 44, 145.

Farnes, P., Barker, B. E., Brownhill, L. E., & Fanger, H. (1964). Mitogenic activity to *Phytolacca americana* (Poke weed). *Lancet*, ii, 1100.

Fawcett, D. W. (1956). Fine structure of chromosomes in meiotic prophase of vertebrate spermatocytes. *J. biophys. biochem. Cytol.*, ii, 403.

Fenyö, E.-M., Klein, E., Klein, G., & Swiech, K. (1968). Selection of an immunoresistant subline with decreased concentration of tumour specific surface antigens. *J. natn. Cancer Inst.*, 40, 69.

Fialkow, P. J. (1970). Personal communication.

Fialkow, P. J., Klein, G., Gartler, S. M., & Clifford, P. (1970). Clonal origin for individual Burkitt tumours. *Lancet*, i, 384.

Fialkow, P. J., Klein, G., Giblett, E. R., Gothoskar, B. & Clifford, P. (1971). Evidence for foreign cell contamination in Burkitt tumours. *Lancet*, 1, 883.

Galton, D. (1970). Personal communication.

Goldstein, G., Klein, G., Pearson, G., & Clifford, P. (1969). Direct membrane immunofluorescence reaction of Burkitt's Lymphoma cells in culture. *Cancer Res.*, 29, 749.

GREEN, I., INKELAS, M., & ALLEN, L. B. (1960). Hodgkin's Disease: a maternal to foetal lymphocyte chimera. *Lancet*, **i**, 30.

GRIPENBERG, U., LEVAN, A., & CLIFFORD, P. (1969). Chromosomes in Burkitt's Lymphoma. Serial studies in a case with bilateral tumours showing different chromosomal stemlines. *Int. J. Cancer*, **4**, 334.

GROSS, L. (1961). *Oncogenic Viruses*. Oxford, London, New York, Paris: Pergamon Press.

GUNVÉN, P., KLEIN, G., HENLE, G., HENLE, W., & CLIFFORD, P. (1970). Antibodies to (EBV)-associated membrane and viral capsid antigens in Burkitt Lymphoma patients. *Nature, Lond.* **228**, 1053.

HADDOW, A. J. (1961). Malignant lymphoma in African children: bioclimatic distribution. *East African Virus Research Institute, Annual Report for 1960–1961. No. 11*, 30.

HADDOW, A. J. (1963). An improved map for the study of Burkitt's Lymphoma syndrome in Africa. *E. Afr. med. J.*, **40**, 429.

HARRIS, R. J. C. (1970). The Aetiology of Murine Leukaemia—Lymphoma. *Burkitt's Lymphoma*, p. 215. Burkitt, D. P., and Wright, D. H. (Eds.). Edinburgh and London: E. and S. Livingstone.

HASHEM, N., & KABARITY, A. (1966). Mitogenic activity of legumes and other vegetable seeds on peripheral lymphocyte cultures. *Lancet*, **i**, 1428.

HELLSTRÖM, I., HELLSTRÖM, K. E., EVANS, C. A., HEPPNER, G. H., PIERCE, G. E., & YANG, J. P. S. (1969). Serum mediated protection of neoplastic cells from inhibition by lymphocytes immune to their tumour specific antigens. *Proc. natn. Acad. Sci. U.S.A.*, **62**, 362.

HENLE, G., & HENLE, W. (1966). Immunofluorescence in cells derived from Burkitt's Lymphoma. *J. Bact.*, **91**, 1248.

HENLE, G., & HENLE, W. (1967). Immunofluorescence interference and complement fixation techniques in the detection of Herpes type virus in Burkitt tumour cell lines. *Cancer Res.*, **27**, 2442.

HENLE, G., HENLE, W., & DIEHL, V. (1968). Relation of Burkitt's tumour associated Herpes type virus to infectious mononucleosis. *Proc. natn. Acad. Sci. U.S.A.*, **59**, 94.

HENLE, G., HENLE, W., CLIFFORD, P., DIEHL, V., KAFURO, G. W., KIRYA, B. G., KLEIN, G., MORROW, R. H., MANUBE, G. M. R., PIKE, M. C., TUKEI, P. M., & ZEIGLER, J. L. (1969). Antibodies to Epstein-Barr virus in Burkitt's Lymphoma and control groups. *J. natn. Cancer Inst.*, **43**, 1147.

HENLE, W., & HENLE, G. (1969). The relation between Epstein Barr virus and infectious mononucleosis, Burkitt's Lymphoma and cancer of the post-nasal space. *E. Afr. med. J.*, **46**, 402.

HENLE, W., HENLE, G., ZAJAC, B. A., PEARSON, G., WAUBKE, R., & SCRIBA, M. (1970). Differential reactivity of human sera with EBV induced 'early antigens'. *Science*, **169**, 188.

HENLE, G., HENLE, W., KLEIN, G., GUNVÉN, P., CLIFFORD, P., MORROW, R. H. & ZEIGLER, J. L. (1971). Antibodies to early EBV induced antigen in Burkitt's Lymphoma. *J. Nat. Cancer Inst.*, in press.

HERSHKO, C. (1970). Personal communication.

HOWARD, J. P., CEVIK, N., & MURPHY, M. L. (1966). Cytosine arabinoside (NSC-63878) in acute leukaemia in children. *Cancer Chemother. Rep.*, **50**, 287.

IRIARTE, P. V., HANANIAN, J., & CARTNER, J. A. (1966). Central nervous system leukaemia and solid tumours of childhood: treatment with 1,3-bis(2-chloroethyl)-1-nitrosourea (BCNU). *Cancer*, **19**, 1187.

JACOBS, P. A., TOUGH, I. M., & WRIGHT, D. H. (1963). Cytogenic studies in Burkitt's Lymphoma. *Lancet*, **ii**, 1144.

JOHANNSON, B. (1969, 1970). Personal communication.

KAFUKO, G. W., & BURKITT, D. P. (1970). Burkitt's Lymphoma and Malaria. *Int. J. Cancer*, **6**, 1.

KALISS, N. (1958). Immunological enhancement of Tumour Homografts in mice: A review. *Cancer Research*, **18**, 992.

KLEIN, E., CLIFFORD, P., KLEIN, G., & HAMBERGER, C. A. (1967). Further studies on the membrane immunofluorescence reaction of Burkitt Lymphoma cells. *Int. J. Cancer*, **2**, 27.

KLEIN, G., CLIFFORD, P., KLEIN, E., & STJERNSWÄRD, J. (1966). Search for tumour specific immune reaction in Burkitt Lymphoma patients by the membrane immunofluorescence reaction. *Proc. natn. Acad. Sci. U.S.A.*, **55**, 1628.

KLEIN, G., KLEIN, E., & CLIFFORD, P. (1967a). Search for host defences in Burkitt's Lymphoma. Membrane immunofluorescence tests on biopsies and tissue culture lines. *Cancer Res.*, **27**, 2510.

KLEIN, G., CLIFFORD, P., KLEIN, E., SMITH, T., MINOWADA, J., KOURILSKY, F. M., & BURCHENAL, J. H. (1967b). Membrane immunofluorescence reactions of Burkitt Lymphoma cells from biopsy specimens and tissue culture. *J. natn. Cancer Inst.*, **39**, 1027.

KLEIN, G., CLIFFORD, P., KLEIN, E., & STJERNSWÄRD, J. (1967c). Search for tumour specific immune reactions in Burkitt Lymphoma patients by membrane immunofluorescence reaction. *Treatment of Burkitt's Tumour*, p. 209. Burchenal, J. H., and Burkitt, D. P. (Eds.). Berlin, Heidelberg, New York: Springer-Verlag.

KLEIN, G., PEARSON, G., HENLE, G., HENLE, W., DIEHL, V., & NIEDERMAN, J. C. (1968a). Relation between Epstein Barr viral and cell immunofluorescence in Burkitt tumour cells. II. Comparison of cells and sera from patients with Burkitt's Lymphoma and infectious mononucleosis. *J. exp. Med.*, **128**, 1021.

KLEIN, G., PEARSON, G., NADKARNI, J. S., NADKARNI, J. J., KLEIN, E., HENLE, G., HENLE, W., & CLIFFORD, P. (1968b). Relation between Epstein Barr viral and cell membrane immunofluorescence of Burkitt tumour cells. I. Dependence of cell membrane immunofluorescence on presence of EB virus. *J. exp. Med.*, **128**, 1011.

KLEIN, G., PEARSON, G., HENLE, G., HENLE, W., GOLDSTEIN, G., & CLIFFORD, P. (1969a). Relation between Epstein Barr viral and cell membrane immunofluorescence in Burkitt tumour cells. III. Comparison of blocking of direct membrane immunofluorescence and anti EBV reactivity of different sera. *J. exp. Med.*, **129**, 697.

KLEIN, G., CLIFFORD, P., HENLE, G., HENLE, W., GEERING, G., & OLD, L. J. (1969b). EBV associated serological patterns in a Burkitt Lymphoma patient during regression and recurrence. *Int. J. Cancer*, **4**, 416.

KLEIN, G. (1970). Some Immunological Studies. *Burkitt's Lymphoma*, p. 172. Burkitt, D. P., and Wright, D. H. (Eds.). Edinburgh and London: E. and S. Livingstone.

KLEIN, G., GEERING, G., OLD, L. J., HENLE, G., HENLE, W., & CLIFFORD, P. (1970). Comparison of anti EBV titre and the EBV associated membrane reactive and precipitating antibody levels in the sera of Burkitt Lymphoma and nasopharyngeal carcinoma patients and controls. *Int. J. Cancer*, **5**, 185.

KLEIN, G., GERGELY, L., & GOLDSTEIN, G. (1971). Two coloured immunofluorescence studies on EBV determined antigens. *Clin. exper. Immunol.*, **8**, 593.

KOHN, G., MELLMAN, W. J., MOORHEAD, P. S., LOFTUS, J., & HENLE, G. (1967). Involvement of C group chromosomes in five Burkitt Lymphoma cell lines. *J. natn. Cancer Inst.*, **38**, 202.

Lancet. (1970). Editorial, 'Single cell origin for Burkitt's Tumour', **i**, 400.

LEVAN, A., & MANOLOV, G. (1970). Personal communication.

LEVY, J. A., TANABE, E., & CURNEN, E. C. (1968). Occurence of Rheovirus antibodies in healthy African children and in children with Burkitt's Lymphoma. *Cancer*, **21**, 53.

LILLY, F., BOYSE, E. A., & OLD, L. J. (1964). Genetic basis of susceptibility to viral leukaemogenesis. *Lancet*, **ii**, 1207.

MANOLOV, G., LEVAN, A., NADKARNI, J. S., NADKARNI, J. J. & CLIFFORD, P. (1970). Burkitt's Lymphoma with female karyotype in African male child. *Heredity*, **66**, 79.

MATHÉ, G., SCHWARZENBERG, L., AMIEL, J. L., SCHNEIDER, M., CATTAN, A., & SCHLUMBERGER, J. R. (1967). The role of immunology in the treatment of leukaemias and hematosarcomas. *Cancer Res.*, **27**, 2542.

MATHÉ, G., AMIEL, J. L., SCHWARZENBERG, L., SCHNEIDER, M., CATTAN, A., SCHLUMBERGER, J. R., HAYAT, M., & DE VASSIL, F. (1969). Active Immunotherapy for centre lymphoblastic leukaemia. *Lancet*, **i**, 697.

McCORMICK, K. J., STENBACK, W. A., TRENTIN, J. J., KLEIN, G., NADKARNI, J. S., NADKARNI, J. J., & CLIFFORD, P. (1969). Complement fixation test for detection of herpes like viruses in cell cultures of Burkitt's Lymphoma. *J. Virol.*, **3**, 525.

MILES, C. P., & O'NEILL, F. (1967). Chromosome studies of 8 *in vitro* lines of Burkitt's Lymphoma. *Cancer Res.*, **27**, 392.

MÖLLER, E. (1965). Interaction between tumour and host during progressive neoplastic growth in histoincompatible recipients. *J. natn. Cancer Inst.*, **35**, 1053.

MÖLLER, G. (1961). Demonstration of mouse isoantigens at the cellular level by the fluorescent antibody technique. *J. exp. Med.*, **114**, 415.

MORROW, R. H., PIKE, M. C., & KISUULE, A. (1967). Survival of Burkitt's Lymphoma patients at Mulago Hospital, Uganda. *Br. med. J.*, **4**, 323.

MUELLER, G. C. (1969). The G_1—S conversion; a target for cancer chemotherapy. *Cancer Res.*, **29**, 2394.

NADKARNI, J. S., NADKARNI, J. J., CLIFFORD, P., MANOLOV, G., FENYO, E.-M., & KLEIN, E. (1969). Characteristics of new cell lines derived from Burkitt's Lymphoma. *Cancer*, **23**, 64.

NGU, V. A. (1967a). Clinical Experience in the Therapy of Burkitt Tumour. *Treatment of Burkitt's Tumour*, pp. 71–6. Burchenal, J. H., and Burkitt, D. P. (Eds.). Berlin, Heidelberg, New York: Springer-Verlag.

NGU, V. A. (1967b). Clinical Evidence of Host Defences in Burkitt Tumour. *Treatment of Burkitt's Tumour*, pp. 204–8. Burchenal, J. H., and Burkitt, D. P. Berlin, Heidelberg, New York: Springer-Verlag.

NGU, V. A., BURKITT, D. P., & OSUNKOYA, B. O. (1970). Clinical and Related Evidence of Host Defence Mechanisms. *Burkitt's Lymphoma*, pp. 158–63. Burkitt, D. P., and Wright, D. H. (Eds.). Edinburgh and London: E. and S. Livingstone.

NORIN, T., CLIFFORD, P., EINHORN, N., JOHANSSON, B., KLEIN, G., ONYANGO, J., DE SCHRYVER, A., WALSTAM, R., & EINHORN, J. (1971). Conventional and superfractionated radiotherapy in Burkitt's Lymphoma—submitted for publication.

NOWELL, P. C. (1960). Phytohaemagglutinin: an initiator of mitosis in cultures of normal human leukocytes. *Cancer Res.*, **20**, 462.

O'CONOR, G. T. (1961). Malignant lymphoma in African children: a pathological entity. *Cancer*, **14**, 270.

OETTGEN, H. F., AOKI, T., GEERING, G., BOYSE, E. A., & OLD, L. J. (1967). Definition of an antigenic system associated with Burkitt's Lymphoma. *Cancer Res.*, **27**, 2532.

OLD, L. J., BOYSE, E. A., OETTGEN, H. F., DE HARVEN, E., GEERING, G., WILLIAM-SON, B., & CLIFFORD, P. (1966). Precipitating antibodies in human serum to an antigen present in cultured Burkitt Lymphoma cells. *Proc. natn. Acad. Sci. U.S.A.*, **56**, 1699.

OMMAYA, A. K. (1963). Subcutaneous reservoir and pump for sterile access to ventricular cerebrospinal fluid. *Lancet*, **ii**, 983.

PEARSON, G., KLEIN, G., HENLE, W., & CLIFFORD, P. (1969). Relation between EB viral and cell immunofluorescence in Burkitt tumour cells. IV. Differentiation between antibodies responsible for membrane and viral immunofluorescence. *J. exp. Med.*, **129**, 707.

PEARSON, G., DEWEY, F., KLEIN, G., HENLE, G., & HENLE, W. (1970). Correlation between antibodies to Epstein Barr virus (EBV) induced membrane antigens and neutralization of EBV infectivity. *J. natn. Cancer Inst.*, **45**, 989.

PIKE, M. C. (1966). Chemotherapy in Burkitt's tumour. *Lancet*, **ii**, 856.

PIKE, M. C., WILLIAMS, E. H., & WRIGHT, B. (1967). Burkitt's tumour in the West Nile district of Uganda 1961–5. *Br. med. J.*, **ii**, 395.

PULVERTAFT, R. J. V. (1964). Phytohaemagglutinin in relation to Burkitt's tumour (African lymphoma). *Lancet*, **ii**, 552.

RABSON, A. S., O'CONOR, G. T., BARON, S., WHANG, J. J., & LEGALLAIS, F. Y. (1966). Morphologic, cytogenetic, and virologic studies *in vitro* of a malignant lymphoma from an African child. *Int. J. Cancer*, **1**, 89.

RABSON, A. S., CHU, E. W., BEREZESKY, I. K., LEGALLAIS, F. Y., & GRIMLEY, P. M. (1970). Morphologic and cytogenetic studies *in vitro* of surface adherent lymphoreticulo cells derived from Burkitt lymphoma tissue. *Int. J. Cancer*, **5**, 217.

RALL, D. P., RIESELBACH, R. E., OLIVERIO, V. T., & MORSE, E. (1962). Pharmacology of folic acid antagonists as related to brain and cerebrospinal fluid. *Cancer Chemother. Rep.*, **16**, 187.

RAMALINGASWAMI, V., (1969). Interface of protein nutrition and medicine in the tropics. *Lancet*, **ii**, 733.

SCANLON, E. F., HAWKINS, R. A., FOX, W. W., & SMITH, W. S. (1965). Fatal homotransplanted melanoma. *Cancer*, **18**, 782.

SCHABEL, F. M. Jr. (1969). The use of tumour growth kinetics in planning curative chemotherapy of advanced solid tumours. *Cancer Res.*, **29**, 2384.

SCHAMBEL, F. M., JOHNSTON, T. P., MACCABEB, G. S., MONTGOMERY, J. A., LASTER, L. P., & SKIPPER, H. E. (1963). Experimental evaluation of potential anticancer agents. VIII. Effects of certain nitrosoureas on intracerebral L1210 leukemia. *Cancer Res.*, **23**, 725.

DE SCHRYVER, A. (1969). Personal communications.

DE SCHRYVER, A., FRIBERG, S., KLEIN, G., HENLE, W., HENLE, G., DE THE, G., CLIFFORD, P., & HO, H. C. (1969). Epstein Barr virus associated antibody patterns in carcinoma of the post-nasal space. *Clin. exper. Immunol.*, **5**, 443.

TEN SELDAM, R. E. J., COOKE, R., & ATKINSON, L. (1966). Childhood lymphoma in the territories of Papua and New Guinea. *Cancer*, **19**, 437.

SKIPPER, H. E., SCHABEL, F. M., Jr., & WILCOX, W. S. (1967). Experimental evaluation of potential anticancer agents. XXI. Scheduling of arabinosylcytosine to take advantage of its S-phase specificity against leukemic cells. *Cancer Chemother. Rep.*, **51**, 125.

SMITH, R. T., KLEIN, G., KLEIN, E., & CLIFFORD, P. (1967). Studies of the Membrane Phenomenon in Cultured and Biopsy Cell Lines from Burkitt's Lymphoma. *Advances in Transplantation*, Vol. 779, pp. 483–93. Dausset, J., Hamburger, J., and Mathé, G. (Eds.). Copenhagen: Munksgaard.

STEWART, A. M. (1970). Burkitt's Lymphoma and Malaria. *Lancet*, **ii**, 771.

STEWART, S. E., LOVELACE, E., WHANG, J. J., & NGU, V. A. (1965). Burkitt tumour: tissue culture, cytogenetic and virus studies. *J. natn. Cancer Inst.*, **34**, 319.

STJERNSWÄRD, J., CLIFFORD, P., SINGH, S., & SVEDMYR, E. (1968). Indications of cellular immunological reactions against autochthonous tumour in cancer patients studied *in vitro*. *E. Afr. med. J.*, **45**, 484.

STJERNSWÄRD, J., CLIFFORD, P., & SVEDMYR, E. (1970). General and Tumour Distinctive Cellular Immunological Reactivity. *Burkitt's Lymphoma*, pp. 164–71. Burkitt, D. P., and Wright, D. H. (Eds.). Edinburgh and London: E. and S. Livingstone.

STJERNSWÄRD, J., & CLIFFORD, P. (1970). Tumour distinctive cellular immune reactions against autochthonous cancer. *Proceedings of the Fourth Quadrennial International Perugia Conference on Cancer*, pp. 742–580. Severi, L. (Ed.). University of Perugia, Italy.

SVEDMYR, A., DEMISSIE, A., KLEIN, G., & CLIFFORD, P. (1970). Antibody patterns in different human sera against intracellular and membrane antigen complexes associated with Epstein Barr Virus. *J. natn. Cancer. Inst.*, **44**, 595.

DE THÉ, G., HO, H. C., KWAN, H. C., DESGRANGES, C., & FAVRE, M. C. (1970). Nasopharyngeal Carcinoma (NPC). 1. Types of culture derived from tumour biopsies and non tumourous tissues of Chinese patients with general reference to lymphoblastoid transformation. *Int. J. Cancer*, **6**, 189.

TOMKINS, G. A. (1968). Chromosome studies on cultured lymphoblast cell lines from cases of New Guinea Burkitt's Lymphoma, myeloblastic and lymphoblastic leukaemia and infectious mononucleosis. *Int. J. Cancer*, **3**, 644.

TOSHIMA, S., TAKAGI, N., MINOWADA, J., MOORE, G. E., & SANDBERG, A. (1967). Electron microscopic and cytogenic studies of cells derived from Burkitt's Lymphoma. *Cancer Res.*, **27**, 753.

TURNER, J. H., WALD, N., & QUINLIVAN, W. L. G. (1966). Cytogenetic evidence concerning possible transplacental transfer of leukocytes in pregnant women. *Am. J. Obstet. Gynec.*, **95**, 831.

WEBB, J. S., COSULICH, D. B., MOWAT, J. H., PATRICK, J. B., BROSCHARD, R. W., MEYER, W. E., WILLIAMS, R. P., WOLF, C. F., FULMOR, W., PIDACHS, C., & LANCESTER, J. E. (1962). Structures of mitomycin A, B and C and porfiromycin. *J. Am. chem. Soc.*, **84**, 3185.

WHITTAKER, L. (1970). Intravenous pyelography in Burkitt's tumour. *Australasian Radiology*, **14**, 197.

WRIGHT, D. H. (1967). The epidemiology of Burkitt's tumour. *Cancer Res.*, **27**, 2424.

WRIGHT, D. H. (1970). Gross Distribution and Haematology. *Burkitt's Lymphoma*, pp. 64–81. Burkitt, D. P., and Wright, D. H. (Eds.). Edinburgh and London: E. and S. Livingstone.

ZEIGLER, J. L., MORROW, R. H., FASS, L., KYALWAZI, S. K., & CARBONE, P. P. (1970). Treatment of Burkitt's Lymphoma with cyclophosphamide. *Cancer*, **26**, 474.

6 Transplantation and Cancer

P. R. F. BELL

INTRODUCTION

In the past ten years the study of tissue transplantation has changed from being a purely scientific discipline to a subject which is of direct clinical relevance. Much of the basic work in transplantation immunology had its beginnings in cancer research and now at both clinical and research levels the two are closely related and are being studied with similar techniques.

The central problems in transplantation research concern the rejection of transplanted tissue and the mechanisms by which rejection can be overcome. Those of cancer research are first, why the host does not destroy the malignant cell, and second, how the host's defences might be stimulated to effect destruction of the tumour. In essence these problems are complementary and any advance in one will be reflected in the other. Space does not allow an extensive review of both transplantation and cancer; instead topics of common interest to both will be discussed. Recent success with renal transplantation has produced a large number of patients on long-term immunosuppression. Since experimental immunosuppression is known to increase the oncogenic effect of various agents (Cerilli & Treat, 1969), these patients present an opportunity to assess its effect on the development of spontaneous human cancer.

THE RECOGNITION OF FOREIGN AND ABERRANT CELLS

The mechanism of recognition of foreign cells is basic to both transplantation and cancer and has been termed the surveillance system by Burnet (1959). Surveillance is one of the functions of the reticuloendothelial system which recognizes foreign cells by virtue of their antigenic differences. The need to minimize rejection of normal tissue in clinical organ transplantation has led to the discovery of a number of tissue antigens which are of importance in the rejection of transplanted cells. These antigens are now called transplantation (Histocompatibility or H) antigens. They have been found in most human tissues including white cells, spleen, kidney, liver, muscle and brain and are genetically inherited (Ceppellini, 1969). In addition they appear to be located on the cell membrane (Baldwin and Moore, 1968). Snell and Stimpfling (1966) defined the laws of histocompatibility in the mouse and showed that homografts could be successfully transplanted, without rejection, if the recipient had all the antigens present in the donor tissue. Recent international agreement (International Histocompatibility Conference, 1970) has resulted in the acceptance of 13 major transplantation antigens comprising the H-LA system in man.

Although it is not proven that these antigens are important in cell recognition, it would seem likely that they are, as the greater the genetic difference (and hence H-LA incompatibility) between donor and recipient, the greater is the intensity of rejection (Converse and Rapaport, 1969). Retrospective and prospective studies on human renal transplants have reinforced this view. Patients with identical antigen matching achieve longer survival with fewer rejection crises than those who are poorly matched with their donors (Van Rood *et al.*, 1969; Dausset, Rapaport and Legrand, 1968; Batchelor and Joysey, 1969).

Medawar (1956) suggested that the small lymphocyte was the cell which recognized foreign antigens and two theories have been advanced to explain the process of recognition. Burnet (1959) put forward a clonal selection theory of acquired immunity. He suggested that immunity and antibody production are functions of clones of mesenchymal cells. Each clone is able to react immunologically with a very small number of antigens and each cell is immunologically competent because it carries on its surface a receptor which is able to react with a given antigen. The adult immune system contains only cells bearing patterns which correspond to antigens not present among the normal constituents of the body. During embryonic life, clones of cells complementary to body constituents are eliminated by coming into contact with tissue antigen. As a result, at birth, all such potentially harmful clones will have been destroyed. The remaining cells congregate in the thymus and from there they migrate out and establish themselves in lymph nodes and spleen and give rise to a progeny bearing the particular antigen reactivity of the original clones. According to this theory, the introduction of an antigen leads to its recognition by those cells bearing that particular antigen reactivity. These cells then proliferate and produce a progeny of sensitized lymphocytes which later attack and destroy the antigen (Burnet, 1962).

A different hypothesis was put forward by Burwell (1963), who suggested that lymphocytes act as buffers in a system of tissue specific control mechanisms. Lymphocytes were visualized as having specific macro-molecular groupings, which could react with specific tissue control proteins, keeping these substances at a certain level in order to maintain a steady state. The lack of an exact fit of foreign macromolecules led to recognition and an immune response. In other words the lymphocyte was held to be endowed with a dictionary with which it recognized antigens specific to itself. Thus if the lymphocyte met an antigen, not recorded in the dictionary, it would react against it (Burch and Burwell, 1965), and an immunological reaction would occur.

No definite evidence exists at present to say with any certainty that the lymphocytes are endowed with recognition units by which they can recognize self and non-self, but some recent work with haptene conjugated antigens suggests that lymphocytes may have this property (Siskind, Dunn and Walker, 1968; Mitchison, 1967). Mitchison (1969) has suggested that these hypothetical recognition units will have "combining sites made up of variable amino acid sequences generated by the same mechanism as applies to immunoglobulin, parts of their constant regions in common with immunoglobulins, a multichain structure and multiple combining sites". Before we can accept the existence of these recognition units, it is essential that antibody in significant quantity should be demonstrated on lymphocytes.

In summary then, each individual is endowed with a series of genetically determined transplantation antigens which play a part in recognition of foreign cells. Burnet has suggested that lymphocytes are endowed with self-recognition units (antibody macromolecules) which recognize any antigen as foreign, because self-recognizing clones have been eliminated before birth. In contrast Burwell has suggested that lymphocytes recognize foreign antigens because they are not represented in a dictionary of self-determinants carried by the cell.

THE DESTRUCTION OF FOREIGN AND ABERRANT CELLS

Transplantation of foreign cells into a genetically dissimilar recipient results in the destruction of these cells by a process known as rejection. In general the destructive process is accompanied by a cellular infiltrate consisting mainly of lymphocytes (Medawar, 1956). In the previous section, the small lymphocyte was discussed as the only cell able to recognize foreign tissue. As far as organ homografts and solid tissue are concerned, however, the actual site of recognition is not known. Grafts which do not receive an immediate vascular supply, become sensitized via local lymphatics (Barker and Billingham, 1968). Antigenic material in the form of cellular debris from the graft may pass along lymphatics to the regional lymph nodes and sensitize lymphocytes (Hall, 1967). In contrast lymphatics do not appear to be essential in revascularized allografts which may become sensitized by release of antigenic material into the venous outflow of the organ (Najarian et al., 1966). A second possibility is that host lymphocytes may enter the graft and establish direct contact with antigens (Medawar, 1957). Fishman and Adler (1963) have suggested that macrophages may enhance sensitization by engulfing antigens and presenting them to the lymphocyte in a more acceptable form.

After sensitization, a variable latent period follows. During this period sensitized lymphocytes multiply and antibody molecules are formed. The whole process is terminated when the graft is invaded by mononuclear cells and destroyed. This sequence of events occurs with all tranplanted organs but can be modified in a number of ways.

Holman (1924) was the first to demonstrate that a second skin graft from the same donor to the same recipient resulted in an accelerated destruction of the graft. This observation was later confirmed and expanded by Medawar and his colleagues (Gibson and Medawar, 1943; Medawar, 1944 and 1945; Billingham et al., 1954) which firmly established the destruction of foreign tissue as an immunological phenomenon. These studies also showed that the small lymphocyte once sensitized, maintained its immunological memory against the particular sensitizing antigen.

Rejection is also modified in the presence of preformed antibodies. Under these circumstances, hyperacute destruction of the graft occurs (Altmann, 1963; Goodwin, 1964; Kissmeyer-Nielsen et al., 1966). This type of rejection is particularly dramatic when it occurs in revascularized grafts such as the kidney. The organ never perfuses well and rapidly assumes a dark cyanotic colour due to vascular occlusion caused by fibrin deposition within it (Starzl et al., 1968).

Foreign cells can also be destroyed by a process called allogeneic inhibition (Hellström and Hellström, 1966; Möller and Möller, 1966a). This reaction does not seem to require pre-sensitization and appears to be independent of the classical immune response described earlier. When two antigenetically different lymphocytes are cultured in the presence of phytohaemagglutinin (a substance which activates lymphocytes), there is a mutually damaging effect, which is not seen when genetically similar cells come into contact (Richards, 1969). Although no comparable substance to phytohaemagglutinin has been demonstrated in vivo, it may exist and offer a system of rapid destruction of foreign cells based on genetically determined details of the cell's surface structure. This type of destruction could be of great importance in the everyday elimination of aberrant or neoplastic cells before they become established.

The relative importance of the cellular and humoral aspects of actual graft destruction is still not completely clear. It is generally agreed, however, that small lymphocytes are more important than antibodies. This conclusion is based largely on the failure to transfer transplantation immunity passively by means of serum, whereas passive transfer can be effected by sensitized lymphocytes (Billingham and Barker, 1969a). In addition, if these cells are prevented from reaching the graft by surrounding it with a porous membrane, rejection can be postponed or prevented (Weaver, Algire and Prehn, 1955). A similar effect can be obtained if lymphocytes are depleted by thoracic duct drainage (McGregor and Gowans, 1964). Cytotoxic (humoral) antibodies have been demonstrated against both tumour and skin homografts (Gorer, 1955; Gorer and O'Gorman, 1956; Terasaki et al., 1961) and they are probably the main destructive force in hyperacute rejection, but their place in the homograft reaction is uncertain. In practice it is likely that both factors operate in a synergistic manner, (Batchelor, Boyse and Gorer, 1960) the small lymphocyte being the ultimate agent responsible for the destruction of foreign tissue (Brent and Medawar, 1967; Gowans, 1966; Wilson and Billingham, 1967).

Although we know that both cellular and humoral activities are responsible for graft destruction, the precise way in which foreign cells are killed is not known. Rejection probably differs in grafts which have been revascularized at the time of transplantation as opposed to those which acquire a blood supply later. In the former, obliterative vascular changes are important and contribute to cell death by virtue of ischae-mia. Hume and Egdahl (1955) and Porter et al. (1963) demonstrated severe obliterative vascular changes throughout the renal arterial tree in patients undergoing rejection. These observations have also been confirmed experimentally in dogs (Porter, Calne and Zukoski, 1964) where destruction of peritubular capillaries and arteriolar fibrinoid necrosis were seen. The fluorescent antibody technique has shown that these changes are probably brought about by deposition of antigen-antibody complexes in the vessel wall followed by fibrin and clot forma-tion (Horowitz et al., 1965). Vascular disruption of smaller vessels has also been demonstrated by Kountz et al. (1963). These authors examined rejecting dog kidneys using the electron microscope and demonstrated that endothelial damage was preceded by the intimate apposition of large plasma cells and endothelial cells. Apposition was followed by rupture of adjacent cell membranes, establishment of cytoplasmic continuity and destruction of the vessel wall.

In grafts where this type of vascular reaction is not seen, destruction may follow direct contact with lymphocytes. Sensitized lymphocytes have been shown to be capable of killing cells in vitro in the absence of complement or specific antibodies. Available evidence suggests that they do this by coming into direct contact with foreign cells and releasing a cytotoxic antibody which is lethal to both of them. Alternatively they may release a diffusible cytotoxic agent which could also be important in the recruitment of immunologically uncommitted cells such as macrophages which could help in the destructive process (Billingham and Barker, 1969b).

The rejection of tumour cells is in most respects similar to the rejection of skin (Winn, 1961). In general, cancer cells contain roughly the same spectrum of transplantation antigens as the normal cells from which they arose and are rejected by genetically dissimilar hosts. Tumours can, however, overcome minor antigenic differences and grow, presumably because of their innate neoplastic characteristics (Thomson and Gurney, 1960).

PREVENTION OF CELL DESTRUCTION OR REJECTION

The prevention of destruction of foreign cells by the host is a difficult ideal to achieve, but enough clinical success has been gained in the last ten years to allow us to transplant whole organs with a good chance of success (Human Kidney Transplant Registry, 1971). In spite of this, we are as yet unable to totally and safely suppress the immune response in the specific manner ultimately required for really successful organ transplantation. The more important techniques for this purpose include enhancement, tolerance, immunosuppression and tissue typing and it will be useful to discuss each of these in relation to tissue rejection prior to considering them in the light of their possible role in cancer.

Enhancement: The administration of specific antibody to a graft bearing animal can lead to either destruction or prolonged survival of the graft. The outcome probably depends on factors such as the dose of antibody and the density of combining sites on the graft itself. Under appropriate conditions prolonged survival of the graft is called immunological enhancement. Enhancement has been studied extensively in mouse tumours (Kaliss and Bryant, 1958; Möller, 1963a, b, c; Möller and Möller, 1966b; and Batchelor, 1968). In addition enhancement has been demonstrated with non-tumour transplants by Stuart *et al.* (1968) and more recently by French and Batchelor (1969) using rat kidney allografts.

The mechanism of enhancement is not fully understood, but two suggestions have been advanced. The first is that antibody becomes attached to antigen sites on the cell surface and blocks the antigen, rendering it relatively inert (Billingham, Brent and Medawar, 1956). This interference has been referred to as afferent block of the immune response, and prevents recognition of the foreign cell. The second possibility is derived from the observation that specific antibody can prevent immune lymphocytes from destroying target cells *in vivo* and *in vitro* (Möller, 1963a; Brunner *et al.*, 1968; Hellström *et al.*, 1969). Competition for antigenic receptor sites at the time of rejection could prevent close contact between the lymphocyte and target cells which is apparently required for cell destruction. The precise dosage of antibody required to produce enhancement is not known, but the effect may depend upon the number of binding sites on the cell. In cells with a high density of binding sites more antibody can become attached, fix more complement and presumably lyse the cell. Conversely in cells with few binding sites, less complement is fixed and lysis does not occur (*Lancet*, 1969a). Thus the dose of antibody and the availability of binding sites may explain why antibodies sometimes enhance and sometimes inhibit tumour growth (Möller, 1963a, b, c).

Immunological tolerance: If an animal is exposed to antigen before it has developed the capacity to react against it, then the development of that capacity is delayed and, in the continued presence of antigen, can be indefinitely postponed (Medawar, 1961) giving rise to immunological tolerance. The phase of unreactivity varies in different species, but occurs at, or about, the time of birth and lasts for a varying period thereafter. The resulting tolerance is specific (Billingham *et al.*, 1954) and the host will accept a graft from the antigen donor without subsequent immunosuppression, but will reject grafts from other donors.

The mechanism of tolerance induction is not clear, but is related in some way to the thymus. Thymectomy performed during the period of unreactivity will prolong this state almost indefinitely (Miller, 1961, 1965). The lymphocyte appears to be the effector cell in tolerance as the tolerant state can be passively transferred to irradiated isogenic hosts, by means of tolerant lymphocytes (Van Bekkum, 1963). In addition the introduction of isogenic lymphocytes into a tolerant graft bearing animal will result in the destruction of that graft (Billingham, Brent and Medawar, 1953). Tolerance does not appear to be an all or none affair, but an ill-defined relationship between the dose of antigen and the number of immunologically mature stem cells available. Incomplete tolerance can still be induced in the period immediately after the animal becomes immunologically competent. During this period a large dose of antigen may produce tolerance, whereas a smaller dose can excite antibody production (Billingham and Brent, 1957; Brent and Gowland, 1961).

The induction of tolerance would therefore seem to depend on the ratio of antigen-bearing cells to immunologically competent cells and this may give a clue to its induction in the adult. If the number of mature cells can be reduced to a minimum at the time of antigen administration, this may allow tolerance to develop during the recovery phase of the reticulo-endothelial system. This theory has been intensively investigated in experimental animals, because of the obvious attraction this would offer in clinical organ transplantation. Unfortunately on the whole, very large doses of antigen have been required and the tolerant state has been short-lived (Billingham and Barker, 1969b). There are a few notable exceptions however, including the work of Stuart *et al.* (1968). These authors produced almost indefinite survival of renal homografts in the rat with donor spleen cells given intravenously one day prior to transplant, combined with passive immunization with antiserum prepared by inoculating rats of the same strain with donor lymphocytes. These results are probably an example of a combination of tolerance and enhancement. Perhaps of more importance was the finding of Owen *et al.* (1968) that intravenous administration of exceedingly small doses of donor antigen daily for 5 weeks prior to renal transplantation and daily thereafter prolonged graft survival in rabbits from 12·6 days to 10 weeks. The same author (Owen, 1968) was able to extend the life of guinea pig to rabbit renal heterografts from 24 hours to 25 days.

There is evidence therefore that it is possible to induce a degree of tolerance in adults but the state is unstable and terminated by the cessation of antigen administration.

Immunosuppression: The response of the reticulo-endothelial system to foreign tissues can be extensively modified by means of a variety of techniques aimed at reducing the response of the host's lymphocytes. Therapy with azathioprine and steroids now forms the cornerstone for prevention of tissue rejection and is used routinely in clinical organ transplantation. Azathioprine (an imidazole derivative of 6-mercaptopurine) was first found to delay the onset of rejection in dogs with renal transplants (Calne, 1960, 1961; Zukoski, Lee and Hume, 1960) and although its action lacked consistency, it did produce 10% long term canine survivors (Calne, 1967a). Since that time it has been extensively employed in human renal transplantation with greater success. The mechanism of action of this agent is still in doubt, but its inhibitory effect on nucleic acid synthesis (Elion, Singer and Hitchings, 1954; Berenbaum, 1965) may account for its immunosuppressive actions. Azathioprine appears to be most effective if given at or before the time of exposure to antigen (Sterzl, 1960; Schwartz, Eisner and Dameshek, 1959) and produces a temporary state of lymphoid unreactivity. In addition it prevents or delays the typical infiltrate of lymphoid cells seen in tissue rejection (Calne, 1967b).

Steroids depress antibody production and the cellular response of sensitized lymphocytes (Moeschlin, Baguena and Baguena, 1953) and are actively lympholytic (Creger, Tulley and Hansen, 1956). These effects are probably brought about by a decreased synthesis of nucleic acids (Makman and Nakagawa, 1967). Steroids were first used by Dempster (1953) in an attempt to prolong canine renal homograft survival and although he was able to reduce cellular infiltration, he was unable to prolong survival of the graft. Since that time many authors have demonstrated the ability of this agent to prolong graft survival and even to reverse rejection episodes in dogs (Zukoski, Callaway and Rhea, 1965; Marchioro *et al.*, 1964) and man (Goodwin *et al.*, 1963, Kountz and Cohn, 1967; Bell *et al.*, 1971). The mechanism of action of steroids is not fully understood but evidence suggests that they may act either by retarding antigen release (Billingham, Krohn and Madawar, 1951), destroying lymphocytes (Creger, Tulley and Hansen, 1956) or retarding the development of immunity (Calne, 1967c).

A variety of other techniques are available to abolish or reduce homograft rejection and these include total body irradiation, thymectomy, thoracic duct drainage, extracorporeal irradiation of the blood, and antilymphocyte globulin administration. All of these techniques are capable of extending homograft survival in the experimental animal. Irradiation of the blood by means of an extracorporeal phosphate source surrounding an external arterio-venous shunt (Cronkite et al., 1962) is capable of reducing the frequency of early graft rejection (Persson et al., 1969). This technique allows the destruction of radio-sensitive circulating cells and reduces the immune response by depleting the number of circulating lymphocytes.

Antilymphocyte serum (ALS) was first shown to prolong homograft survival by Woodruff and Anderson (1963). This substance is produced by immunizing an animal of a different species with lymphocytes derived from thymus, lymph nodes or peripheral lymphocytes. After a suitable antibody response has been obtained, the animal is bled and the gamma globulin component extracted from the serum to give anti-lymphocyte globulin (ALG). Since Woodruff and Anderson's original description, ALS has been used in a number of animal studies and found to be a very potent immunosuppressive agent for all types of tissue grafts (Gray, Monaco and Russell, 1964; Abaza et al., 1966). In addition it is the only substance which is able to prevent second set reactions, thereby erasing immunological memory (Levey and Medawar, 1966a and b). Unlike other immunosuppressive agents, ALS seems to act preferentially against cell mediated (homograft) immunity and does not significantly affect the ability of the animal to mount a conventional antibody response. It will also allow successful heterografting, as recently demonstrated by Lance and Medawar (1968). These authors were able to transplant skin from rats, guinea pigs, rabbits and humans to mice. With the aid of ALS these heterografts survived for long periods of time.

Antilymphocyte serum has however several disadvantages. Animal recipients seem to be more susceptible to virus infections such as distemper and hepatitis (Abaza et al., 1966) and hypersensitivity reactions to the serum are not uncommon. Starzl has used ALG in human renal (Starzl et al., 1967) and liver homografts (Starzl et al., 1969) with apparent good effect but on the whole ALG has proved less effective in clinical practice than in experimental animal studies.

Tissue typing: In an earlier part of this chapter, transplantation antigens were discussed as an integral part of the surveillance system of the host. Experimental transplantation has since shown that the intensity of tissue rejection is related to the degree of incompatibility between donor and recipient. With minor antigen differences, transplants can survive for long periods of time without immunosuppression. Tissue typing between donor and recipient has improved the results in clinical renal transplantation (Starzl *et al.*, 1965; Terasaki *et al.*, 1966; Porter *et al.*, 1966; Van Rood *et al.*, 1969) and reduced the severity of rejection reactions. Minor antigenic differences between donor and recipient may also allow the development of tolerance or enhancement which could in turn increase graft survival with or without additional immunosuppression.

THE RELATIVE IMMUNITY OF THE CANCER CELL

The mechanisms involved in recognition and destruction of foreign cells, and the methods available to prevent their destruction, have already been discussed. We can now turn to the apparent immunity of the cancer cell. Enhancement or tolerance could play a part in preventing destruction of the cancer cell, antigens could be modified or the host immune system compromised in such a way that it cannot react normally against the aberrant cell.

Enhancement: Pre-treatment of the host with donor anti-serum or antigen prior to tumour transplantation produces enhancement of tumour growth in animals which are genetically dissimilar (Kaliss and Bryant, 1958; Möller, 1963a, b and c). If pre-treatment with serum is omitted, however, in the same donor-recipient combinations the tumour is usually rejected. The dose of anti-serum used is critical, and may explain why anti-sera sometimes produce inhibition of tumour growth rather than enhancement (Möller, 1963a). High doses may actively destroy cancer cells whereas doses small enough to block antigen receptor sites may protect the cells from immunological attack (Möller, 1963a). Enhancement has also been demonstrated with tumours growing in their strains of origin (Möller, 1964, 1965; Bubenik and Koldovsky, 1965). This observation may be more pertinent to spontaneous human tumour development where antigenic differences between normal and cancer cells are likely to be small. Enhancement is therefore capable of promoting tumour growth and may be an important factor in the induction and spread of spontaneously arising human tumours. Minor antigenic differences could lead to the production of small quantities of antibody which could coat the tumour cell, thereby preventing its recognition and allowing it to assume malignant characteristics.

Tolerance: From the definition set out earlier, it would be reasonable to assume that tolerance as a mechanism for cancer induction would only be of importance if the oncogenic agent was introduced during the period of immunological incompetence at, or about, the time of birth.

We have already seen that the induction of tolerance probably depends on the ratio of antigen to immunologically competent cells. If the number of competent cells is reduced in some way at the time of tumour induction or grafting, it is conceivable that during recovery of the reticulo-endothelial system, tolerance may occur.

Immunological immaturity and viral oncogenesis are complicated subjects, but seem to be related. The effect attributable to the virus itself, or cellular antigen change induced by the virus, or the development of tolerance, seem to differ in different systems (Anthony, 1967a). Examples of immunological tolerance to virus induced carcinoma during the neonatal period, include the Rous virus which induces tumours in neonatal but not adult turkeys, (Harris, 1963) and the polyoma virus which produces far more tumours in neonatal than in adult hamsters (Defendi and Roosa, 1965). In the latter study it was also demonstrated that the injection of isogenic adult lymphocytes could prevent neonatal susceptibility to polyoma virus. In contrast Klein and Klein (1966) reported that administration of the moloney virus to neonatal mice produced tolerance without increased incidence of tumour.

Attempts to produce tolerance to carcinogens have also produced conflicting results. Anderson (1962) injected rat fetuses with 3-methylcholanthrene and subsequently painted the rats with the same carcinogen from 6 weeks of age, and noted no increased incidence of skin tumours. In contrast Anthony (1962) painted mice with dibenzanthracene from birth and compared them with a control group treated from 3 months of age. He noted an increased incidence and size of tumour in the group painted from birth.

Finally, the demonstration by Owen (1968) that an injection of extremely small amounts of antigen before and after homografts or xenografts can result in prolonged survival of the grafts, is probably of great importance in relation to cancer induction. Antigen modification which may occur during cancer induction could presumably act in this way to produce a tolerant state, thereafter allowing the tumour to assume its well-known malignant characteristics.

Possible antigen modifications in cancer: In general, tumours are characterized by the same set of antigens (transplantation antigens) as the animal in which they arose, and are rejected by genetically dissimilar hosts (Anthony, 1967b). Repeated passage of the tumour in inbred animals or following prolonged tissue culture can, however, allow subsequent successful transplantation. This phenomenon could be due to genetic mutation of the cell with subsequent antigen change, blocking of antigen sites on the tumour by antibody (enhancement), or an increased resistance of the tumour to rejection mechanisms (Hellström and Möller, 1965). Antigen changes can, however, occur in cancer cells without the necessity to invoke genetic mutations. Recent observations

have brought to light the existence of tumour specific antigens in experimentally induced tumours, which are not found in normal tissues
(Sjörgen, 1965; Old and Boyse, 1965; Prehn, 1965; Klein, 1966a and b).
Evidence for the existence of such antigens in spontaneously arising
animal tumours is, however, more equivocal. Baldwin (1966) was unable
to detect specific antigens in spontaneous rat reticulum cell sarcoma or
squamous carcinoma. Révész (1960) failed to induce resistance to
spontaneous mouse adenocarcinoma or lymphomas following implantation of irradiated tumour cells into isogenic recipients. Resistance
can, however, always be produced if this procedure is adopted with
methyl cholanthrene induced mouse sarcomas (Klein et al., 1960).

So far there is no unequivocal evidence that all human tumours contain specific antigens (Morton et al., 1968) but evidence that they may
exist has recently been produced in studies with malignant melanoma
(Lewis et al., 1969). These authors, using in vitro tests, found evidence
of tumour specific antibodies in one third of their patients. These antibodies were confined to those patients with localized disease and tended
to disappear with dissemination. Specific antigens have also been found
in spontaneously arising human osteogenic sarcomas (Morton and
Malmgren, 1968). Abnormal antigens, which are not necessarily specific,
have been found in a number of other human tumours such as stomach
(Itakura, 1963), colon (Gold and Freedman, 1965), breast (Tee, Wang
and Watkins, 1965; Loisillier, et al., 1965), lung (de Carvalho and Rand,
1963), ovary (Levi, 1965) and liver (Perez-Cudrado et al., 1965).

If all spontaneously occurring human tumours do contain specific
antigens, it is difficult to imagine how they could be instrumental in
increasing the growth of a tumour. In the presence of a normal immune
system, one would assume that they would increase the chance of
defensive antibody production. However, the antigens could theoretically represent a subtle change, which could increase tumour growth by
the mechanisms of enhancement or tolerance already discussed. Green
(1967) does not believe that these antigenic gains in tumours are important in the aetiology or aggressive nature of cancer, but they may have
some relevance in the overall clinical response of the patient to his
disease.

Paradoxically, it may seem, antigen loss or deletion has also been
demonstrated in cancer cells and forms the basis of Green's immunolo-
logical theory of cancer (1954). It has, however, been pointed out that
the term antigen in this context, does not refer to the histocompatibility
antigens discussed earlier. It refers to tissue specific, or organ specific
substances present on cell membranes. Green (1957; Green and
Anthony, 1963) has suggested that tumour cells are malignant because
they have lost these tissue specific substances and argues that these
substances are essential in normal tissue homeostasis. Evidence for

antigen deletion has mainly been studied in experimentally induced hepatic tumours (Hiramoto *et al.*, 1961; Fischer and Weiler, 1962; Abelev, 1965; Kitagawa *et al.*, 1966) but has also been demonstrated in kidney tumours (Weiler, 1956), muscle tumours (Fel and Tsikarishvili, 1964) and squamous carcinoma (Carruthers and Baumler, 1965). Similar evidence for antigen loss has been found in a variety of spontaneously occurring human tumours including skin (Nairn *et al.*, 1960), thyroid (Goudie and McCallum, 1962), cervix (Hillemanns, 1962), colon (Nairn and Richmond, 1962) and kidney (Nairn *et al.*, 1966).

The central point of the immunological theory of cancer as put forward by Green is that loss of these tissue specific antigens allows the cell to escape from normal tissue homeostatic mechanisms. Relatively little is known of the factors responsible for normal cell growth but several differences between normal and malignant cells have been noted. For example, contact between normal cells in tissue culture is known to prevent movement and mitosis, but malignant cells are not similarly inhibited (Abercrombie *et al.*, 1957). Lowenstein and Kanno (1966) found that the insertion of microelectrodes between adjacent normal cells resulted in a flow of ions between the cells, a phenomenon which was markedly reduced in malignant cells. Stoker (1966) has suggested that the basic defect in the cancer cell is its inability to emit stimuli although it can still respond to stimuli emitted by adjacent normal cells. Normal cells have been shown to emit locally diffusing tissue specific substances called chalones, which may be important in the control of mitosis and organization of tissues. Bullough (1965) demonstrated that normal epidermal cells which have been damaged, emit a specific chalone which is capable of inhibiting mitosis in epidermal, but not other cells. Similar specific mitotic inhibitor substances have been demonstrated for other tissues, for instance liver and kidney (Saëtren, 1956) and bone marrow (Rytömaa and Kiviniemi, 1968). The cancer cell may differ from normal cells by losing these specific growth regulating substances and thus becoming malignant.

The mechanism by which antigen loss occurs is not known, but evidence suggests that it may be intimately connected with the carcinogenic effect of various oncogenic agents. One explanation for antigen loss or change, could be genetic mutation of the cellular DNA, or an alteration in messenger RNA. Orgel (1965) has shown that mutations can be induced by chemical alteration of DNA, and Kidson and Kirby (1965) have demonstrated a decreased synthesis of messenger RNA in the livers of rats fed with a carcinogenic aminoazo dye. Since there is experimental evidence of incorporation of many carcinogenic agents into DNA or RNA (Brookes and Lawley, 1964; Brookes, 1966; Marroquin and Farber, 1962; Colburn and Boutwell, 1966), mutation or alteration in messenger RNA could explain the mechanism of antigen loss. Similar considerations could apply to radiation carcinogenesis in view of the profound effects produced by ionizing radiation (Alexander and Bacq, 1961; Upton, 1963). Viral carcinogenesis differs in that exogenous DNA or RNA is injected into the cell (Stoker, 1964), but precisely how the genetic information coded in viral nucleic acids alters the cell is not yet known (Zamecnik, 1966). It is conceivable that viral oncogenesis may be a result of competitive suppression of cell proteins, essential for cellular activity resulting in neoplastic transformation.

Another explanation of antigen deletion rests upon the observation that many carcinogens are covalently bound to cell protein (Miller and Miller, 1952; Miller, Miller and Hartmann, 1961; Colburn and Boutwell, 1966; Pullman, 1964). More importantly, those carcinogens so far investigated have shown a degree of specificity in protein binding (Sorof et al., 1963; Abell and Heidelberger, 1962), becoming bound to particular protein fractions in the cell. Tumours on the other hand are deficient in these specific protein fractions and are not able to bind the carcinogens which originally produced the tumour (Abell and Heidelberger, 1962; Sorof et al., 1963; Miller and Miller, 1952). These observations reinforced the protein deletion hypothesis of carcinogenesis put forward by Miller and Miller (1952). The deletion of these proteins as a result of carcinogen binding could also explain antigen loss. Protein bound carcinogen has been found in cell nuclei (Bakay and Sorof, 1964; Rees, Rowland and Varcoe, 1965) and the microsomal fraction of the cell. The major binding site, however, is the surface membrane of the cell (Hultin, 1956a and b; Arcos and Arcos, 1958; Westrop and Green, 1960; Green and Ghose, 1964).

The binding of carcinogens to cell membranes may be of particular importance in view of the behavioural characteristics of cancer cells. These cells exhibit continued growth in cell culture in spite of apposition to other cells (Abercrombie et al., 1957), have an increased surface elasticity (Mateyko and Kopac, 1964) and a decreased mutual adhesiveness (Coman, 1960). These findings coupled with the knowledge that chemical carcinogens after binding with protein are capable of altering their antigenicity (Creech, 1952; Creech, Havas and Andre, 1955; Korosteleva, 1957) tie in well with Green's concept of cancer induction. The alteration of normal tissue specific protein could lead to the production of an antigenetically different one, so that the cell would lose a normal tissue specific factor and also gain one. The loss of this factor (antigen deletion), especially if it occurred on the cell membrane, could lead to the escape of the cell from normal homeostatic mechanisms and render it malignant.

Further evidence for antigen change was recently provided by an elegant study carried out by Mathé (1969). Mice were injected with dimethylbenzanthracene (DMBA), and the injected skin grafted after 5–30 days to isogenic animals. These grafts were rejected at the usual time, but a second graft from the same donor (taken from a site not injected with DMBA) to the same recipient was not rejected in an accelerated fashion suggesting that DMBA had caused antigen change in the original skin graft.

Decreased immune reactivity: Another explanation of neoplasia could be that the immune system of the host is primarily at fault and fails to recognize and prevent the outgrowth of cancer cells. There is no definite evidence that immunosuppression alone increases the incidence of spontaneous tumours in experimental animals, but it is known from animal studies that tumours tend to develop more readily in certain conditions characterized by disturbance of the host immune system (Schwartz *et al.*, 1966). A combination of immunosuppression and viral or chemical carcinogens has been shown to increase the incidence of malignant tumours in experimental animals. For example, Woods (1969) has shown that immunosuppression with antilymphocyte serum enhances the rate and frequency of induction of squamous cancers by dimethylbenzanthracene (DMBA) in hamster cheek pouches and reduces the induction period of cancer. Antilymphocyte serum has also been found to increase the susceptibility to oncogenic viruses (Hirsch and Murphy, 1968; Allison and Law, 1968) and Gaugas *et al.* (1969) found an unexpectedly high incidence of tumours in thymectomized mice treated with antilymphocyte serum and *Mycobacterium leprae*. In contrast Law, Ting and Allison (1968) found no difference between control animals injected with murine sarcoma virus and those given antilymphocyte serum. The animals, however, were injected with murine sarcoma virus at birth and probably developed tolerance to the virus in question. From this evidence it is clear that antilymphocyte serum given with an oncogenic agent increases the risk of cancer production and this effect has also been seen with other modes of immunosuppression which include thymectomy (Martinez, Dalmasso and Good, 1964; Davis and Lewis, 1967) and azathioprine (Casey, 1968).

It is also known that immunosuppression increases the incidence of neoplasia and allows the establishment of tumour transplants which would otherwise not have survived (Cerilli, 1969). In addition these agents have been shown to increase the incidence of metastasis in established animal tumours (Anthony, 1967c).

Just as rejection can be prevented or modified by depressing the immune response, the discovery of specific antigens in human melanomas has provided a means of augmenting the immune response. Killed melanoma cells excised from the patient and usually conjugated with a foreign protein such as rabbit gamma globulin (Czajkowski *et al.*, 1967) are reinjected. This procedure is often followed by the appearance of specific anti-tumour antibodies and is sometimes accompanied by regression of the neoplasm (Lewis *et al.*, 1969).

Melanoma is the only spontaneously occurring human tumour in which immunotherapy has so far proved to be of significant benefit but it seems likely that a similar result will eventually be achieved with other types of neoplasia (see Chapter 7).

Spontaneous tumours in immunosuppressed patients: The necessary immunosuppression in human renal transplantation has inadvertently provided a situation which compares in some ways with the animal studies already described, except of course that no carcinogen is administered at the same time. These patients therefore provide us with an opportunity to assess the incidence of spontaneously occurring human tumours in immunosuppressed patients. Evidence is already available which suggests that patients with spontaneously depressed immune responses due to agammaglobulinaemia or hypoglobulinaemia have a high incidence of malignancy (Fialkow, 1967; Schwartz, 1964) as do patients with autoimmune disease (Good, 1967).

Confirmation of earlier experimental work on the homotransplantability of tumours was provided early in the history of human transplantation. Patients were given organs taken from donors dying of metastatic carcinoma and although the organs were macroscopically free of metastases, subsequent events showed that they did in fact contain viable cancer cells. In 6 recipients of kidneys transplanted from donors dying of cancer of the bronchus (Martin *et al.*, 1965), kidney (Hume *et al.*, 1966), thyroid (Muiznieks *et al.*, 1968) and larynx (McPhaul and McIntosh, 1965), the same tumour arose in the recipients 7–18 months after transplantation. In one case, however, where the donor died of bronchial carcinoma, termination of immunosuppression resulted in rejection of kidney and cancer (Wilson *et al.*, 1968).

Hepatoma has been treated by excision of the recipient's own liver and replacement with a transplanted organ (Starzl *et al.*, 1969). One of the longest survivors after this procedure died at 13 months with disseminated tumour which was detectable within 3 months of transplantation. Further experience with these tumours suggests that transplantation combined with immunosuppression nearly always results in the recurrence and dissemination of the original cancer.

Spontaneous neoplasms have also been reported in patients following renal transplantation with immunosuppression (Lancet, 1969b; Doak *et al.*, 1968; Penn *et al.*, 1969; Siegel *et al.*, 1969; Deodhar *et al.*, 1969; Schneck and Penn, 1971). All of these patients have received immunosuppression with azathioprine and steroids and in addition, at least 5 of them have received antilymphocyte globulin. The majority of tumours so far described have been lymphatic in origin with an incidence of 9 such tumours in 2,500 transplants (Penn and Starzl, 1970). In addition there has been one dysgerminoma (Good, 1967), one squamous cell carcinoma (Hume *et al.*, 1966), two anaplastic carcinomata, one carcinoma of cervix (Penn and Starzl, 1970), and one case of disseminated visceral Kaposi's sarcoma (Siegel *et al.*, 1969). Of particular interest was the case of reticulum cell sarcoma arising at the site of injections of antilymphocyte globulin in the buttock (Deodhar *et al.*, 1969). As the authors point out, reticulum cell sarcoma very rarely arises at this site. They suggest that it may have done so as a result of oncogenic viruses present in the injected serum or because of attraction of precursors of tumour cells by the relatively high concentration of foreign antigens at the site of the injection. This particular case confirms clinically, the experimental observations of Allison and Law (1968) who found an extremely high incidence of reticulum cell sarcoma at the site of injection in mice injected with leukaemogenic virus and anti-lymphocyte serum. Two examples of a reticulum cell sarcoma arising in transplant patients are shown in Figs. 1 and 2. In the first patient (Fig. 1) the tumour was localized to the brain and in the second (Fig. 2) the neoplasm was widely disseminated.

The observed increase in spontaneous tumours in immunosuppressed patients could be due to several factors. It may be argued that at least in some cases the tumour swere present prior to transplantation. Except in one case (Penn *et al.*, 1969) this possibility seems unlikely as the tumours arose several months after the onset of immunosuppression. A second possibility is that immunosuppression reduces the surveillance and defence mechanisms against spontaneously arising malignant cells which are thereby allowed to proliferate. This is in some ways similar to the observation that cancer patients do in fact have a reduced immune responsiveness (Grace and Kendo, 1958; Kelly *et al.*, 1958) which is only demonstrable in the presence of metastasis (Soloway and Rapaport, 1965) and could be an effect, rather than a cause of cancer. A third possibility is that the immunosuppressive drugs used are themselves carcinogenic. Azathioprine is known to cause structural and chromosome abnormalities in man (Jensen and Soborg, 1966) and could therefore be carcinogenic. The fourth possibility is that immunosuppression reduces the host resistance to viral infections thereby allowing a greater opportunity for oncogenic viruses to produce neoplasia.

Many experimental viral tumours develop only if the virus is induced during the neonatal period prior to the development of immunological tolerance (Stewart, Eddy and Stanton, 1959) unless the host defences are first reduced (Koldovsky and Svoboda, 1965). Burkitt's lymphoma (see Chapter 5) is thought to be particularly susceptible to host control mechanisms as complete regression is not unusual and remissions have been obtained with specific and non-specific immunotherapeutic methods. These methods have included passive immunization with sera

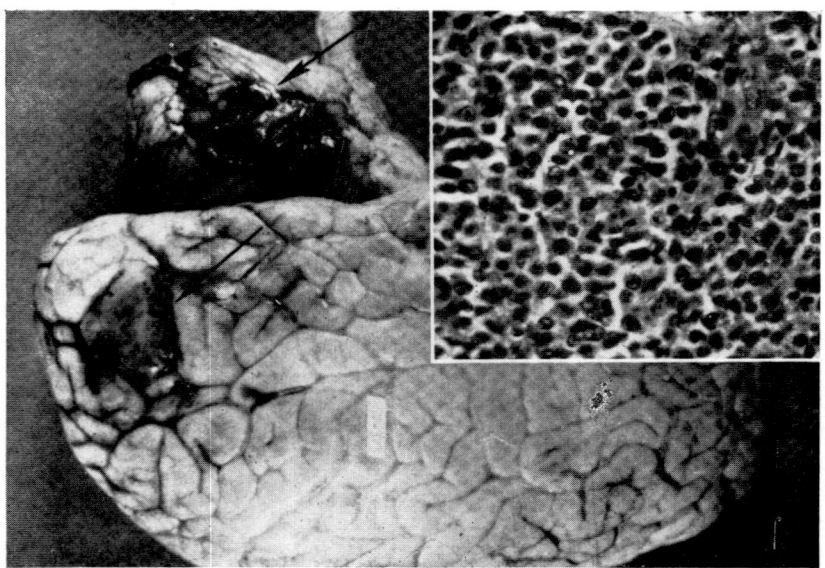

FIG. 6.1. Nodules of tumour are visible in the occipital lobes and cerebellum. Inset—histological picture typical of reticulum cell sarcoma. (By courtesy of *Transplantation Proceedings*.)

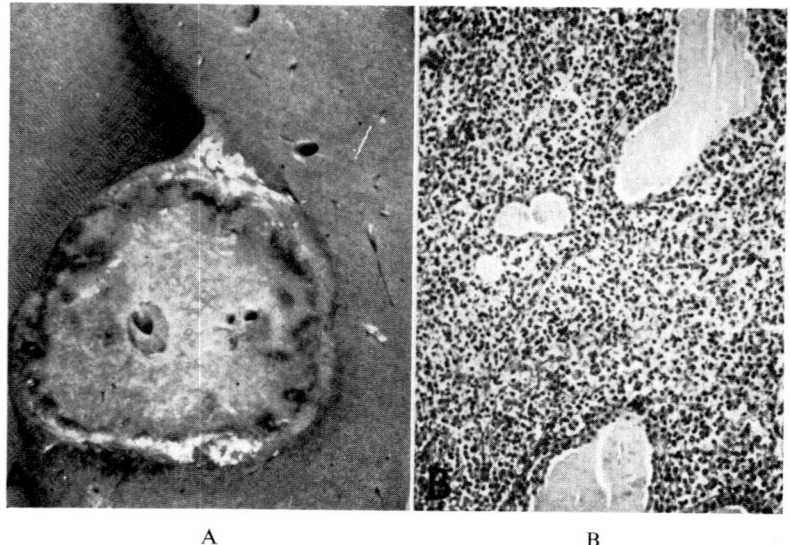

A   B

FIG. 6.2. A—Tumour nodule in the liver. B—Infiltration of the thyroid by malignant reticulum cells. (By courtesy of *Transplantation Proceedings*.)

from patients whose tumours have regressed, or by smallpox vaccination (*B.M.J.*, 1966). Epstein-Barr virus is a distinct member of the herpes group and may be concerned in the induction of Burkitt's lymphoma (*Lancet*, 1969b) as every patient with this disease has antibody against this virus (*B.M.J.*, 1969). Whether this virus is merely a passenger or an oncogenic agent remains to be seen, but if it is oncogenic then the result may depend upon the timing of infection. If infection and neoplastic transformation occurs in infancy or childhood prior to the development of immunological competence, a lymphoma may be the result. In contrast an infection during adult life may produce either no effect or a disease such as mononucleosis (*Lancet*, 1968). A further explanation for the possible difference in the outcome of infection has been suggested by Burkitt (1969). In the absence of chronic lymphoreticular proliferation caused by parasites such as malaria, contact with Epstein-Barr virus may result in subclinical infection with a few cases of infectious mononucleosis and rare cases of lymphoma. In the presence of chronic lymphoreticular proliferation, however, lymphoma becomes more common and infectious mononucleosis rare. This theory has interesting implications when applied to the transplant situation where lymphoreticular proliferation is commonly produced either by ALS administration or by the antigen in the graft itself. Consequently it will be of interest if Epstein-Barr virus has any relationship to the induction of lymphomas in transplant patients. Viral particles have been looked for in at least one post-transplant lymphoma (Deodhar *et al.*, 1969) but none have so far been found.

The extraordinarily high incidence of lymphoid tumours may be related to chronic antigen stimulation of the reticulo-endothelial system by either foreign protein in anti-lymphocyte globulin or by the graft itself without the need to invoke additional viral infection. There is experimental evidence (Dameshek and Schwartz, 1959; Metcalf, 1963; Schwartz *et al.*, 1966; Walford and Hildemann, 1965) which suggests that chronic antigenic stimulation may increase the incidence of experimental lymphomas. Penny and Hughes (1970) reviewed 87 cases of plasma cell dysplasia, 32 of which had been receiving allogen injections for over 5 years and found no increased incidence of neoplasia. This observation does not, however, exclude the possibility that neoplasia can be caused by a combination of immunosuppression and antigen administration.

TRANSPLANTATION AS A THERAPY FOR CANCER

The application of routine surgical techniques to the treatment of cancer arising in vital organs has been limited by the need to preserve as much of these organs as possible. The advent of successful clinical transplantation raises the possibility of complete excision and replacement of organs by healthy homografts as a therapeutic measure in cancer surgery. This apparently extreme method of treatment has received attention because of the poor results obtained with conventional methods of cancer therapy in organs such as the liver and kidney.

In the case of non-vital organs, the success of cancer surgery depends on two factors. First, removal of the primary tumour with adjacent tissue, in the hope that neoplasm has not spread beyond the limits of resection. Secondly, removal by the reticulo-endothelial system of malignant cells, outside the area of excision. From the surgical point of view the most important factor is probably the latter. Any interference with the host defence mechanisms might therefore be expected to bias survival in favour of the cancer cell and the necessary immuno-suppression which accompanies organ transplantation may therefore increase the survival capabilities of circulating cancer cells. In the preceding sections of the chapter we have already seen that clinical and experimental immunosuppression increases the incidence of tumour production. Unless all malignant cells can be removed prior to transplantation the chances of recurrent tumour would therefore be expected to be high. Clinical results have so far borne out this hypothesis.

For obvious reasons the liver has been the commonest target for replacement therapy. Unlike many other vital organs it is unpaired and cannot be removed without replacement. In addition tumours of the liver are rapidly fatal and difficult to control by other means. Several attempts have been made to resect hepatic neoplasms and replace them with normal organs; so far the greatest success has been achieved by Starzl and his collaborators (1969). In their series, patients received liver transplants for hepatomas thought to be confined to the liver. All of those that survived the operation died of recurrent cancer. The longest survivor lived for 13 months before dying of widespread recurrence but was shown to have pulmonary metastases as early as 4 months after transplantation. This experience would seem to confirm that immunosuppression apparently favours the survival and establishment of disseminated malignant cells and suggests that this type of therapy is of limited value in the treatment of hepatic neoplasia.

Because the kidney is a paired organ, relatively few patients require a transplant following resection of a tumour unless it occurs in a solitary organ. This unusual situation has, however, arisen in at least two patients (Woodruff, 1970). In one of them a hypernephroma arose in a solitary kidney and in the second a small tumour was found in the recipient's own functionless kidneys which were removed for other reasons prior to transplantation. Neither of these patients has had recurrence of tumour 5 years and 18 months after transplantation. Why these patients should have done so much better than those with liver cancer is difficult to explain. It may be that renal carcinoma is a less aggressive disease, but it is far more likely that all tumour cells were removed during nephrectomy.

Several transplants (Hardy, 1963) have been performed for carcinoma of the lung but all of these patients have died a short time after transplantation so that the effect of this procedure on ultimate survival and tumour recurrence cannot be judged.

Recent advances in transplantation of bone marrow have raised the possibility of marrow transplants in patients suffering from primary marrow cancer. This procedure has been limited by the occurrence of what is termed graft versus host disease. In this syndrome, the transplanted immune cells mount a rejection reaction against the recipient which eventually ends in death. This type of reaction is particularly severe if the recipient's bone marrow has been destroyed by total body irradiation. Recent techniques of donor marrow separation (Dicke, Van Hooft and Van Bekkum, 1968) aimed at eliminating immuno-competent cells have, however, allowed successful short term transplantation in patients with primary marrow aplasias (Bach et al., 1968; de Koning et al., 1969). Mathé et al. (1970) treated 6 cases of acute myeloblastic leukaemia and 4 with acute lymphatic leukaemia using marrow transplants. The recipients were given anti-lymphocyte serum prior to transplantation and the graft versus host reaction eliminated. None of these cases received any benefit from the procedure and succumbed to their original disease. The improved methods of marrow separation already referred to may in future allow successful marrow transplantation without producing a graft versus host reaction. Transplantation can then be preceded by radiation therapy to destroy leukaemic cells. This avenue of marrow transplantation has yet to be fully explored.

Broadly speaking therefore, transplantation as a therapy for patients with cancer of vital organs has yielded disappointing results. The liver is the only organ in which sufficient transplants have been performed to draw any conclusions. The results with this organ have been very depressing with a recurrence within a few months. It would seem therefore that a combination of viable cancer cells and immunosuppression weighs the chances of survival distinctly in favour of the malignant cell. When it becomes possible to apply more selective immunosuppression in organ transplantation, replacement therapy for cancer may become a useful therapeutic approach to this problem.

CONCLUSIONS

Foreign cells are recognized by the host's surveillance system by virtue of their transplantation antigens and rejected if not recognized as self. The stronger the histocompatibility barrier, the greater the rejection response. Rejection can, however, be overcome in a variety of ways, which include antigen matching of donor and host coupled with immunosuppression aimed at crippling the surveillance system. In general these measures prolong the life of the graft but eventual rejection occurs unless the donor and recipient are genetically identical.

The cancer cell is rejected in much the same way if it is transplanted across a strong histocompatibility barrier, but can become established even under these circumstances, and once established continues to grow. Immunosuppression allows greater survival of tumour cells and increases the risk of metastasis.

What part then does the immune response of the host play in controlling a cancer, is the immune response deficient and therefore a primary cause of cancer or does the change occur in the cancer cell allowing it to avoid recognition and destruction? Cancer research has unearthed many potential carcinogens which no doubt continuously exert an effect on human cells because they form a part of our environment. A current theory of cancer induction as postulated by Green (1954) suggests that all tissues possess tissue specific substances located on the cell membrane. These substances are vital in control of normal cell homeostasis and loss of them leads to malignancy. The Millers (1953) proposed a protein deletion hypothesis for neoplasia which fits in well with Green's theory. Carcinogens have been shown to react with specific cellular proteins, located mainly on the cell membrane and in doing so change the antigenicity of the cell so that it loses normal tissue specific factors and becomes malignant. At the same time, it gains a different antigen which may or may not be recognized as such by the host (Hamilton Fairley, 1969). If recognized, in the face of a normal immune response it is destroyed, but in the face of a depressed immune response it will divide and establish itself (Burnet, 1967). Even if the immune response is normal a cancer cell could establish itself by means of enhancement or tolerance.

The relationship between the immune response and the altered cell which has been released from normal homeostatic mechanisms is a delicate one, relatively minor changes meaning the difference between survival and death. In patients with organ transplants we have a situation in which we have theoretically balanced the scales in favour of the potential cancer cell and already an increased incidence of neoplasia has been reported. It will be of interest to observe these patients carefully over the years to see if this susceptibility to cancer increases with the length of immunosuppression. In return, the knowledge gained from cancer immunology may be of benefit to the organ transplanter as a more rewarding future may be to try and alter the transplant rather than suppress the immune response of the recipient.

It has been demonstrated clinically (Robinson et al., 1965; Amos et *al.*, 1965) and experimentally (Ben-Hur *et al.*, 1966; Marchant, 1966) that skin grafts from donors suffering from cancer are less susceptible to rejection than normal tissues. More recently, Ben-Hur (1969) found that immersion of skin homografts in heated Ehrlich's tumour resulted in a prolonged survival of grafts compared to controls. He suggested that an 'antigen loss factor' was released from the malignant cells and was responsible for altering in some way the antigenicity of the graft without causing tumour formation. This type of treatment of the graft may be more promising than trying to depress the host immune response and thus exposing him to a series of potential dangers such as infection and cancer.

A more promising future approach to cancer may lie in immuno-therapy aimed at awakening the apparently dormant immune response. The demonstration of specific tumour antigens in human melanomas and the success, albeit limited, so far achieved by immunizing the patient with his own tumour, point to the fact that we should try and augment the defence mechanisms of the host as much as possible and not deplete them with potentially immunosuppressive drugs.

REFERENCES

ABAZA, H. M., NOLAN, B., WATT, J. G., & WOODRUFF, M. F. A. (1966). Effect of anti-lymphocyte serum on the survival of renal homotransplants in dogs. *Transplantn*, **4**, 618.

ABELEV, G. I. (1965). Antigenic structure of chemically induced hepatomas. *Prog. exp. tumor res.*, **7**, 104.

ABELL, C. W., & HEIDELBERGER, C. (1962). Interaction of carcinogenic hydrocarbons with tissues. VIII. Binding of tritium labelled hydrocarbons to the soluble proteins of mouse skin. *Cancer Res.*, **22**, 931.

ABERCROMBIE, M., HEAYSHAM, J. E. M., & KARTHAUSER, H. M. (1957). Social behaviour of cells in tissue culture. III. Mutual influence of sarcoma cells and fibroblasts. *Expl Cell Res.*, **13**, 276.

ALEXANDER, P., & BACQ, Z. M. (1961). *Fundamentals of Radiobiology.* 2nd edition. London: Pergamon Press.

ALLISON, A. C., & LAW, L. W. (1968). Effects of anti-lymphocyte serum on virus oncogenesis. *Proc. Soc. exp. Biol. Med.*, **127**, 207.

ALTMANN, B. (1963). Tissue transplantation: circulating antibody in the homo-transplantation of kidney and skin. *Ann. R. Coll. Surg.*, **33**, 79.

AMOS, D. N., HATTLER, B. G., & SHINGLETON, W. W. (1965). Prolonged survival of skin grafts from cancer patients on normal recipients. *Lancet*, **i**, 414.

ANDERSON, M. R. (1962). Induction of partial acquired tolerance to a carcinogen. *Nature, Lond.*, **194**, 290.

ANTHONY, H. M. (1962). Immunological phenomenon associated with carcino-genesis. *Rep. Br. Emp. Cancer Campn*, **40**, 443.

ANTHONY, H. M. (1967a). *An Immunological Approach to Cancer*, p. 136. London: Butterworths.

ANTHONY, H. M. (1967b). *An Immunological Approach to Cancer*, p. 40. London: Butterworths.

ANTHONY, H. M. (1967c). *An Immunological Approach to Cancer*, pp. 115–32. London: Butterworths.

ARCOS, J. C., & ARCOS, M. (1958). Fine structural alterations in cell particles during chemical carcinogenesis. I. Influence of the feeding of aminoazo dyes on the swelling and solubilisation of rat liver microsomes. *Biochim. biophys. Acta*, **28**, 9.

BACH, F. H., ALBERTINI, R. J., ANDERSON, J. L., JOO, P., & BORTIN, M. M. (1968). Bone marrow transplantation in a patient with the Wiskott–Aldrich syndrome. *Lancet*, **ii**, 1364.

BAKAY, B., & SOROF, S. (1964). Soluble nuclear proteins of liver and tumour in azo dye carcinogenesis. *Cancer Res.*, **24**, 1814.

BALDWIN, R. W. (1966). Tumour specific immunity against spontaneous rat tumours. *Int. J. Cancer*, **1**, 257.

BALDWIN, R. W., & MOORE, M. (1968). Isolation of membrane associated tumour specific antigens from rat hepatomas induced by aminoazo dye. *Nature, Lond.* **220**, 287.

BARKER, C. F., & BILLINGHAM, R. E. (1968). The role of afferent lymphatics in the rejection of skin homografts. *J. exp. Med.*, **128**, 197.

BATCHELOR, J. R., BOYSE, E. A., & GORER, P. A. (1960). Synergic action between iso-antibody and immune cells in graft rejection. *Trans. plantn Bull*, **26**, 449.

BATCHELOR, J. R. (1968). The use of enhancement in studying cancer antigens. *Cancer Res.*, **98**, 1410.

BATCHELOR, J. R., & JOYSEY, V. C. (1969). Influence of HL–A incompatibility on cadaveric renal transplantation. *Lancet*, **ii**, 790.

VAN BEKKUM, D. W. (1963). Determination of specific immunological tolerance in radiation chimeras. *Transplantn*, **1**, 39.

BELL, P. R. F., BRIGGS, J. D., CALMAN, K. C., PATON, A. M., WOOD, R. F. M., MACPHERSON, S. G., & KYLE, K. (1971). Reversal of acute clinical and experimental organ rejection using large doses of intravenous Prednisolone. *Lancet*, **i**, 876.

BEN-HUR, N., BIRAN, S., & ROBINSON, E. (1966). Comparison of the survival of skin grafts from normal mice and mice with Ehrlich Ascites tumour. *Transplantn*, **4**, 205.

BEN-HUR, N. (1969). Experiments with 'antigen loss factor'. *Plastic reconstr. Surg.*, **43**, 61.

BERENBAUM, M. C. (1965). Immunosuppressive agents. *Br. med. Bull.*, **21**, 140.

BILLINGHAM, R. E., KROHN, P. L., & MEDAWAR, P. B. (1951). Effect of cortisone on survival of skin homografts in rabbits. *Br. med. J.*, **i**, 1157.

BILLINGHAM, R. E., BRENT, L., & MEDAWAR, P. B. (1953). Actively acquired tolerance to foreign cells. *Nature, Lond.*, **172**, 603.

BILLINGHAM, R. E., BRENT, L., MEDAWAR, P. B., & SPARROW, E. M. (1954). Quantitative studies on tissue transplantation immunity. I. The survival times of skin homografts exchanged between members of different inbred strains of mice. *Proc. R. Soc.* (B), **143**, 43.

BILLINGHAM, R. E., BRENT, L., & MEDAWAR, P. B. (1956). Enhancement in normal homografts with a note on its possible mechanisms. *Transplantn, Bull.*, **3**, 84.

BILLINGHAM, R. E., & BRENT, L. (1957). A simple method for inducing tolerance of skin homografts in mice. *Transplantn Bull.*, **4**, 67.

BILLINGHAM, R. E., & BARKER, C. F. (1969a). Recent developments in transplantation immunology. *Plastic reconstr. Surg.*, **43**, 559.

BILLINGHAM, R. E., & BARKER, C. F. (1969b). Recent developments in transplantation immunology. *Plastic reconstr. Surg.*, **44**, 20.

BRENT, L., & GOWLAND, G. (1961). Cellular dose and age of host on the induction of tolerance. *Nature, Lond.*, **192**, 1265.

BRENT, L., & MEDAWAR, P. B. (1967). Cellular immunity and the homograft reaction. *Br. med. Bull.*, **23**, 55.

Br. med. J. (1966). Leading article. **i**, 1043.

Br. med. J. (1969). Lymphomas and glandular fever. **2**, 445.

BROOKES, P., & LAWLEY, P. D. (1964). Evidence for the binding of polynuclear aromatic hydrocarbons to the nucleic acids of mouse skin: relation between carcinogenic power of hydrocarbons and their binding to deoxyribonucleic acid. *Nature, Lond.*, **202**, 781.

BROOKES, P. (1966). Quantitative aspects of the reaction of some carcinogens with nucleic acids and the possible significance of such reactions in the process of carcinogenesis. *Cancer Res.*, **26**, 1994.

BRUNNER, K. T., MAUEL, J., CEROTTINI, J. C., & CHAPIUS, B. (1968). Quantitative assay of the lytic action of immune lymphoid cells on ^{51}Cr labelled allogeneic target cells *in vitro*; inhibition by iso-antibody and by drugs. *Immunology*, **14**, 181.

BUBENIK, J., & KOLDOVSKY, P. (1965). Factors influencing the induction of enhancement and resistance to methyl cholanthrene induced tumours in a syngeneic system. *Folia. biol., Praha*, **11**, 258.

BULLOUGH, W. S. (1965). Mitotic and functional homeostasis: a speculative review. *Cancer Res.*, **25**, 1683.

BURCH, P. R. J., & BURWELL, R. G. (1965). Self and non-self: a clonal induction approach to immunology. *Q. Rev. Biol.*, **40**, 252.

BURKITT, D. P. (1969). Etiology of Burkitt's Lymphoma—alternative hypothesis to a vectored virus. *J. natn. Cancer Inst.*, **42**, 19.

BURNET, F. M. (1959). The Clonal Selection Theory of Acquired Immunity. Cambridge: University Press.

BURNET, F. M. (1962). *The Integrity of the Body*. London: Oxford University Press.

BURNET, F. M. (1967). Immunological aspects of malignant disease. *Lancet*, **i**, 1171.

BURWELL, R. G. (1963). The role of lymphoid tissue in morphostasis. *Lancet*, **ii**, 69.

CALNE, R. Y. (1960). The rejection of renal homografts: inhibition in dogs by 6-mercaptopurine. *Lancet*, **i**, 417.

CALNE, R. Y. (1961). Observations on renal homotransplantation. *Brit. J. Surg.*, **48**, 384.

CALNE, R. Y. (1967a). *Renal Transplantation*, p. 107. London: Arnold.

CALNE, R. Y. (1967b). *Renal Transplantation*, p. 115. London: Arnold.

CALNE, R. Y. (1967c). *Renal Transplantation*, p. 137. London: Arnold.

CARRUTHERS, C., & BAUMLER, A. (1965). Immunochemical staining with fluorescein labelled antibodies as an aid in the study of skin cancer formation. *J. natn. Cancer Inst.*, **34**, 191.

DE CARVALHO, S., & RAND, H. J. (1963). Antigens in human tumours revealed in suppressed rabbits rendered tolerant to normal human tissues. *Exp. molec. Path.*, **2**, 32.

CASEY, T. P. (1968). The development of lymphomas in mice with autoimmune disorders treated with azathiporine. *Blood*, **31**, 396.

CEPPELLINI, R. (1969). Genetics of transplantation. Organ transplantation today. *Excerpta med.*, Amsterdam, p. 26.

CERILLI, G. J., & TREAT, R. C. (1969). The effect of anti-lymphocyte serum on the induction and growth of tumour in the adult mouse. *Transplantn*, **8**, 774.

COLBURN, N. H., & BOUTWELL, R. K. (1966). The binding of β-propiolactone to mouse skin DNA *in vivo*; its correlation with tumour initiating activity. *Cancer Res.*, **26**, 1701.

COMAN, D. R. (1960). Reduction in cellular adhesiveness upon contact with a carcinogen. *Cancer Res.*, **20**, 1202.

CONVERSE, J. M., & RAPAPORT, F. T. (1969). The development of tissue typing. *Plastic reconstr. Surg.*, **44**, 9.

CREECH, H. J. (1952). Chemical and immunologic properties of carcinogen protein conjugates. *Cancer Res.*, **12**, 557.

CREECH, H. J., HAVAS, F., & ANDRÉ, J. (1955). Immunological properties of carcinogen protein conjugates containing polycyclic hydrocarbons and substituted stilbenes. *Cancer Res.*, **15**, 726.

CREGER, W. P., TULLEY, E. H., & HANSEN, D. G. (1956). A note on the effect of hydrocortisone on the microelectrophoretic characteristics of human red cell antibody unions. *J. Lab. clin. Med.*, **47**, 686.

CRONKITE, E. P., JANSEN, C. R., MATHER, G. C., NIELSON, N. O., USENIK, E. R., & SIPE, C. R. (1962). Studies on lymphocytes. I. Lymphopaenia produced by prolonged extracorporeal irradiation of circulating blood. *Blood*, **20**, 203.

CZAJKOWSKI, N. P., ROSENBLATT, M., WOLF, P. L., & VASZQUEZ, M. T. (1967). A new method of active immunisation to autologous human tumour tissue. *Lancet*, **ii**, 905.

DAMESHEK, W., & SCHWARTZ, R. S. (1959). Leukaemia and auto-immunisation— some possible relationships. *Blood*, **14**, 1151.

DAUSSET, J., RAPAPORT, F. T., & LEGRAND, L. (1968). Choice of Donors by Tissue Groups in The HU–I Systems. *Advances in Transplantation*. Dausset, J., Hamburger, J., and Mathé, G. (Eds.). Copenhagen: Munksgaard.

DAVIS, R. C., & LEWIS, J., Jr. (1967). Effect of thymectomy on an anti-lymphocyte serum treated human tumour xenograft. *Surg. Forum*, **18**, 229.

DEFENDI, V., & ROOSA, R. A. (1965). The effect of thymectomy on induction of tumours and on the transplantability of polyoma induced tumours. *Cancer Res.*, **25**, 300.

DEMPSTER, W. J. (1953). Kidney homotransplantation. *Br. J. Surg.*, **40**, 447.

DEODHAR, S. D., KUKLINCA, A. D., VIDT, D. G., ROBERTSON, A. L., & HAZARD, J. B. (1969). Development of reticulum cell sarcoma at the site of anti-lymphocyte globulin injection in a patient with renal transplant. *New Engl. J. Med.*, **280**, 1104.

DICKE, K. A., VAN HOOFT, J. I. M., & VAN BEKKUM, D. W. (1968). The selective elimination of immunologically competent cells from bone marrow and lymphatic cell mixtures. *Transplantn*, **6**, 562.

DOAK, P. B., NORTH, J. D. K., MONTGOMERIE, J. Z., & SMITH, F. (1968). Reticulum cell sarcoma after renal homotransplantation and azathioprine and prednisone therapy. *Br. med. J.*, **2**, 746.

ELION, G. B., SINGER, S., & HITCHINGS, G. H. (1954). The fate of 6-mercaptopurine in mice. *Ann. N.Y. Acad. Sci.*, **60**, 297.

HAMILTON FAIRLEY, G. (1969). The relationship between immunity and malignant disease. *Br. med. J.*, **2**, 467.

FEL, V. J., & TSIKARISHVILI, T. N. (1964), Reduction of normal muscle antigens in rat tumours of muscle origin induced by intramuscular injections of 20-methyl cholanthrene. *Cancer Res.*, **24**, 1675.

FIALKOW, P. J. (1967). Immunologic oncogenesis. *Blood*, **30**, 388.

FISCHER, C., & WEILER, E. (1962). Histological demonstration of liver specific antigen and its disappearance in hepatomas by means of fluorescein labelled anti-complement. *Z. Krebsforsch.*, **64**, 441.

FISHMAN, M., & ADLER, F. L. (1963). Antibody formation initiated *in vitro*. II. Antibody synthesis in X-irradiated recipients of diffusion chambers containing nucleic acid derived from macrophages incubated with antigen. *J. exp. Med.*, **117**, 595.

FRENCH, M. E., & BATCHELOR, J. R. (1969). Immunological enhancement of rat kidney grafts. *Lancet*, **ii**, 1103.

GAUGAS, J. M., CHESTERMAN, F. C., HIRSCH, M. S., REES, R. W. J., HARVEY, J. J., & GILCHRIST, C. (1969). Unexpected high incidence of tumours in thymectomised mice treated with anti-lymphocyte globulin and *Mycobacterium leprae*. *Nature, Lond.*, **221**, 1033.

GIBSON, T., & MEDAWAR, P. B. (1943). Fate of skin homografts in man. *J. Anat.*, **77**, 299.

GOLD, P., & FREEDMAN, S. O. (1965). Demonstration of tumour specific antigens in human colonic carcinomata by immunological tolerance and absorption techniques. *J. exp. Med.*, **121**, 439.

GOOD, F. A. (1967). Experimental and Clinical Experiences with Chemical Suppression of Immunity. A Personal Review. *Immunopathology Fifth International Symposium*, pp. 366–416. Miescher, P. A., and Graber, P. (Eds.). New York: Grune and Stratton.

GOODWIN, W. E., KAUFMAN, J. J., MIMS, M. M., TURNER, R. D., GLASSOCK, R., GOLDMAN, R., & MAXWELL, M. M. (1963). Human renal transplantation. I. Clinical experiences with six cases of renal homotransplantation. *J. Urol.*, **89**, 13.

GOODWIN, W. E. (1964). Discussion at the Human Kidney Transplant Conference (Washington, 1963). *Transplantn*, **2**, 584.

GORER, P. A. (1955). The antibody response to skin homografts in mice. *Ann. N.. Y Acad. Sci.*, **59**, 365.

GORER, P. A., & O'GORMAN, P. (1956). The cytotoxic activity of isoantibodies in mice. *Transplantn Bull.*, **3**, 142.

GOWANS, J. L. (1966). Life span, recirculation and transformation of lymphocytes. *Int. Rev. exp. Path.*, **5**, 1.

GRACE, J. T., & KENDO, T. (1958). Investigations of host resistance in cancer patients. *Ann. Surg.*, **148**, 633.

GRAY, J. G., MONACO, A. P., & RUSSELL, P. S. (1964). Heterologous mouse anti-lymphocyte serum to prolong skin homografts. *Surg. Forum*, **15**, 142.

GREEN, H. N. (1954). An immunological concept of cancer: a preliminary report. *Br. med. J.*, **ii**, 1374.

GREEN, H. N. (1957). The absence of immunologic identity on neoplastic cells. *Ann. N. Y. Acad. Sci.*, **68**, 268.

GREEN, H. N., & ANTHONY, H. M. (1963). The immunological theory of cancer. *Practitioner*, **190**, 705.

GREEN, H. N., & GHOSE, T. (1964). Localisation of liver specific antibody in normal and 3-methyl-DAB treated rats. *Nature, Lond.*, **201**, 308.

GREEN, H. N. (1967). *An Immunological Approach to Cancer*, p. 284. London: Butterworths.

GOUDIE, R. B., & McCALLUM, H. M. (1962). Loss of tissue specific auto-antigens in thyroid tumours. *Lancet*, **i**, 348.

HALL, J. G. (1967). Studies of the cells in the afferent and efferent lymph nodes draining the site of skin homografts. *J. exp. Med.*, **125**, 737.

HARDY, J. D., WEBB, W. R., DALTON, M. L., Jr., & WALKER, G. (1963). Lung homotransplantation in man. *J. Am. med. Ass.*, **186**, 1065.

HARRIS, R. J. (1963). Recent Progress in Tumour Virology. *Cancer Progress*, **1**, 5.

HELLSTRÖM, K. E., & MÖLLER, G. (1965). Immunological and immunogenetic aspects of tumour transplantation. *Proc. Allergy*, **9**, 158.

HELLSTRÖM, I., & HELLSTRÖM, K. E. (1966). Recent studies on the mechanisms of the allogeneic inhibition phenomenon. *Ann. N.Y. Acad. Sci.*, **129**, 724.

HELLSTRÖM, I., HELLSTRÖM, K. E., EVANS, C. A., HEPPNER, G. H., PIERCE, G. E., & YANG, J. P. S. (1969). Serum mediated protection of neoplastic cells from inhibition by lymphocytes immune to their tumour specific antigens. *Proc. natn. Acad. Sci., U.S.A.*, **62**, 362.

HILLEMANNS, H. G. (1962). Serologische und immunhistologische Untersuchungen zur Entstehung des Portiokrebses. *Z. Naturf.*, **17b**, 240.

HIRAMOTO, R., BERNECKY, J., JURANDOWSKI, J., & PRESSMAN, D. (1961). Immuno-histochemical staining properties of the N-2-FAA rat hepatoma. *Cancer Res.*, **21**, 1372.

HIRSCH, M. S., & MURPHY, F. A. (1968). Effects of anti-lymphoid sera on viral infections. *Lancet*, **ii**, 37.

HOLMAN, E. (1924). Protein sensitisation in iso-skin grafting: is the latter of practical value? *Surgery Gynec. Obstet.*, **38**, 100.

HOROWITZ, R. E., BURROWS, L., PARONETTO, F., DREILING, D., & KARK, A. E. (1965). Immunologic observations on homografts. II. The canine kidney. *Transplantn*, **3**, 318.

HULTIN, T. (1956a). The distribution of protein bound azodye in subfractions of liver cytoplasm fractions. *Expl Cell Res.*, **10**, 697.

HULTIN, T. (1956b). The intracellular distribution of protein bound azodye in rat liver. *Expl Cell Res.*, **10**, 71.

HUMAN KIDNEY TRANSPLANT REGISTRY (1971). Eighth Report. *Transplantn*, **11**, 328.

HUME, D. M., & EGDAHL, R. H. (1955). Progressive destruction of renal homografts isolated from the regional lymphocytes of the host. *Surgery*, **38**, 194.

HUME, D. M. (1966). Progress in Clinical Renal Homotransplantation. *Advances in Surgery*, Vol. 2, p. 419. Welch, C. E. (Ed.). Chicago: Year Book Medical Publishers.

INTERNATIONAL HISTOCOMPATIBILITY CONFERENCE, 1970. Los Angeles.

ITAKURA, K. (1963). Studies on human cancer antigens by the gel diffusion method. *Gann (Japanese Journal of Cancer Research)*, **54**, 93.

JENSEN, M. K., & SOBORG, M. (1966). Chromosome aberrations in human cells following treatment with imuran: preliminary report. *Acta med. scand.*, **179**, 249.

KALISS, N., & BRYANT, B. F. (1958). Factors determining homograft destruction and immunological enhancement in mice receiving successive tumour inocula. *J. natn. Cancer Inst.*, **20**, 691.

KELLY, W. D., GOOD, R. A., & VARCO, R. L. (1958). Allergy and skin homograft survival in Hodgkin's disease. *Surgery Gynec. Obstet.*, **107**, 565.

KIDSON, C., & KIRBY, K. S. (1965). Selective alteration of rapidly labelled RNA synthesis in rat liver during aminoazodye carcinogenesis. *Cancer Res.*, **25**, 472.

KISSMEYER-NIELSEN, F., OLSEN, S., PETERSEN, V. P., & FJELDBÖRG, O. (1966). Hyperacute rejection of kidney allografts, associated with pre-existing humoral antibodies against donor cells. *Lancet*, **ii**, 662.

KITAGAWA, M., TANIGAKI, N., YAGI, Y., PLANINSEK, J., & PRESSMAN, D. (1966). Carcinogen binding antigens in rat liver microsomes. *Cancer Res.*, **26**, 752.

KLEIN, G., SJÖGREN, H. O., KLEIN, E., & HELLSTRÖM, K. E. (1960). Demonstration of resistance against methyl cholanthrene-induced sarcomas in the primary autochthonous host. *Cancer Res.*, **20**, 1561.

KLEIN, G. (1966a). Recent trends in tumour immunology. *Israel J. med. Sci.*, **2**, 135.

KLEIN, G. (1966b). Tumour antigens. *A. Rev. Microbiol.*, **20**, 723.

KLEIN, E., & KLEIN, G. (1966). Immunological tolerance of neonatally infected mice to the Moloney leukaemia virus. *Nature, Lond.*, **209**, 163.

KOLDOVSKY, P., & SVOBODA, J. (1965). Induction of tumours by Rous sarcoma virus in adult mice. *Folia biol., Praha*, **11**, 203.

DE KONING, J., VAN BEKKUM, D. W., DICKE, K. A., DOOREN, L. J., VAN ROOD, J. J., & RADL, J. (1969). Transplantation of bone marrow cells and fetal thymus in an infant with lymphopenic immunological deficiency. *Lancet*, **ii**, 1223.

KOROSTELEVA, T. A. (1957). The action of carcinogenic substances upon proteins. *Vop. Onkol.*, **3**, 641.

KOUNTZ, S. L., WILLIAMS, M. A., WILLIAMS, P. L., KAPROS, C., & DEMPSTER, W. J. (1963). Mechanism of rejection of homotransplanted kidneys. *Nature, Lond.*, **199**, 257.

KOUNTZ, S. L., & COHN, R. (1967). *Advances in Transplantation*, p. 617. Dausset, J., Hamburger, J., and Mathé, G. (Eds.). Copenhagen: Munksgaard.

LANCE, J. E. M., & MEDAWAR, P. B. (1968). Survival of skin heterografts under treatment with anti-lymphocyte serum. *Lancet*, **i**, 1174.

Lancet (1968). Leading Article, **ii**, 1381.

Lancet (1969a). Graft survival and immunological enhancement. **ii**, 1111.

Lancet (1969b). Immunosuppression and cancer. **i**, 505.

LAW, L. W., TING, R. C., & ALLISON, A. C. (1968). Effects of ALS on induction of tumours and leukaemia by murine sarcoma virus. *Nature, Lond.*, **220**, 612.

LEVI, M., & MANDL, I. (1965). Specific antibody produced in response to sonified tissue culture cells of ovarian tumour. *Fedn Proc. Fedn Am. Socs exp. Biol.*, **24**, 177.

LEVEY, R. H., & MEDAWAR, P. B. (1966a). Some experiments on the action of anti-lymphoid anti-sera. *Ann. N. Y. Acad. Sci.*, **129**, 164.

LEVEY, R. H., & MEDAWAR, P. B. (1966b). Nature and mode of action of anti-lymphocytic anti-serum. *Proc. natn. Acad. Sci. U.S.A.*, **56**, 1130.

LEWIS, M. G., IKONOPISOV, R. L., NAIRN, R. C., PHILLIPS, T. M., HAMILTON FAIRLEY, G., BODENHAM, D. C., & ALEXANDER, P. (1969). Tumour specific antibodies in human malignant melanoma and their relationship to the extent of the disease. *Br. med. J.*, **2**, 549.

LOISILLIER, F., BUFFE, D., TAN K. B., BURTIN, P., & GRABAR, P. (1965). Étude immunologique des epithéliomas mammaires humains. *Annls Inst. Pasteur, Paris*, **109**, 1.

LOWENSTEIN, W. R., & KANNO, Y. (1966). Intercellular communication and control of tissue growth: lack of communication between cancer cells. *Nature, Lond.*, **209**, 1248.

MAKMAN, M. H., & NAKAGAWA, S. (1967). Studies of the mode of action of adrenal steroids on lymphocytes. *Recent Prog. Horm. Res.*, **23**, 195.

MARCHANT, J. (1966). Prolonged survival of allogenetic skin from tumour bearing mice. *Int. J. Cancer*, **1**, 557.

MARCHIORO, T. L., AXELL, H. K., LAVIA, M. F., WADDELL, W. R., & STARZL, T. E. (1964). The role of adrenocortical steroids in reversing established homograft rejection. *Surgery*, **55**, 412.

MARROQUIN, R. F., & FARBER, E. (1962). The apparent binding of radioactive 2-acetylaminofluorene to rat liver ribonucleic acid, *in vivo*. *Biochim. biophys. Acta*, **55**, 403.

MARTIN, D. C., RUBINI, M., & ROSEN, V. J. (1965). Cadaveric renal homotransplantation with inadvertent transplantation of carcinoma. *J. Am. med. Ass.*, **192**, 752.

MARTINEZ, C., DALMASSO, A. P., & GOOD, R. A. (1964). Homotransplantation of Normal and Neoplastic Tissue in Thymectomised Mice. *The Thymus in Immunobiology*, p. 465. Good, R. A., and Gabrielsen, A. E. (Eds.). New York: Hoeber Medical Division, Harper & Row.

MATEYKO, G. M., & KOPAC, M. J. (1964). Physical properties of human gynaecological tumours: microsurgical and centrifugation studies of living cells. *Prog. exp. Tumour Res.*, **4**, 27.

MATHÉ, G., AMIEL, J. L., SCHWARZENBERG, L., CHOAY, J., TROLARD, P., SCHNEIDER, M., HAYAT, M., SCHLUMBERGER, J. R., & JASMIN, Cl. (1970). Bone marrow graft in man after conditioning by antilymphocyte serum. *Br. med. J.*, **2**, 131.

MATHÉ, G. (1969). Are the neoantigens induced by chemical carcinogens or by leukaemogenic viruses particular to cancer cells? *Transplantn Proc.*, **1**, 113.

McGREGOR, D. D., & COWANS, J. L. (1964). Survival of homografts of skin in rats depleted of lymphocytes by chronic drainage from the thoracic duct. *Lancet*, **i**, 629.

MEDAWAR, P. B. (1944). Behaviour and fate of skin autografts and skin homografts in rabbits. *J. Anat.*, **78**, 176.

MEDAWAR, P. B. (1945). A second study of the behaviour and fate of skin homografts in rabbits. *J. Anat.*, **79**, 157.

MEDAWAR, P. B. (1956). A discussion on immunological tolerance. *Proc. R. Soc.* (B), **146**, (922), 1.

MEDAWAR, P. B. (1957). The homograft reaction. *Proc. R. Soc.* (B), **149**, 145.

MEDAWAR, P. B. (1961). Mechanisms of Immunological Tolerance, p. 17. Hašek, M., Lengerová, A., and Vojtišková, N. (Eds.). London: Academic Press.

METCALF, D. (1963). Induction of reticular tumours in mice by repeated antigenic stimulation. *Acta Un. int. Cancr.*, **19**, 657.

MILLER, E. C., & MILLER, J. A. (1952). *In vivo* combinations between carcinogens and tissue constituents and their possible role in carcinogenesis. *Cancer Res.*, **12**, 547.

MILLER, J. A., & MILLER, E. C. (1953). The carcinogenic aminoazo dyes. *Adv. Cancer Res.*, **1**, 339.

MILLER, E. C., MILLER, J. A., & HARTMANN, H. A. (1961). N-hydroxy-2-acetylaminofluorene. A metabolite of 2-acetylaminofluorene. *Cancer Res.*, **18**, 469.

MILLER, J. F. A. P. (1961). Immunological function of the thymus. *Lancet*, **ii**, 748.

MILLER, J. F. A. P. (1965). The thymus and transplantation immunity. *Br. med. Bull.*, **21**, 111.

MITCHISON, N. A. (1967). Antigen recognition responsible for the induction *in vitro* of the secondary response. *Cold Spr. Harb. Symp. quant. Biol.*, **32**, 431.

MITCHISON, N. A. (1969). Organ Transplantation Today, pp. 14–17. Mitchison, N. A., Creep, J. M., and Hattinga Verschure, J. C. M. (Eds.). Amsterdam: Excerpta Medica Foundation.

MOESCHLIN, S., BAGUENA, R., & BAGUENA, J. (1953). The influence of ACTH and cortisone on experimental antibody production in rabbits. *Int. Archs Allergy appl. Immun.*, **4**, 83.

MOLLER, G. (1963a). Studies on the mechanism of immunological enhancement of tumour homografts. I. Specificity of immunological enhancement. *J. natn. Cancer Inst.*, **30**, 1153.

MOLLER, G. (1963b). Studies on the mechanism of immunological enhancement of tumour homografts. II. Effect of isoantibodies on various tumour cells. *J. natn. Cancer Inst.*, **30**, 1177.

MOLLER, G. (1963c). Studies on the mechanism of immunological enhancement of tumour homografts. III. Interaction between humoral isoantibodies and immune lymphoid cells. *J. natn. Cancer Inst.*, **30**, 1205.

MOLLER, G. (1964). Effect on tumour growth in syngeneic recipients of antibodies against tumour specific antigens in methyl cholanthrene induced mouse sarcomas. *Nature, Lond.*, **204**, 846.

MOLLER, E. (1965). Antagonistic effects of humoral isoantibodies on the *in vitro* cytotoxicity of immune lymphoid cells. *J. exp. Med.*, **122**, 11.

MOLLER, G., & MOLLER, E. (1966a). Interaction between allogeneic cells in tissue transplantation. *Ann. N.Y. Acad. Sci.*, **129**, 735.

MOLLER, G., & MOLLER, E. (1966b). Antibodies to Biologically Active Molecules, p. 349. Cinader, B. (Ed.). Oxford University Press.

MORTON, D. L., MALMGREN, R. A., HOLMES, E. C., & KETCHAM, A. S. (1968). Demonstration of antibodies against human malignant melanoma by immunofluorescence. *Surgery*, **64**, 233.

MCPHAUL, J. J., & MCINTOSH, D. A. (1965). Tissue transplantation still vexes. (Letter to Editor.) *New Engl. J. Med.*, **272**, 105.

MUIZNIEKS, H. W., BERG, J. W., LAWRENCE, W., & RANDALL, H. T. (1968). Suitability of donor kidneys from patients with cancer. *Surgery*, **64**, 871.

NAIRN, R. C., RICHMOND, H. G., MCENTEGART, M. G., & FOTHERGILL, J. E. (1960). Immunological differences between normal and malignant cells. *Br. med. J.*, **ii**, 1335.

NAIRN, R. C., & RICHMOND, H. G. (1962). Loss of gastrointestinal specific antigen in neoplasia. *Br. med. J.*, **i**, 1791.

NAIRN, R. C., GHOSE, T., & TANNENBERG, A. E. G. (1966.) Kidney specific antigen depletion in human renal carcinoma. *Br. J. Cancer*, **20**, 756.

NAJARIAN, J. S., MAY, J., COCHRUM, K. C., BARONBERG, N., & WAY, L. W. (1966). Mechanism of antigen release from canine kidney homotransplants. *Ann. N.Y. Acad. Sci.*, **129**, 76.

OLD, L. J., & BOYSE, E. A. (1965). Antigens of tumours and leukaemias induced by viruses. *Fedn Proc. Fedn Am. Socs exp. Biol.*, **24**, 1009.

ORGEL, L. E. (1965). The chemical basis of mutation. *Adv. Enzymol.*, **27**, 289.

OWEN, E. R., SLOME, D., & WATERSON, D. (1968). *Advances in Transplantation*, pp. 385–92. Copenhagen: Munksgaard.

OWEN, E. R. (1968). Prolonged survival in heterografted kidneys with transplantation antigen pre-treatment. *Nature, Lond.*, **219**, 970.

PENN, I., HAMMOND, W., BRETTSCHNEIDER, L., & STARZL, T. E. (1969). Malignant lymphomas in transplantation patients. *Transplantn Proc.*, **1**, 106.

PENN, I., & STARZL, T. E. (1970). Malignant lymphomas in transplant patients: a review of the world literature. *Int. J. Pharmacol.*, in press.

PENNY, R., & HUGHES, S. (1970). Repeated stimulation of the reticulo-endothelial system and the development of plasma cell dyscrasias. *Lancet*, **i**, 77.

PERSSON, B., ROSEGREN, B., BERGENTZ, S. E., & HOOD, B. (1969). Evaluation of preoperative extracorporeal irradiation of the blood in human renal transplantation. *Transplantn*, **7**, 534.

PEREZ-CUDRADO, S., HUBERMAN, S., & RACE, G. J. (1965). Cancerous and normal tissue antigens studied by immunohistochemical and ultrastructural methods. *Cancer, N.Y.*, **18**, 73.

PORTER, K. A., OWEN, K., MOWBRAY, J. F., THOMSON, W. B., KENYON, J. R., & PEART, W. S. (1963). Obliterative vascular changes in four human kidney transplants. *Br. med. J.*, **ii**, 639.

PORTER, K. A., CALNE, R. Y., & ZUKOSKI, C. F. (1964). Vascular and other changes in 200 canine renal homotransplants treated with immunosuppressive drugs. *Lab. Invest.*, **13**, 810.

PORTER, K. A., RANDALL, J. M., STOLINSKI, C., TERASAKI, P. I., MARCHIORO, T. L., & STARZL, T. E. (1966). Light and electron microscope study of biopsies from 33 renal allografts and an isograft $1\frac{3}{4}$ to $2\frac{1}{2}$ years after transplantation. *Ann. N.Y. Acad. Sci.*, **129**, 615.

PREHN, R. T. (1965). Cancer antigens in tumours induced by chemicals. *Fedn Proc. Fedn Am. Socs exp. Biol.*, **24**, 1018.

PULLMAN, B. (1964). Electronic aspects of the interactions between the carcinogens and possible cellular sites of their activity. *J. cell. comp. Physiol.*, **64**, Suppl. 1, 91.

REES, K. R., ROWLAND, G. F., & VARCOE, J. S. (1965). Studies on the binding of tritiated p-methylaminoazobenzine in rat liver and the role of intranuclear binding sites in the early stages of carcinogenesis. *Br. J. Cancer*, **19**, 903.

RÉVÉSZ, L. (1960). Detection of antigenic differences in isologous host tumour systems by pre-treatment with heavily irradiated tumour cells. *Cancer Res.*, **20**, 443.

RICHARDS, V. (1969). Immunology of cancer. *Am. J. Surg.*, **118**, 498.

ROBINSON, E., BEN-HUR, N., SHULMAN, J., HOCHMAN, A., & NEUMAN, Z. (1965). Comparative study of skin homografts of normal donors and donors with malignant neoplasia in a host with malignant disease. *J. natn. Cancer Inst.*, **24**, 185.

RYTÖMAA, T., & KIVINIEMI, K. (1968). Control of DNA duplication in rat chloroleukaemia by means of the granulocytic chalone. *Eur. J. Cancer*, **4**, 595.

SAÉTREN, H. (1956). A principle of autoregulation of growth production of organ specific mitose-inhibitors in kidney and liver. *Expl Cell Res.*, **11**, 229.

SCHNECK, S. A., & PENN, I. (1971). De-novo brain tumours in renal-transplant recipients. *Lancet*, **i**, 983.

SCHWARTZ, R., EISNER, A., & DAMESHEK, W. (1959). The effect of 6-mercaptopurine on primary and secondary immune responses. *J. clin. Invest.*, **38**, 1394.

SCHWARTZ, R. (1964). *Immunologic Disorders in Malignant Lymphomas. Proceedings of the Fifth National Cancer Conference*, p. 645. Philadelphia: J. B. Lippincott Company.

SCHWARTZ, R., ANDRE-SCHWARTZ, J., ARMSTRONG, M. Y. K., & BELDOTTI, L. (1966). Neoplastic sequelae of allogenic disease. I. Theoretical considerations and experimental design. *Ann. N.Y. Acad. Sci.*, **129**, 804.

SIEGEL, J. H., JANIS, R., ALPER, J. C., SCHUTTE, H., ROBBINS, L., & BLAUFOX, J. (1969). Disseminated visceral Kaposi's Sarcoma appearing after human renal homograft operation. *J. Am. med. Ass.*, **207**, 1493.

SISKIND, G. W., DUNN, P., & WALKER, J. G. (1968). Studies on the control of antibody synthesis. *J. exp. Med.*, **127**, 55.

SJÖRGEN, H. (1965). Transplantation methods as a tool for detection of tumour specific antigens. *Prog. exp. Tumor Res.*, **6**, 289.

SNELL, G. D., & STIMPFLING, J. H. (1966). Genetics of Tissue Transplantation. *Biology of the Laboratory Mouse*, p. 457. Green, E. L. (Ed.). New York: Dover Publications Inc.

SOLOWAY, A. C., & RAPAPORT, F. T. (1965). Immunologic responses in cancer patients. *Surgery Gynec. Obstet.*, **121**, 756.

SOROF, S., YOUNG, E. M., McCUE, M. M., & FETTERMAN, P. L. (1963). Zonal electrophoresis of the soluble proteins of liver and tumour in azodye carcinogenesis. *Cancer Res.*, **23**, 685.

STARZL, T. E., MARCHIORO, T. L., TERASAKI, P. I., PORTER, T. D., FARIS, T. J., HERRMANN, D. L., VREDEVOE, D. L., HUTT, M. P., OGDEN, D. A., & WADDELL, W. R. (1965). Chronic survival after human renal homotransplantation. Lymphocyte antigen matching, pathology and influence of thymectomy. *Ann. Surg.*, **162**, 749.

STARZL, T. E., MARCHIORO, T. L., PORTER, K. A., IWASAKI, Y., & CERILLI, G. J. (1967). The use of heterologous antilymphoid agents in canine renal and liver homotransplantation and in human renal transplantation. *Surgery Gynec. Obstet.*, **123**, 301.

STARZL, T. E., LERNER, R. A., DIXON, F. J., GROTH, C. G., BRETTSCHNEIDER, L., & TERASAKI, P. I. (1968). Schwartzman reaction after human renal homotransplantation. *New Engl. J. Med.*, **278**, 642.

STARZL, T. E., BRETTSCHNEIDER, L., PENN, I., BELL, P., GROTH, C. G., BLANCHARD, H., KASHIWAGI, N., & PUTNAM, C. W. (1969). Orthotopic liver transplantation in man. *Transplantn Proc.*, **1**, 216.

STĚRZL, J. (1960). Inhibition of the inductive phase of antibody formation by 6-mercaptopurine examined by the transfer of isolated cells. *Nature, Lond.*, **185**, 256.

STEWART, S. E., EDDY, B. E., & STANTON, M. F. (1959). *Proceedings of the 3rd Canadian Cancer Conference*, p. 287. New York.

STOKER, M. (1964). Cell virus relationships with tumour viruses. *Br. med. Bull.*, **2**, 145.

STOKER, M. (1966). *Mechanisms of Viral Carcinogenesis. Proc. 6th Canadian Cancer Congress*, p. 357. New York: Pergamon.

STUART, F. P., SAITOH, T., FITCH, F. W., & SPARGO, B. H. (1968). Immunologic enhancement of renal allografts in the rat. *Surgery*, **64**, 17.

TEE, D. E. H., WANG, M., & WATKINS, J. (1965). Antigenc properties of human tumours, 'Tumour Specific Antigens'. *Eur. J. Cancer*, **1**, 315.

TERASAKI, P. I., BOLD, E. J., CANON, J. A., & LONGMIRE, W. P., Jr. (1961). Antibody response to homografts. VI. *In vitro* cytotoxins produced by skin homografts in rabbits. *Proc. Soc. exp. Biol. Med.*, **106**, 133.

TERASAKI, P. I., VREDEVOE, D. L., STARZL, T. E., PORTER, K. A., MARCHIORO, T. L., FARIS, T. D., & HERMANN, T. J. (1966). Serotyping for homotransplantation. *Transplantn*, **4**, 688.

THOMPSON, J. S., & GURNEY, C. W. (1960). Heterologous transplantation of mouse tumours into the new born albino rat. *Cancer Res.*, **20**, 1365.

UPTON, A. (1963). Biological effects of ionising radiation. *Int. Rev. exp. Path.*, **2**, 199.

VAN ROOD, J. J., VAN LEEUWEN, A., BRUNING, J. W., & PORTER, K. A. (1969). *The Importance of Leukocyte Antigens in Renal Transplantation. Proceedings of the First International Congress of the Transplantation Society*, p. 213. Copenhagen: Munksgaard.

WALFORD, R. L., & HILDEMANN, W. H. (1965). Life span and lymphoma incidence of mice injected at birth with spleen cells across a weak histocompatibility locus. *Am. J. Path.*, **46**, 713.

WEAVER, J. M., ALGIRE, G. H., & PREHN, R. T. (1955). The growth of cells *in vivo* in diffusion chambers. II. The role of cells in the destruction of homografts in mice. *J. natn Cancer Inst.*, **15**, 1737.

WEILER, E. (1956). Antigenic differences between normal hamster kidney and stilboestrol induced kidney carcinoma: complement fixation on reactions with cytoplasmic particles. *Br. J. Cancer*, **10**, 553.

WESTROP, J. W., & GREEN, H. N. (1960). Binding of a hepatocarcinogen to the structural lipoprotein of rat liver: its bearing on the immunological theory of cancer. *Nature, Lond.*, **186**, 350.

WILSON, D. B., & BILLINGHAM, R. E. (1967). Lymphocytes and transplantation immunity. *Adv. Immunol.*, **7**, 189.

WILSON, R. E., HAGER, E. B., HAMPERS, C. L., CORSON, J. M., MERRILL, J. P., & MURRAY, J. E. (1968). Immunologic rejections of human cancer transplanted with a renal allograft. *New Engl. J. Med.*, **278**, 479.

WINN, H. J. (1961). Immune mechanisms in homotransplantations. II. Quantitative assay of the immunologic activity of lymphoid cells stimulated by tumour homografts. *J. Immunol.*, **86**, 228.

WOODS, D. A. (1969). Influence of antilymphocyte serum on DMBA induction of oral carcinogens. *Nature, Lond.*, **224**, 276.

WOODRUFF, M. F. A., & ANDERSON, N. A. (1963). Effect of lymphocyte depletion by thoracic duct fistula and administration of antilymphocyte serum on the survival of skin homografts in rats. *Nature, Lond.*, **200**, 702.

WOODRUFF, M. F. A. (1970). Personal communication.

ZAMECNIK, P. C. (1966). The mechanism of protein synthesis and its possible alteration in the presence of oncogenic RNA viruses. *Cancer Res.*, **26**, 1.

ZUKOSKI, C. F., LEE, H. M., & HUME, D. M. (1960). The prolongation of functional survival of canine renal homografts by 6-mercaptopurine. *Surg. Forum*, **11**, 470.

ZUKOSKI, C. F., CALLOWAY, J. M., & RHEA, W. G. (1965). Prolonged acceptance of a canine renal allograft achieved with prednisolone. *Transplantn*, **3**, 380.

7 Immunotherapy of Cancer

J. MAXWELL ANDERSON

INTRODUCTION

The most efficient cures of diseases that our philosophy can conceive involve the *potentiation of normal,* biophysical or biochemical processes or the *countering of abnormal* processes which lead to, or accompany, disease. Cancer presents very few examples of this ideal at present but studies of what has become known as 'host resistance' are clearly an early step in this apparently logical direction. Of the multitudinous factors, such as intercellular communication, metabolic peculiarity, biochemical epicurism and hormonal requirement, possibly involved in host resistance only one, the immune activities of the lymphoreticular system, will be considered in this chapter. Moreover we shall focus in as simple jargon-free language as possible* upon that small area of this subject, recently sharing in the huge expansion of scientific investigation, which concerns the treatment of human cancer. The paucity of experimental data in man necessitates reference to laboratory animal studies which are here placed in the human context without attempting a comprehensive evaluation of them.

First the concepts of ablationary treatment and autonomous growth are criticized in the light of modern attitudes to cancer biology, leading into a statement of basic immunological mechanisms involved in res-

---

* *Immunity* is the property whereby the lympho-reticular system makes a memorized response to an antigenic stimulus. This may result in a state of positive reaction known as sensitization, or in one of negative reaction (diminished or absent) known variously as immunological tolerance, immunological paralysis or immunosuppression. It is not strictly correct therefore to follow common usage of the word immunization as synonymous with sensitization or stimulation (see Gell and Coombs, 1968).

Cancer is used for any malignant growth in man, rodent or other experimental animal. Although this word is often synonymous with carcinoma, it will be used in the general manner because there is no other satisfactory single word for all categories of malignancies.

Autochthonous refers to tissues of any sort originating in the same host.

Syngeneic refers to tissues originating in an animal of the same inbred strain.

Allogeneic refers to tissues originating in different individuals of the same species or in members of a different inbred strain.

Allograft (homograft in the old terminology) is a portion of tissue of any type transplanted from one individual to another of the same species or between individuals of different inbred strains.

Autograft is a portion of tissue of any type transplanted from one site to another upon the same individual.

193

ponses to cancer and of recent discoveries in this field which appear relevant to treatment. There follows a tentative formulation of indications for immunotherapy and a description of possible methods of treatment and their recent applications.

Ignorance of the fundamental nature of cancer has fostered the development of two inter-related and apparently all-embracing doctrines which studies of the past two decades have shown to have very limited application. They are those of (1) treatment by ablation and (2) autonomous growth.

Until efficient early diagnostic tests are developed, we will have the problem of treating cancers which have invaded vital neighbouring parts or have metastasized widely making complete excision impossible. Intra-abdominal metastases from a cancer of the stomach or colon and distant metastases occurring some time after an apparently successful regime of mastectomy and irradiation for mammary cancer are two exasperatingly common situations demonstrating some of the inadequacies of surgical, and radiotherapeutic, ablation. More extensive excisions of cancer-bearing bowel or breast and the lymph-draining tissues have often reduced survival rates (Gilbertsen, 1969) or failed to improve them (Kaae and Johansen, 1967). The mistaken and still widely held view that cancers grow rapidly, which permeates these attitudes to treatment, should now be replaced by the concept of maturation of growth controls which are regarded as properties of the *whole organization* of an individual animal as well as characters of its component cells and organs. Growth of tissues may proceed with positive accretionary rapidity, or it may be slow, absent or even negative. Shifts within this physiological spectrum occur in the normal pre- and post-natal growth of young animals, in liver regeneration and in cancer growth; the rates of growth varying with the cell cycles of the tissues at different times. The cell cycles of rodent intestinal mucosa and bone marrow are approximately 10 hours whilst those of rodent cancers are rarely less than this. Thus the increased proliferation of cancers appears to be incidental to a failure to limit growth rate and to an impairment of differentiation, so that expansive growth is the result of accumulation of proliferating cells and not of an increased rate of proliferation. The normal restrictions upon growth and the stimuli for differentiation are unknown so that there is a vast field of biology in need of elucidation; it involves the characterization of cell cycles and trigger mechanisms as well as the study of cell populations as a whole to establish patterns of proliferation and the laws governing the architecture of specific organs. Enquiry along these lines is a logical approach to the problems of inadequacy and irrelevance that ablation necessarily presents.

Autonomy implies that the growth of a cancer is determined by certain (unknown) characteristics of the cancer itself, and is not influenced by any of the systems of the organism as a whole. It has been favoured, although evidence for hormonal control of mammary cancer has been available since 1896 (Beatson), and generally regarded as the norm with a few outstanding exceptions. The simple, though technically difficult, observation of cancer cells in the brachial venous blood of between 10 and 40% of patients, and in almost 100% of blood samples withdrawn from the venous effluent of cancer-bearing organs, by many workers, presented one of the most strongly discordant challenges to autonomy. Since the occurrence of metastases does not match this outpouring of presumably viable cells, comprehensive inhibitors of growth must be widespread. This reasoning, in association with observations of prolonged dormancy with subsequent growth and of spontaneous regressions such as the 176 cases—half were one of either choriocarcinoma, hypernephroma, melanoma or neuroblastoma, all tumours whose rarity may result from powerful host restraints—described by Everson and Cole (1966), has with gathering momentum propelled medical thought in the direction of systemic controls of growth.

BASIC IMMUNOLOGY

Twenty five years ago the young biology of tissue transplantation borrowed and developed many concepts and techniques from experimental cancer. Now this process is reversed. The relevance to cancer of the concepts of immunity that have evolved in transplantation biology are increasingly obvious, and are the focus of basic studies and of applications to treatment. The mechanisms for removal of foreign (non-self) material which has by accident or artifice passed through the surface or visceral lining of the body are part of the functions of the lympho-reticular system. They often involve *memory* with a depressed or an increased response to second or subsequent exposures to the same material and are therefore considered to be *mechanisms of immunity*. The belief has gradually evolved that the body is continually patrolled by the agents of the lympho-reticular system for the detection and elimination of any foreign material, and this is the essential nature of the well-known rejection of surgical transplants. It is widely accepted that these patrols deal with microorganisms, particulate matter, cells, tissues or organs from other individuals, and most significantly in the present context, with cancer cells. This system was aptly named 'immunological surveillance' by Burnett (1957) and it is the neatest and most comprehensive hypothesis available for explaining the variable natural histories of cancers of the same type, the apparently innocent fate of circulating cancer cells, spontaneous regression, and the vagaries of dormancy.

Specific actions and reactions involved in immunity require to be defined and they are generally described in terms of antigens and antibodies. An antigen is a substance capable of provoking a specific reaction against itself in a potentially reactive individual; its most basic property is a mosaic of molecular configurations, outlines or twists. Many parts of the mosaic are potential antigenic determinants which activate the production of immunoglobulins of a specific type when the antigen is placed in the tissues or circulation of a foreign host. In most mammals including man there are three main classes of immunoglobulin which can function as antibody and are designated A (IgA), G (IgG) and M (IgM). IgG is present in highest concentration in the serum immunoglobulins and in most antibodies. It consists of two light amino-acid chains of low molecular weight (about 22,000) and two heavy chains (molecular weight of about 50,000). It is widely agreed that variation in the sequences of the amino acids constituting these chains is the basis of the specificity of an antibody for a given antigen. Thus antibody may be defined as a population of immunoglobulin molecules specifically capable of uniting at their combining sites with a definable substance which has a more or less unique physico-chemical configuration.

Antibody is produced by the lympho-reticular system in two ways. The well-known circulating antibody in plasma is produced by plasma cells principally located in the medullary cords and germinal centres of lymph nodes and the spleen in response to antigens quite unrelated to the host. A second type of response occurs towards antigens originating in the host or very closely resembling antigens of the host's tissues; in this case antibody is produced by small lymphocytes, now designated 'antigen-reactive', and retained within them until they reach the foreign antigen to destroy it either by releasing antibody into the tissues or directly into the target material. This *cell-mediated immunity* is responsible for delayed hypersensitivity reactions like that following the intradermal injection of tuberculoprotein. The nature of the antigenic determinants is known in only very few of these situations but it is widely believed that they are host antigens modified by a hapten, a skin-reactive chemical, a virus or a somatic mutation. According to this necessarily abbreviated account, which may be taken as acceptable to most students of immunology, it is clear that the reactions towards tissue transplanted from other individuals of the same sort (species) will be dealt with by the mechanisms mediated by cells, as has been indubitably established by many researches during the past two decades. The interchangeability of different cell types of the lympho-reticular system, particularly the roles of the bone marrow stem cells and of the thymus, is the subject of much speculation and study at present.

To postulate immunity related to cancer calls for the demonstration of cancer-specific antigen or antigens, and for evidence that the lympho-reticular system of a cancer-bearing host reacts against these non-self antigens by producing corresponding antibody and or, antigen-reactive small lymphocytes. Immune reactions, whether of the delayed hyper-sensitivity type or not, to common antigens and to cancers of the same and of other sorts, are collateral responses of obvious interest, which will now be reviewed following a statement of the evidence for cancer-specific immunity, making special reference to data of possible thera-peutic interest.

Presumably the existence of cancer-specific antigens was suspected by medical scientists shortly after the discovery of vaccination and the development of the concept of immunity in relation to disease. The idea was certainly accepted by 1895 when Héricourt and Richet attempted passive 'immunization' with antisera produced in animals injected with human tumours. Bashford (1906) claimed in the Fourth Annual Report of the Imperial Cancer Research Fund that prior inoculations of tumour, and of whole blood in mice, prevented the growth of trans-plants of a mammary adenocarcinoma. Although closely inbred mice were not available at that time and the experiments could not be controlled genetically, careful observations appear to have been made upon many thousands of animals, confirming that after spontaneous disappearance of some of the transplanted tumours subsequent trans-plants did not grow despite repeated inoculations. Bashford suggested that the effects of protecting inoculations "must have been primarily produced by way of the body fluids", and he noted that the results showed "only . . . the possibility of rendering normal mice unsuitable for the growth of experimental cancer". Established transplants and spontaneous cancers were not affected. In the intervening 64 years this sort of finding has been repeatedly obtained but, little understood, by workers with more sophisticated techniques and genetically controlled animals, with the result that the present generation has viewed 'cancer immunity' rather sceptically. However, gradual, and latterly rapid, accumulation of knowledge has demanded that scepticism give way to critical optimism.

Cancer-specific antigens were first identified in a little-quoted study by Gross (1943) describing the failure of mice to accept transplants of a specific cancer after they had been immunized with material from the same cancer growing upon syngeneic mice. Similar specificities have been demonstrated in many other systems (Baldwin, 1955; Prehn and Main, 1957; Old and Boyse, 1964; Klein et al., 1960; Baldwin and Moore, 1968). Correlations with three of the characteristics of cancer-specific antigens in laboratory rodents have been made in man. These are (1) their comparability to transplantation antigens of normal tissues and thus their classification as antigens of the delayed-hypersensitivity type invoking cell-mediated immunity; the responses are, however, much weaker than those which follow exposure to normal transplantation antigens. (2) the *group* specificity of all cancers induced by a given virus in any single strain of susceptible rodent and (3) the *individual* specificity of spontaneous (Baldwin, 1966) and of chemical-induced cancers (Prehn and Main, 1957; Klein and Klein, 1962; Baldwin and Barker, 1967a; Baldwin, 1970). Such cancers have different antigenic determinants although induced by the same chemical, and multiple cancers induced in one animal by the same chemical also have specific antigenicity for each cancer. The reasons for this heterogeneity and for the difference from virus-induced cancers are unknown. It is interesting to note that occasionally a chemical-induced cancer has antigens also present in embryonic tissues of the host animal, suggesting that the chemical has allowed the expression of dormant genetic material that was active transiently during embryogenesis, recalling, but not necessarily in accord with, Cohnheim's theory of 'embryonic rests' of cells as the sources of some cancers. In defining human cancer-specific antigens the greatest problem, as with rodent cancers, is the complexity of the mixtures of antigens in all normal and abnormal tissues, and the difficulty of reducing test reactions with unwanted antigens to the minimum. The technique of labelling antibody with fluorescein has solved this problem for colonic cancer, melanoma, osteosarcoma and Burkitt lymphoma. Gold and Freedman (1965) used it to provide the first unequivocal demonstration of cancer-specific antigens in carcinomas of the colon. Morton *et al.* (1968) found that all of 7 melanomas tested contained a common cancer-specific antigen. Similar results were obtained with melanoma by Lewis *et al.* (1969) and with sarcomas (Morton *et al.*, 1969). The sharing of common antigens by each of these and the intra-cellular location of the antigen suggest that viruses are involved in these cases, as is also likely in Burkitt lymphoma in which cancer-specific antigens have been detected upon cell membrane and in cytoplasm (Henle and Henle, 1966; Klein *et al.*, 1967).

These recent successes have been obtained by labelling specific antibody found in the serum of cancer-bearing and of some normal individuals, but the techniques have not been successful in the common cancers, with the exception of carcinoma of the colon, probably because immune reactions mediated principally by cells, rather than by humoral antibody are involved. On this account cutaneous responses of the delayed-hypersensitivity type towards cancer-specific antigens and positive results in other tests of cellular immunity, would be expected. Delayed cutaneous hypersensitivity to extracts of autologous cancers has been demonstrated in approximately one quarter of each of two series (Hughes and Lytton, 1964; Stewart, 1968) in one of which a few patients gave an immediate response. Immediate responses, within 15 or 20 minutes of intradermal injection, were observed in all of another group of 48 patients (Grace and Kondo, 1958) and there were no positive reactions to extracts of unspecified normal tissue from each patient. The differences between these reports probably reside in the heterogeneity of the immune status of each of the groups studied, and further investigation of them in this context is worthwhile, especially since a cellular infiltrate similar to that of delayed cutaneous hypersensitivity is seen around mammary (Cutler *et al.*, 1969) and gastric (Black *et al.*, 1954) cancers with a good prognosis, and since in humans sensitized by allografts of skin delayed cutaneous hypersensitivity to specific cell-free extracts is present (Merrill *et al.*, 1961).

Non-specific delayed hypersensitivity reactions to tuberculin and other bacterial antigens are often absent from cancer-bearing patients in whom skin allografts survive longer than in normal subjects (Snyderman, 1960; Kelly and Lamb, 1960; Miller *et al.*, 1961; Gardner *et al.*, 1962), but these reactions depend upon the uncontrolled natural exposure to microorganisms, and cellular immunity is more adequately assessed by sensitization with a chemical such as dinitrochlorobenzene (DNCB) and subsequent challenge. The simplicity of technique, reproducibility and end-point assessment with DNCB are all superior to skin transplantation and its more complex immunological function of rejection. 95–100% of normal subjects are DNCB-positive. In cancer-bearing patients approximately the same rate of positivity accompanies a good prognosis while approximately the same rate of negativity accompanies a poor prognosis (Eilber and Morton, 1970). A similar condition exists in Hodgkin's disease where half of those patients in good condition have depressed delayed hypersensitivity reactions whereas 88% of those in poor condition are deficient (Lamb *et al.*, 1962). The recovery of absent tuberculin sensitivity following apparently successful treatment noted in cancer of the lung (Hughes and Mackay, 1965) is a thread of evidence favouring assessment of non-specific cellular immunity as a measure of prognosis in cancer. In association with knowledge of specific cell-mediated reactions against autochthonous cancer this type of information may find a place in selection of different regimes of immunotherapy, for a reactive host may benefit from active sensitization and a non-reactive host may require passive or augmentative measures.

Although the bulk of current evidence establishes the antigen-reactive lymphocyte as the major vector of immune responses towards cancer-specific antigens, as well as towards the non-self histocompatibility antigens of normal tissues transplanted from another individual, the importance of humoral antibody must be acknowledged. The history of antibody's significance starts in 1907 when Flexner and Jobling reported unusually rapid growth of cancers transplanted to rats previously injected with cancer material killed by heat. Twenty five years later similar effects were observed in mice and rabbits by Casey (1932) who called it 'enhancement of malignancy'. The term 'enhancement' has been retained by later workers, prominent among whom is Kaliss (1965) who has shown that the phenomenon is due to the presence of humoral antibody and that the effect can be passively transferred to other hosts by injection of serum. Kaliss and other investigators have observed that mixing antisera with cancer cells *in vitro* allows the development of cancers from these cells when reimplanted to hosts under conditions that otherwise preclude growth. A double concept of the paradoxical behaviour of humoral antibody in enhancement has evolved from the many attempts to define it—and it appears that antibody may act upon either (1) the afferent limb of the cellular immunity system by encountering cancer-specific antigens before they reach lymphoid nodes or centres where they would normally initiate the activation of antigen-sensitive lymphocytes, or (2) the efferent limb of the same system by blocking receptors on the tumour cells so that antigen-reactive lymphocytes cannot recognize and attack the cells. The second of these views has received strong support from observations made with a technique of culturing cancer cells and lymphocytes together (Hellström and Sjögren, 1965; Hellström, 1967). This work is remarkable particularly for its reproducibility with different systems of animal cancers and for the correlation between these results and those obtained using human material (Hellström *et al.*, 1968b). Although the methods have been criticized by several workers their validity has apparently been confirmed in studies reported by Barski and Youn (1969), Bubenik and Perlman (1970) and Baldwin and Embleton (1971).

The technique is known as the colony inhibition test (Fig. 1) and it consists of placing the suspension of cells from a cancer into a Petri

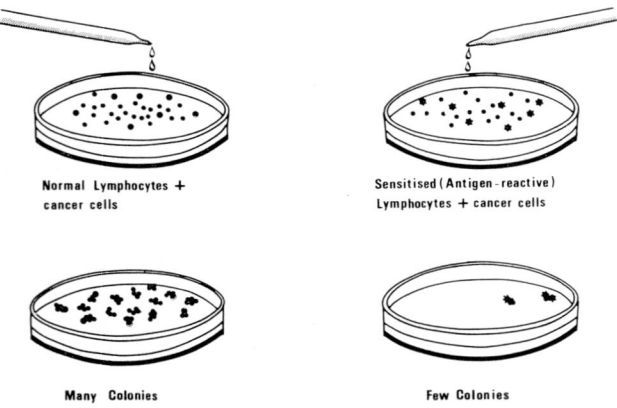

Normal Lymphocytes +   Sensitised (Antigen-reactive)
cancer cells   Lymphocytes + cancer cells

Many Colonies   Few Colonies

FIG. 7.1. The 'colony inhibition' test.

dish and observing the number of colonies formed by dividing cells aggregating into separate clumps, each derived from a single cell. Comparison of the number of colonies formed when antigen-reactive lymphocytes are used and the number of colonies with control lymphocytes gives a measure of the number of cancer cells killed or inhibited by the test lymphocytes. The action of serum alone or combined with lymphocytes has also been measured in this way. Hellström studied four different animal systems with a high incidence of spontaneous regression of cancer growth and the results were in general the same in all situations. Hosts in which cancers grew had factors in their sera which blocked the inhibition of their own cancers' colony formation by their own lymphocytes, presumably by combining with or coating the cancer cells. This factor was located in the 7S fraction of the serum globulins indicating that it was antibody-like material which may in nature defeat the attack of host lymphocytes upon a cancer, in accordance with the hypothetical action of the efferent form of enhancement. Indications that this may be the situation in man were obtained in a study of a large variety of cancers including those of breast, colon, larynx, lung, lip and thyroid, also melanoma, sarcoma and Wilm's tumour (Hellström et al., 1968b, 1971).

Neuroblastoma of childhood has been most extensively studied and may be regarded as a model, evoking a strong, aetiologically obscure immune response, for human cancer in general. It often grows rapidly and sometimes regresses spontaneously like the animal systems already discussed. Lymphocytes from patients with neuroblastoma inhibit colony formation by cells from their own cancers and from the cancers of others but they do not inhibit colony formation by normal cells. Surprisingly lymphocytes from the mothers of the patients and from some relatives inhibited colony formation by neuroblastoma cells from a number of hosts, recalling the cross-reactivity reported in a fluorescent antibody study whereby cancer-specific antigens were demonstrated in melanomas and sarcomas (Morton et al., 1968, 1969). Both cases may be manifestations of involvement, though not necessarily causative, of viruses. Blocking factor which abrogated the colony inhibition of patients' own lymphocytes upon neuroblastoma cells was almost invariably present in the serum from other patients with growing neuroblastomas.

Thus Hellström has advanced understanding of enhancement in man and animals by proposing a role for enhancing or *blocking factor* in natural conditions. The work has also re-affirmed the existence of cancer-specific antigens and established not only the involvement, but also the integration, of humoral and cellular immunity in cancer biology. Another potentially important development of this work is the demonstration of a *de-blocking* factor, in the sera of animals with regressing tumours, which decreases the blocking effect of sera from animals with growing cancers, indicating that it may be worthwhile to pursue the characterization of this material as a possible means of treatment.

INDICATIONS FOR IMMUNOTHERAPY

Application to patient care of the information discussed above, and of background knowledge which cannot be reviewed here in the interests of lucidity and space, is a challenge of some delicacy. The clinical quandary is that terminal patients are unlikely to respond to immunotherapy, and that the best type of therapy devoid of risk for patients with localized cancers is difficult to determine. It is probably unrealistic to expect responses in patients with widespread disease since cure has never been achieved in a comparable animal system; also a high rate of failure would bring into disrepute methods of treatment which show recent promise, after engaging men's minds as being biologically feasible for at least a century. In the case of patients with a reasonably good prognosis many writers on this question have feared that enhancement rather than inhibition of growth might result from immunotherapy, but apart from the two animal preparations of primary inoculation with cancer material killed by heat and the subsequent passive transfer of serum, there are no other well-established reports of growth-stimulating procedures. Thus there is a strong case for the expansion of the few clinical studies of immunotherapy already made. This should be the province of critical investigators with bridled enthusiasm, mature clinical judgment and experience in immunology. It is an ideal point of confluence for the skills of the laboratory and of the clinic, in the well-established pattern of modern medical science.

With our present knowledge it is feasible to make a start upon formulating some indications for immunotherapy in cancer (Table I) always allowing that, at present, immunotherapies can only be adjuncts to established surgery and radiotherapy. Only the broadest outlines of such a system, in the following categories, can be construed.

1. those types of cancers known to *regress spontaneously* are worth intensive investigation such as has been undertaken with neuroblastoma, and with choriocarcinoma (Bagshawe, 1966, 1969). Hypernephroma and possibly melanoma fall into this category. Cancers of the prostate and the thyroid glands are diagnosed in minute form microscopically more frequently than their clinical presentations would suggest, indicating the possibility that growth controls operate in a manner similar to those clinically manifested in tumours that regress.

2. cancers in which *cancer-specific antigenicity has been demonstrated*, cancers of the colon and lung, osteosarcoma, melanoma and Burkitt lymphoma belong to this category.

TABLE I
Possible Indications for Immunotherapy as an Adjunct to Established Treatments

1. Cancers known to regress spontaneously on occasion:
   neuroblastoma
   choriocarcinoma
   hypernephroma
   (melanoma, prostate, thyroid)

2. Cancer-specific antigens demonstrated:
   colon
   lung
   osteosarcoma
   melanoma
   Burkitt lymphoma

3. Combined treatment advantageous:
   radiosensitization
      breast cancer
      colon cancer
      thyroid cancer
      head and neck cancer
      hypernephroma
      neuroblastoma

4. Small cancers with poor prognosis:
   sinuses and nasopharynx
   intracranial
   intraspinal

5. Extensive local spread or nodal metastases outwith feasible excision:
   breast cancer
   lung cancer
   melanoma

3. situations in which *combination of immunotherapy* with already established methods of treatment offers special advantages. The clearest example is radiosensitization by autotransplantation of irradiated tumour (Haddow and Alexander, 1964; Anderson *et al.*, 1970) which may be applicable to cancers of the breast, thyroid, and of the gastro-intestinal tract when unresectable due to local invasion, as well as to neuroblastoma and hypernephroma.

4. patients in whom the mass of a *cancer is small but the prognosis is poor*, because it infiltrates vital parts, for example cancers invading

the base of the skull or placed within the cranium or the spinal canal.

5. where *extension beyond the limits of local resection* has occurred before diagnosis, as is common with cancers of the breast and the lung and with melanoma.

METHODS OF IMMUNOTHERAPY

The central principle of immunotherapy in cancer is to potentiate or strengthen the cancer-specific sensitivity, which may be totally masked in unknown ways, or exist to only a small degree. It is, therefore, highly pertinent to question how sensitization and consequent destruction of cancer-specific antigen so rarely occurs. The three most cogent explanations are: (1) Hellström's proposal that blocking factors counteract the effect of antigen-sensitive lymphocytes; (2) that the inherent cell cycle time of successfully growing cancers allows a growth rate that cannot be contained by the weak sensitivity cancers commonly induce; (3) Alexander's (1970) suggestion that the first line of immune defence, the local lymph nodes draining a cancer-bearing part, are incapable of responding to the cancer-specific antigens, although retaining other immune functions, until the cancer is excised. It may be that continual perfusion of the nodes with antigen interferes with the migration of only those cells immunologically activated by that antigen because the nodal response to other antigens is unaffected. In the rat experiment reported (Alexander *et al.*, 1969) function of the suppressed nodes, as measured by the appearance of immunoblasts in the effluent lymph, had returned within 24 hours after excision of the cancer. Thus the nodal suppression is temporary, it is also localized since distant nodes were able to react to a challenge of lethally X-irradiated autochthonous cancer cells. This hypothesis requires verification in other animal systems and in man. Elimination of such post-excisional activity in regional lymph nodes of human subjects by therapeutic X-irradiation could account for the reduced survival rate in mammary cancer patients so treated, that has been suggested in the extensive, albeit retrospective, analysis of Bond (1967) (but see Chapter 1).

Theoretically an attack may be mounted at each of these possible escape routes, and elsewhere upon the immune system of action and reaction, by at least 4 approaches that promote sensitization (Table II) by:

1. preventing the action of blocking factor by giving de-blocking factor.

2. augmenting cellular immunity by infusing lymphocytes.

TABLE II

POSSIBLE SENSITIZING IMMUNOTHERAPIES

1. Prevent action of blocking factor.
2. Augment cellular immune system.
3. Additional cancer-specific antigenic stimulus.
4. Non-specific antigenic stimulation of lympho-reticular system.

3. providing alternative sources of cancer-specific antigen to increase the stimulus to the weak system of immunity that is apparently a common feature in cancer.

4. non-specific stimulation of the lympho-reticular system.

De-blocking factor. Passive transference of sensitivity in man by the intravenous injection of antiserum raised in animals has been attempted frequently and was the first method of cancer immunotherapy reported (Héricourt and Richet, 1895). The use of de-blocking factor is a particular type of passive immunotherapy that would be indicated if it were determined that a patient was making blocking factor responsible for preventing the action of his antigen-reactive lymphocytes. Further attention should therefore be given to Hellström's studies of colony inhibition with human cancers, and to the characterization of de-blocking factor. An obvious danger of administering an antiserum or antibody of unspecified nature is that it may be of the blocking type which may promote the sort of rapid growth of cancer which has been called 'enhancement of malignancy' in animals (see above). No examples of this have been described in the relevant human studies but these mainly involve heterologous antisera, all types of which are generally toxic to the initiating antigen, whereas enhancement in animals is a property of homologous antisera and only of those raised with certain cancers in specific strains of inbred rodents. Clearly the unqualified term 'antibody' in this context is far too vague and there is a need for definition of those characters and properties of the different immunoglobulins related to the growth of cancers, and possibly of normal tissues.

Not only heterologous antisera have been used in human immunotherapy but also human gamma globulin either pooled (Moore *et al.*, 1957) or from autovaccinated patients (Finney *et al.*, 1960), and whole blood from a patient with spontaneous remission of melanoma (Sumner and Foraker, 1960) have been the subjects of uncontrolled studies with little evidence of benefit. None of these treatments nor any of the other immunotherapies attempted have been encouraging; Southam (1961) presented a comprehensive account up to that time and the field will not be re-reviewed here.

A recent notable report is that of regression of Burkitt lymphoma in otherwise untreated patients, following the infusion of homologous plasma from lymphoma patients in prolonged remission (Ngu, 1967). This claim may be interpreted in Hellström's terms as indicating the presence of de-blocking factor, and it should be investigated further in this context with a view to the development of effective immunotherapy for lymphoma and for the common cancers of Caucasoid peoples although the observation has not been confirmed (Fass et al., 1970).

Cellular augmentation. To accept that lymphoid cells discharge an intimately important role in the rejection of experimentally trans-planted cancers and in the control of growth of naturally occurring cancers implies that these cells are deficient in quality or quantity when cancers grow apace. Augmentation of this phase of immunity by trans-ferring white blood cells or lymphocytes from one individual to another is one obvious possible corrective. Transference of sensitized lymphoid cells is more acceptable since the feasibility of transmitting sensitivity to delayed-type antigens such as normal histocompatibility and cancer-specific antigens by means of lymph nodal or splenic cells (Mitchison, 1954), thoracic duct or peripheral blood cells (Billingham et al., 1962) and by peritoneal cells (Old et al., 1963) is well substantiated. This type of animal experiment can be so designed that the cellular transplant is not rejected by virtue of differing from the recipient in normal histo-compatibility antigens, but such ideal conditions cannot ordinarily be achieved with human subjects. Perhaps this will become possible with improvements in tissue typing, but a simpler possibility is to sensitize the patient's own lymphoid cells *in vitro* and return them to the circu-lation as specifically antigen-reactive cells. The two main types of cellular augmentation are therefore the allografts and the autografts.

(a) *Allografts of lymphoid cells.* Bone marrow grafts given to acci-dentally irradiated patients (Mathé et al., 1959) upon the grounds of comparable animal experiments (Barnes and Loutit, 1953) appeared to have some success and subsequently stimulated attempts to treat leukaemia by intentional irradiation followed by bone marrow grafts (Mathé et al., 1965). Little success attended these efforts. In some cases (Graw and Santos, 1971) the grafted cells appeared to react against the hosts in the manner well known in animals as graft-versus-host disease, secondary disease and runt disease, despite close matching of the trans-plantation antigens of donor and host. Unsensitized splenic cells were given to 8 patients with advanced cancers following courses of chemo-therapy aimed at reducing immune responses which would destroy the grafts (Woodruff and Nolan, 1963). Growth of some of the cancers appeared to be reduced by the immunotherapy but the multiple treatments involved do not allow clear assessments.

Transplantation of sensitized allogeneic lymphoid cells has been attempted and extensively studied by Dr. G. E. Moore at Roswell Park Memorial Institute in the United States of America. Subcutaneous transplants of comparable cancers were exchanged between pairs of patients, and their circulating leucocytes were cross-transfused for 3 weeks starting 10 days after the cancer transplantations. Twenty-six of 40 patients were acceptable for evaluation, all were conventionally incurable with widespread metastases and most were cases of melanoma. Two complete regressions, 3 partial regressions and 2 with regression of some of many metastases were observed. None of these patients had chemotherapy, radiotherapy or other treatment (Nadler and Moore, 1966). Presumably the transplanted cells were rejected since most patients did not respond and since skin sensitivities were stated not to be transferred. Similar results were reported in a larger series of patients with melanoma (Nadler and Moore, 1968) and in a group with melanoma and colonic carcinoma (Humphrey et al., 1968). At present 23 positive responses (all or the majority of lesions decreased by 50% in size) have been observed in the Roswell Park Memorial Institute series of 118 patients with various cancers, mainly melanoma. Metastases disappeared completely in 3 of the 23 responding patients (Moore, 1970).

In general the results with allografts have not been encouraging; presumably the cells are rejected, but this has not been definitely demonstrated, nor has sensitivity to the target cancer.

(b) *Autografts of 'sensitized' lymphoid cells.* Lymphoid cells appear to remain in tissue culture for many weeks without growth and then proliferate rapidly while retaining cytological characters of normality. According to Moore (1969) these cells appear to have an infinite life span, unlike human fibroblasts in culture (Hayflick, 1965). These and other important findings carry implications that demand their study by other workers. There are no animal studies of similar systems involving *in vitro* sensitization to autochthonous cancer but since the concept has a sound theoretical basis clinical trials have been made. Moore and Moore (1969) established a cell line from primary cultures of the peripheral leucocytes of a patient with metastatic melanoma, after a dormant period of 157 days. The proliferating cells had a normal karyotype and produced immunoglobulin. Ten grams of metastatic melanoma were minced, X-irradiated and added to a 15 litre culture of the patient's lymphoid cells; thereafter cells were harvested from the culture repeatedly and returned to the patient by intravenous infusion. During a period of 2 months 115 grams of cultured lymphoid cells were given. Some of the patient's metastases regressed, others did not. The patient returned to his occupation of medical practice. One of another 5 patients similarly treated had a dramatic regression of a huge recurrent melanoma but several other nodules did not regress. Moore has established more than one thousand lymphoid cell lines and he stresses the apparent normality of the cells, which have successfully raised heterologous antisera in horses for use in transplantation immunosuppression (Najarian *et al.*, 1969). Further developments should aim at establishing that these cells are reactive towards autochthonous cancer and at defining the *in vivo* conditions of this reaction, bearing in mind the roles of blocking and de-blocking factors discussed above. It seems feasible that cells from spleen, bone marrow, lymph nodes or the thoracic duct could also be cultured in this way and tested in similar experiments.

Increased specific antigenic stimulus. To impel the patient's natural immune reactions in the direction of sensitization towards his own cancer is analogous to the active 'immunization' procedures of immunoprophylaxis for infectious diseases. This may be attempted by replanting a preparation of the cancer. The following procedures for increasing the antigenicity of such a sample have been studied in man:

(a) rendering down to a suspension of whole cells and X-irradiation to prevent growth. This appeared to be effective in the animal cancers tested by Cohen *et al.* (1956), Haddow and Alexander (1964) and by a number of others. The same may hold for some human cancers since 2 patients inoculated with irradiated cells from their own melanomas developed antibodies to the melanoma cells, which had not been detected previously (Lewis *et al.*, 1969); however, no significant clinical advantage was observed in another group of 10 melanomas so treated (Van den Brenk, 1969) but 3 of these had distant metastases. Anderson *et al.* (1970) copied the rat experiment of Haddow and Alexander (1964), aiming to sensitize a pilot group of 9 patients with early cancer of the breast to subsequent proposed radiotherapy. Inguinal lymph nodes draining the inoculation sites had proliferations of blast cells in the thymus-dependent areas, these were similar to the appearances during rejection of allografts of skin (de Sousa and Anderson, 1970) and typical of cell-mediated responses (Parrott *et al.*, 1966). No clinical evidence of enhancement of malignancy in these patients, nor in another with cancer of the colon similarly treated, was found during observation periods of 2–4 years; however, 3 patients with many distant metastases died without evidence of benefit.

Chemical attenuation of suspensions of whole cancer cells by formalin (Bismanis, 1964) and nitrogen mustard (Kikkawa, 1961) appears to retain antigenicity of animal cancers, and the methods seem worthy of human application.

(b) Homogenization and admixture of the cancer sample with Freund's adjuvant has been a widely successful animal procedure which was applied to 114 patients with gynaecological cancers (Graham and Graham, 1959). Twenty-nine of these were fully evaluated and in 3 of them diminished growth of cancer was observed but each patient had either radiotherapy or surgery, leaving residual cancer, at the time of inoculation. Some melanoma-bearing patients treated similarly developed circulating antibody, but this was not seen in subjects with carcinoma of the colon (Hughes *et al.*, 1970).

(c) Coupling non-antigenic material to a highly antigenic protein makes both components antigenic in animals (Landsteiner, 1945). The technique was reported as producing a compound which consistently raised circulating antibody to human cancer cells (Czajkowski *et al.*, 1967) and was associated with favourable clinical responses. Another report of this technique failed to confirm either of these claims, but 1 of 23 sera (Cunningham *et al.*, 1969) did have cancer-specific precipitating antibody, and the absence of clinical evidence of enhancement of malignancy was noted. Thus the efficiency of coupling has not been established with human material and doubts have been expressed about the possibility of increasing the antigenicity of rodent cancer cells in this way (Baldwin and Barker, 1967b).

Non-specific lympho-reticular stimulation. The Calmette-Guérin bacillus (Stjernswärd, 1966), Zymosan (Martin *et al.*, 1968), *Corynebacterium parvum* (Woodruff and Boak, 1966) and vaccinia virus (Old *et al.*, 1961) are agents believed to stimulate the lympho-reticular system in a general non-specific way, thereby limiting growth of animal cancers. The Calmette-Guérin bacillus has produced temporary regression of skin nodules of melanoma when injected *locally*, in a manner similar to the response seen in primary cancers of skin treated by local application of a sensitizing chemical such as dinitrochlorobenzene (Klein, 1968). Both of these responses appear to be localized forms of sensitization but the part played by chemical toxicity of the agents is not fully evaluated. Vaccinia virus applied locally to skin nodules of melanoma is reported as producing regression of treated nodules and of distant melanoma (Belisario and Milton, 1961; Burdick *et al.*, 1964; Milton and Brown, 1966; Hunter-Craig *et al.*, 1970) but the mode of action is unknown. Controlled human studies of these agents which show convincing evidence of effectiveness against animal and human cancers are urgently needed.

CONCLUSION

Although it has been said that "prophecy is the most gratuitous form of error" I shall hazard the prediction that elucidation of the physiology of immunity will lead to exploitation of normal and pathological mechanisms in the diagnosis and treatment of cancer during the next decade or two. The clear establishment of antigenic specificity in animal cancers along with the early successful steps towards this goal in human cancers, the discovery of blocking and de-blocking factors in animal and human systems, and the few regressions of melanoma after infusion of cultured autologous and homologous lymphocytes are the principal pillars of this prediction. More experiments are clearly warranted with the aim of adding benefits of immunotherapy to the methods of surgery, radiotherapy and chemotherapy already known to eliminate or control cancers, and can be expected to add to our general understanding of human biology.

There can be little doubt that study of the whole cancer-bearing organism is a necessity where therapeutic applications are the driving forces. Until recent years fundamental knowledge has been inadequate to allow research workers to cope directly with cancers and it has been common to find that an investigator, after expending much time and energy upon study of a cancer, has turned to basic research in a particular discipline. It now seems that in many fields (including immunology, microbiology, biochemistry, cybernetics and epidemiology) the painstaking establishment of basic facts has set the stage for a new approach to the direct study of cancers. The interdisciplinary attitudes required for this sort of work are now common amongst progressive investigators and they can be confidently expected to open up the routes to successful treatment, and the prevention (Roe, 1967) of cancer. There is at times, however, a lack of vigour in the application of available knowledge. This must be corrected, investigation should be promoted, and the common attitude of hopeless inertia that many doctors take towards cancer should be discarded.

REFERENCES

ALEXANDER, P. (1970). Defeat of the Immune Defences of the Host in Primary Sarcomata. *The Biology and Surgery of Tissue Transplantation*, pp. 153–62. Anderson, J. M. (Ed.). Oxford and Edinburgh: Blackwell Scientific Publications.

ALEXANDER, P., BENSTED, J., DELORME, E. J., HALL, J. G., & HODGETT, J. (1969). Cellular immune responses to primary sarcomata in rats. Part II. Abnormal responses of nodes draining the tumour. *Proc. R. Soc.* (B), **174**, 237.

ANDERSON, J. M., DE SOUSA, M. A. B., HALNAN, K. E., KELLY, F., & HANNAH, G. (1970). Assessment of immunisation by autotransplantation of human cancer. *Br. J. Surg.*, **57**, 557.

BAGSHAWE, K. D. (1966). Immunotherapy of cancer. *Br. med. J.*, **ii**, 463.

BAGSHAWE, K. D. (1969). *Choriocarcinoma. The Clinical Biology of the Trophoblast and Its Tumours*, pp. 293–7. London: Edward Arnold.

BALDWIN, R. W. (1955). Immunity to methylcholanthrene induced tumours in inbred rats following atrophy and regression of the implanted tumours. *Br. J. Cancer*, **9**, 652.

BALDWIN, R. W. (1966). Tumour-specific immunity against spontaneous rat tumours. *Int. J. Cancer*, **1**, 257.

BALDWIN, R. W. (1970). Tumour specific antigens associated with chemically induced tumours. *Revue eur. Étud. clin. biol.*, **15**, 1.

BALDWIN, R. W., & BARKER, C. R. (1967a). Tumour-specific antigenicity of amino-azo-dye induced rat hepatomas. *Int. J. Cancer*, **2**, 355.

BALDWIN, R. W., & BARKER, C. R. (1967b). Immunization against human tumours. *Lancet*, **ii**, 1090.

BALDWIN, R. W., & EMBLETON, M. J. (1971). Demonstration by colony inhibition methods of cellular and humoral immune reactions to tumour-specific antigens associated with amino-azo-dye-induced rat hepatomas. *Int. J. Cancer*, **7**, 17.

BALDWIN, R. W., & MOORE, M. (1969). Isolation of membrane-associated tumour-specific antigen from an amino-azo dye-induced rat hepatoma. *Int. J. Cancer*, **4**, 753.

BARNES, D. W. H., & LOUTIT, J. F. (1953). Protective effects of implants of splenic tissue. *Proc. R. Soc. Med.*, **46**, 251.

BARSKI, G., & YOUN, J. K. (1969). Evolution of cell-mediated immunity in mice bearing an antigenetic tumour. Influence of tumour growth and surgical removal. *J. natn. Cancer Inst.*, **43**, 111.

BASHFORD, E. F. (1906). Report of the general superintendent. *Fourth Annual Report of the Imperial Cancer Research Fund*, pp. 5–11.

BEATSON, G. T. (1896). On the treatment of inoperable cases of carcinoma of the mamma: suggestions for a new method of treatment, with illustrative cases. *Lancet*, **ii**, 104 and 162.

BELISARIO, J. C., & MILTON, G. W. (1961). The experimental local therapy of cutaneous metastases of malignant melanoblastomas with cowpox vaccine or colcemid (demecolcine or omaine). *Aust. J. Derm.*, **6**, 113.

BILLINGHAM, R. E., SILVERS, W. K., & WILSON, D. B. (1962). Adoptive transfer of transplantation immunity by means of blood-borne cells. *Lancet*, **i**, 512.

BISMANIS, J. E. (1964). Immunisation of mice against Ehrlich ascites carcinoma with formalinised tumour cells grown in tissue culture. *J. Path. Bact.*, **87**, 444.

BLACK, M. M., OPLER, S. R., & SPEER, F. D. (1954). Microscopic structure of gastric carcinoma and the regional lymph nodes in relation to survival. *Surgery Gynec. Obstet.*, **98**, 725.

BOND, W. H. (1967). The Influence of Various Treatments on Survival Rates in Cancer of the Breast. *The Treatment of Carcinoma of the Breast*, pp. 24–39. Jarrett, A. S. (Ed.). Published for Syntex Pharmaceuticals Limited by Excerpta Medica Foundation.

BUBENICK, J., PERLMANN, P., HELMSTEIN, K., & MOBERGER, G. (1970). Immune response to urinary bladder tumours in man. *Int. J. Cancer*, **5**, 39.

BURDICK, K. H., & HAWK, W. A. (1964). Vitiligo in a case of vaccinia virus-treated melanoma. *Cancer, Philad.*, **17**, 708.

BURNET, F. M. (1957). Cancer—a biological approach. *Br. med. J.*, **i**, 779.

CASEY, A. E. (1932). Experimental enhancement of malignancy in the Brown–Pearce rabbit tumor. *Proc. Soc. exp. Biol. Med.*, **29**, 816.

COHEN, A., & COHEN, L. (1956). Radiobiology of the C3H mouse mammary carcinoma: increased radiosensitivity of the tumour induced by inoculation of the host with radiation-attenuated isografts. *Br. J. Cancer*, **10**, 312.

CUNNINGHAM, T. J., OLSON, K. B., LAFFIN, R., HORTON, J., & SULLIVAN, J. (1969). Treatment of advanced cancer with active immunization. *Cancer*, **24**, 932.

CUTLER, S. J., BLACK, M. M., MORK, T., HARVEI, S., & FREEMAN, C. (1969). Further observations on prognostic factors in cancer of the female breast. *Cancer*, **24**, 653.

CZAJKOWSKI, N. P., ROSENBLATT, M., WOLF, P. L., & VAZQUEZ., J. (1967). A new method of active immunisation to autologous human tumour tissue. *Lancet*, **ii**, 905.

DE SOUSA, M. A. B., & ANDERSON, J. M. (1970). A Study of Human Lymph Node Biopsies. *The Biology and Surgery of Tissue Transplantation*, pp. 175–83. Anderson, J. M. (Ed.). Oxford and Edinburgh: Blackwell Scientific Publications.

EILBER, F. R., & MORTON, D. L. (1970). Impaired immunologic reactivity and recurrence following cancer surgery. *Cancer*, **25**, 362.

EVERSON, T. C., & COLE, W. H. (1966). *Spontaneous Regression of Cancer.* Philadelphia: W. B. Saunders Company.

FASS, L., HERBERMAN, R. B., ZIEGLER, J., & MORROW, R. H., Jr. (1970). Evaluation of the effect of remission plasma on untreated patients with Burkitt's lymphoma. *J. nat. Canc. Inst.*, **44**, 145.

FINNEY, J. W., BYERS, E. H., & WILSON, R. H. (1960). Studies in tumour auto-immunity. *Cancer Res.*, **20**, 351.

FLEXNER, S., & JOBLING, J. W. (1907a). On the promoting influence of heated tumour emulsions on tumor growth. *Proc. Soc. exp. Biol. Med.*, **4**, 156.

FLEXNER, S., & JOBLING, J. W. (1907b). Restraint and promotion of tumour growth. *Proc. Soc. exp. Biol. Med.*, **5**, 16.

GARDNER, R. J., & PRESTON, F. W. (1962). Prolonged skin homograft survival in advanced cancer and cirrhosis of the liver. *Surgery Gynec. Obstet.*, **115**, 399.

GELL, P. G. H., & COOMBS, R. R. A. (1968). *Clinical Aspects of Immunology*, 2nd edition. Oxford and Edinburgh: Blackwell Scientific Publications.

GILBERTSEN, V. A. (1969). Results of treatment of stomach cancer. *Cancer*, **23**, 1305.

GOLD, P. (1967). Circulating antibodies against carcino-embryonic antigens of the human digestive system. *Cancer*, **20**, 1663.

GOLD, P., & FREEDMAN, S. O. (1965). Demonstration of tumor-specific antigens in human colonic carcinomata by immunological tolerance and absorption techniques. *J. exp. Med.*, **121**, 439.

GRACE, J. T., & KONDO, T. (1958). Investigations of host resistance in cancer patients. *Ann. Surg.*, **148**, 633.

GRAHAM, J. B., & GRAHAM, R. M. (1959). The effect of vaccine on cancer patients. *Surgery Gynec. Obstet.*, **109**, 131.

GRAW, R. G., Jr. & SANTOS, G. W. (1971). Bone marrow transplantation in patients with leukaemia. *Transplantation*, **11**, 197.

GROSS, L. (1943). Intradermal immunization of C3H mice against a sarcoma that originated in an animal of the same line. *Cancer Res.*, **3**, 326.

HADDOW, A., & ALEXANDER, P. (1964). An immunological method of increasing the sensitivity of primary sarcomas to local irradiation with X-rays. *Lancet*, **i**, 452.

HAYFLICK, L. (1965). The limited *in vitro* lifetime of human diploid cell strains. *Expl Cell Res.*, **37**, 614.

HELLSTRÖM, I. (1967). A colony inhibition (CI) technique for demonstration of tumour cell destruction by lymphoid cells *in vitro*. *Int. J. Cancer*, **2**, 65.

HELLSTRÖM, I., HELLSTRÖM, K. E., PIERCE, G. E., & BILL, A. H. (1968a). Demonstration of cell-bound and humoral immunity against neuroblastoma cells. *Proc. natn. Acad. Sci. U.S.A.*, **60**, 1231.

HELLSTRÖM, I., HELLSTRÖM, K. E., PIERCE, G. E., & YANG, J. P. S. (1968b). Cellular and humoral immunity to different types of human neoplasms. *Nature, Lond.*, **220**, 1352.

HELLSTRÖM, I., & SJÖGREN, H. O. (1965). Demonstration of H-2 isoantigens and polyoma specific tumor antigens by measuring colony formation *in vitro*. *Expl Cell Res.*, **40**, 212.

HELLSTRÖM, I., HELLSTRÖM, K. E., SJÖGREN, H. O., & WARNER, G. A. (1971). Demonstration of cell-mediated immunity to human neoplasms of various histological types. *Int. J. Cancer*, **7**, 1.

HENLE, G., & HENLE, W. (1966). Immunofluorescence in cells derived from Burkitt's lymphoma. *J. Bact.*, **91**, 1248.

HÉRICOURT, J., & RICHET, C. (1895). De la sérothérapie dans le traitement du cancer. *C. r. Acad. Sci.*, **121**, 567.

HUGHES, L. E., KEARNEY, R., & TULLY, M. (1970). A study in clinical cancer immunotherapy. *Cancer*, **26**, 269.

HUGHES, L. E., & LYTTON, B. (1964). Antigenic properties of human tumours: delayed cutaneous hypersensitivity reactions. *Br. med. J.*, **i**, 209.

HUGHES, L. E., & MACKAY, W. D. (1965). Suppression of the tuberculin response in malignant disease. *Br. med. J.*, **ii**, 1346.

HUMPHREY, L. J., LINCOLN, P. M., & GRIFFEN, W. O., Jr (1968). Immunologic response in patients with disseminated cancer. *Ann. Surg.*, **168**, 374.

HUNTER-CRAIG, I., NEWTON, K. A., WESTBURY, G., & LACEY, B. W. (1970). Use of vaccinia virus in the treatment of metastatic malignant melanoma. *Br. med. J.*, **2**, 512.

KAAE, S., & JOHANSEN, H. (1967). Simple versus Radical Mastectomy in Primary Breast Cancer. *Prognostic Factors in Breast Cancer, Proceedings of the First Tenovus Symposium, Cardiff, April 1967*, pp. 93–102. Forrest, A. P. M., and Kunkler, P. B. (Eds.). E. and S. Livingstone.

KALISS, N. (1965). Immunological enhancement and inhibition of tumour growth: relationship to various immunological mechanisms, *Fedn Proc. Fedn Am. Socs exp. Biol.*, **24**, 1024.

KELLY, W. D., LAMB, D. L., VARCO, R. L., & GOOD, R. A. (1960). An investigation of Hodgkin's disease with respect to the problem of homotransplantation. *Ann. N.Y. Acad. Sci.*, **87**, 187.

KLEIN, E. (1968). Tumors of the skin. X. Immunotherapy of cutaneous and mucosal neoplasms. *N.Y. St. J. Med.*, **68**, 900.

KLEIN, G., & KLEIN, E. (1962). Antigenic properties of other experimental tumors. *Cold Spring Harb. symp. quant. Biol.*, **27**, 463.

KLEIN, G., KLEIN, E., & CLIFFORD, P. (1967). Search for host defences in Burkitt lymphoma: membrane immunofluorescence tests on biopsies and tissue culture lines. *Cancer Res.*, **27**, 2510.

KLEIN, G., SJÖGREN, H. O., KLEIN, E., & HELLSTRÖM, K. E. (1960). Demonstration of resistance against methylcholanthrene-induced sarcomas in the primary autochthonous host. *Cancer Res.*, **20**, 1561.

KIKKAWA, K. (1961). Does inoculation of the attenuated or dead cells of Walker 256 tumor cause any inhibitory effects on tumor takes? (Preliminary study). *Osaka Cy med. J.*, **7**, 15.

LAMB, D., PILNEY, R., KELLY, W. D., & GOOD, R. A. (1962). Comparative study of the incidence of anergy in patients with carcinoma, Hodgkin's disease and other lymphomas. *J. Immunol.*, **89**, 555.

LANDSTEINER, K. (1945). *The Specificity of Serological Reactions*. Cambridge, Mass., Harvard University Press.

LEWIS, M. G., IKONOPISOV, R. L., NAIRN, R. C., PHILLIPS, T. M., FAIRLEY, G. H., BODENHAM, D. C., & ALEXANDER, P. (1969). Tumour-specific antibodies in human malignant melanoma and their relationship to the extent of the disease. *Br. med. J.*, **3**, 547.

MARTIN, D. S., & HAYWORTH, P. (1968). Life-time results of immunotherapy, combination chemotherapy, and surgery upon spontaneous breast cancer. *Proc. Am. Ass. Cancer Res.*, **9**, 45.

MATHÉ, G., AMIEL, J. L., SCHWARZENBERG, L., CATTAN, A., & SCHNEIDER, M. (1965). Adoptive immunotherapy of acute leukemia: experimental and clinical results. *Cancer Res.*, **25**, 1525.

MATHÉ, G., JAMMET, H., PENDIC, B., SCHWARZENBERG, L., DUPLAN, J. F., MAUPIN, B., LATARJET, R., LARRIEU, M. J., KALIC, D., & DJUKIC, Z. (1959). Transfusions et greffes de moelle osseuse homologue chez des humains irradiés à haute dose accidentellement. *Revue fr. Étud. clin. biol.*, **4**, 226.

MCNEER, G. P., CANTIN, J., CHU, F., & NIXON, J. J. (1968). Effectiveness of radiation therapy in the management of sarcoma of the soft somatic tissues. *Cancer*, **22**, 391.

MERRILL, J. P., FRIEDMAN, E. A., WILSON, R. E., & MARSHALL, D. C. (1961). Production of 'delayed type' cutaneous hypersensitivity to human donor leukocytes as a result of the rejection of skin homografts. *J. clin. Invest.*, **40**, 631.

MILLER, D. G., LIZARDO, J. G., & SNYDERMAN, R. K. (1961). Homologous and heterologous skin transplantation in patients with lymphomatous disease. *J. natn. Cancer Inst.*, **26**, 569.

MILTON, G. W., & BROWN, M. M. L. (1966). The limited role of attenuated smallpox virus in the management of advanced malignant melanoma. *Aust. N.Z. J. Surg.*, **35**, 286.

MITCHISON, N. A. (1954). Passive transfer of transplantation immunity. *Proc. R. Soc.* (B), **142**, 72.

MOORE, G. E. (1969). Lymphoblastoid cell lines from normal persons and those with nonmalignant diseases. *J. surg. Res.*, **9**, 139.

MOORE, G. E., & MOORE, M. B. (1969). Auto-inoculation of cultured human lymphocytes in malignant melanoma. *N.Y. St. J. Med.*, **69**, 460.

MOORE, G. E., SANDBERG, A., & AMOS, D. B. (1957). Experimental and clinical adventures with large doses of gamma and other globulins as anticancer agents. *Surgery*, **41**, 972.

MOORE, M., & PRICE, C. H. G. (1970). Personal communication.

MORTON, D. L., MALMGREN, R. A., HALL, W. T., & SCHIDLOVSKY, G. (1969). Immunological and virus studies with human sarcomas. *Surgery*, **66**, 152.

MORTON, D. L., MALMGREN, R. A., HOLMES, E. C., & KETCHAM, A. S. (1968). Demonstration of antibodies against human malignant melanoma by immunofluorescence. *Surgery*, **64**, 233.

NADLER, S. H., & MOORE, G. E. (1966). Clinical immunologic study of malignant disease: response to tumor transplants and transfer of leukocytes. *Ann. Surg.*, **164**, 482.

NADLER, S. H., & MOORE, G. E. (1968). Immunotherapy of malignant melanoma. *Geriatrics*, **23**, 150.

NAJARIAN, J. S., SIMMONS, R. L., GEWURZ, H., MOBERG, A., MERKEL, F., & MOORE, G. E. (1969). Anti-serum to cultured human lymphoblasts: preparation, purification and immunosuppressive properties in man. *Ann. Surg.*, **170**, 617.

NGU, W. A. (1967). Clinical Evidence of Host Defences in Burkitt Tumour. *UICC Symposium on the Treatment of Burkitt Tumour*, pp. 204–8. New York: Springer-Verlag.

OLD, L. J., BENACERRAF, B., CLARKE, D. A., CARSWELL, E. A., & STOCKERT, E. (1961). The role of the reticuloendothelial system in the host reaction to neoplasia. *Cancer Res.*, **21**, 1281.

OLD, L. J., & BOYSE, E. A. (1964). Immunology of experimental tumours. *A. Rev. Med.*, **15**, 167.

OLD, L. J., BOYSE, E. A., BURNETT, B., & LILLY, F. (1963). *Cell Bound Antibodies*, pp. 89–99. Philadelphia: Wistar Institute Press.

PARROTT, D. M. V., & DE SOUSA, M. A. B. (1966). Changes in the thymus-dependent areas of lymph nodes after immunological stimulation. *Nature, Lond.,* **212,** 1316.

PREHN, R. T., & MAIN, J. M. (1957). Immunity to methylcholanthrene induced sarcomas. *J. natn. Cancer Inst.,* **18,** 769.

ROE, F. J. C. (1967). *The Prevention of Cancer,* London: Butterworths.

SNYDERMAN, R. K., MILLER, D. G., & LIZARDO, J. G. (1960). Prolonged skin homograft and heterograft survival in patients with neoplastic disease. *Plastic reconstr. Surg.,* **26,** 373.

SOUTHAM, C. M. (1961). Applications of immunology to clinical cancer. Past attempts and future possibilities. *Cancer Res.,* **21,** 1302.

STEWART, T. H. M. (1968). The immunological reactivity of patients with cancer: a preliminary report. *Can. med. Ass. J.,* **22,** 342.

STJERNSWÄRD, J. (1966). Effect of bacillus-Calmette-Guérin and/or methylcholanthrene on antibody-forming cells measured at cellular level by hemolytic plaque test. *Cancer Res.* **26,** 1591.

SUMNER, W. C., & FORAKER, A. G. (1960). Spontaneous regression of human melanoma, clinical and experimental studies. *Cancer,* **13,** 79.

VAN DEN BRENK, H. A. S. (1969). Autoimmunization in human malignant melanoma. *Br. med. J.,* **4,** 171.

WOODRUFF, M. F. A., & BOAK, J. L. (1966). Inhibitory effect of injection of *Corynebacterium parvum* on the growth of tumour transplants in isogeneic hosts. *Br. J. Cancer,* **20,** 345.

WOODRUFF, M. F. A., & NOLAN, B. (1963). Preliminary observations on treatment of advanced cancer by injection of allogeneic spleen cells. *Lancet,* **ii,** 426.

8 Prospects from Radiobiology

N. M. BLEEHEN

INTRODUCTION

The application of critical investigative methods to the study of the effects of ionizing radiation on biological material was long delayed after its initial use in the therapy of patients. The development of a suitable method for assessing the viability of cells *in vitro* by Puck and Marcus (1956) provided the impetus for a rapid advance in our understanding of the effects of ionizing radiation at a cellular level. This has been associated with much work using other methods, so that we now have a considerable understanding of the effects of radiation at a molecular, cellular and tissue level. Simultaneously, our understanding of the growth pattern of normal and malignant tissues on a morphological and functional basis has helped to integrate this data in a coherent manner. Radiobiology is beginning to provide a rational explanation for the long observed results of radiotherapy and to suggest prospects for future improvements.

Radiotherapy has evolved numerous techniques, partly as a result of empirical clinical experience and partly as a development of current scientific thought. It has been found that the biological effect may depend on numerous factors. These include the quality of the radiation which may vary, either from the point of view of the energy spectrum of the electromagnetic radiation (X or γ rays) or the mass and charge of particles (electrons, neutrons, negative π mesons and protons); the dose rate at which the cells are exposed; the number of fractions into which the total dose is divided and the overall duration of the course of treatment. The presence or absence of dose-modifying factors (radio-protectors or sensitizers) presents possibilities for improving the therapeutic response.

This chapter will attempt to summarize some selected aspects of current radiobiological knowledge, indicating their relevance to radiotherapy and their potential for further practical developments. No attempt has been made to provide a detailed comprehensive discussion of the subject as there have been numerous recent reviews of the relevant literature and for further information readers are referred to Andrews, 1968; Deeley and Wood, 1967; Pizzarello and Witcofski, 1967.

CURRENT TECHNIQUES AND RESULTS

The goal of any curative radiation treatment of a cancer is the reduction of the number of viable tumour cells capable of sustained divisions (i.e. clonogenic cells) to below the number from which clinical recurrence will be likely. This should be performed without permanent incapacitating damage to the normal tissues of the host. Regaud (1923) provided some experimental evidence of the value of dividing the total dose of radiation into several smaller doses (fractionation) with his experiments on ram and rabbit testicles. This was applied by Coutard (1932) and others to the treatment of patients and has provided extensive empirical clinical experience. Whereas these methods yielded much practical information they were very difficult to quantitate accurately in terms of scientific criteria. Only recently have such observations been revived, with careful quantitative measurements of reactions of the normal and tumour tissues, to yield valuable information about the actions of the ionizing radiations.

ASSESSMENT OF CELL SURVIVAL FOLLOWING IRRADIATION

Puck and Marcus (1956) developed a simple method for measuring the effect of radiation on the reproductive viability of cells. They were able to grow HeLa cells on culture media so that viable cells would continue to divide and form visible colonies (clones). This technique enabled them to demonstrate the fraction of the total number of cells exposed which survived a single dose of radiation, and to relate this surviving fraction to the magnitude of exposure dose. A graphical plot of radiation dose and the log of the surviving fraction gave a straight line relationship for values other than those at the lowest doses (Fig. 1). This method has been utilized and extended by numerous

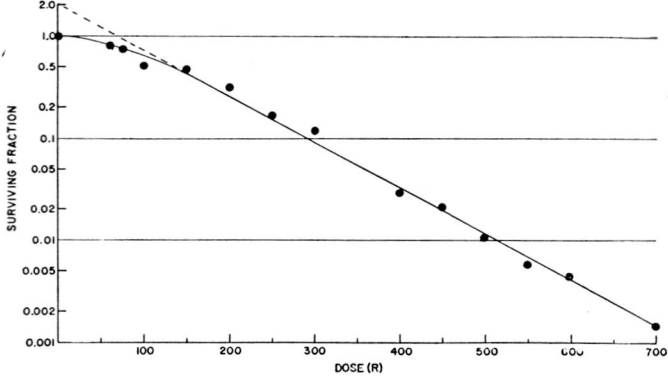

FIG. 8.1. Survival of reproductive capacity in HeLa cells as a function of X-ray dose.
(From Puck and Marcus, 1956.)

workers to a variety of cell lines derived from human and animal tissues (reviewed by Elkind and Whitmore, 1967).

Other cells and tissues investigated have yielded similar relationships, and methods of defining the parameters of the curve have been evolved. The slope of the straight part of the graph is known as the D_0. The point at which the straight part of the survival curve when extrapolated backwards reaches the ordinate defines N, the extrapolation number. As can be seen from the typical curve in Fig. 1, the slope of the curve does not usually extrapolate back to a surviving fraction of 1 (that is all the cells surviving), but frequently predicts greater numbers at zero dose. There is much theoretical discussion of the shape of these curves based on the target theory. The basis for this theory is that these curves can be explained if it is assumed that it may be necessary for the radiation to damage more than one target (multi-target theory), or damage one target more than once (multi-hit theory), and that repair of sublethal intracellular damage may occur. The curved initial part of the plot is known as the 'shoulder' and is the low dose range in which much of the radiation energy is dissipated on sublethal damage.

Elkind and Sutton (1959) showed that recovery from sublethal doses of irradiation could occur when Chinese hamster cells in culture were exposed to two doses of X-radiation separated by varying intervals of time (Fig. 2). This observation has been extended and confirmed in other cell lines in culture (see Elkind and Whitmore, 1967, for

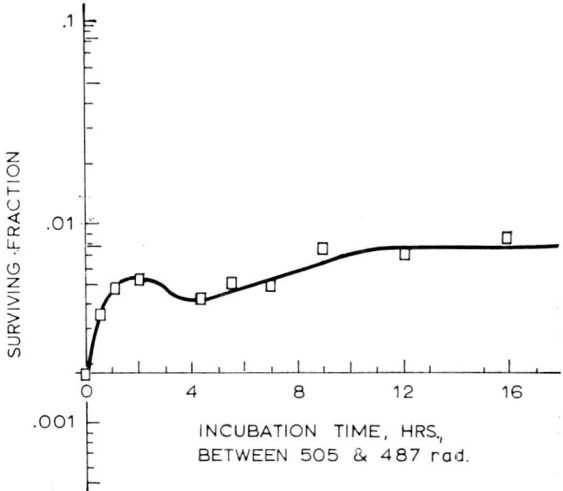

Fig. 8.2. Recovery of X-irradiated cells as a function of time following the irradiation. Cells exposed to a first dose of irradiation of 505 rads at 0 hr and tested with a second dose of 487 rads after varying incubation times. (From Elkind and Sutton, 1959.)

references). The result of this recovery is such that by about 12 hours following a single dose of irradiation those cells which have received only sublethal radiation damage will appear to have completely recovered from that damage when tested with a further radiation exposure.

In vivo methods have been developed to complement the studies made on *in vitro* systems since they are more easily identified with the human situation. However, analysis of the results becomes more difficult because of the less easily defined situations. Hewitt and Wilson (1959) employed a dilution assay for estimating the viability of mouse leukaemia cells *in vivo*. Varying numbers of cells obtained by serial dilutions of a suspension of leukaemic cells were injected into groups of mice and the number of cells needed to kill 50% of the mice (T.D.$_{50}$) ascertained. Leukaemic cells could be irradiated *in vivo* and the proportion of the total number of cells that remained viable could be assessed. Survival curves similar to those of cells in culture were found. This method has been extended to solid tumours by a similar method using homogenization of the tumour into single cell suspensions (e.g. Reinhold, 1965).

Other methods used in assaying the viability of tumour cells following irradiation have included the estimation of the dose required to cure 50% of the tumours irradiated (the T.C.D.$_{50}$ of Suit and Shalek, 1963). Thomlinson (1960) used the time taken for an experimental tumour to regrow to a specified volume after X-radiation as an iso-effect method for comparing results.

Cloning techniques have been adapted to *in vivo* studies. Till and McCulloch (1961) were able to assay the viability of haematopoietic cells growing *in vivo* when injected into heavily irradiated recipient mice. The viable clonogenic cells grow into nodules in the spleen which can then be counted and survival curves plotted. Hill and Bush (1969) have been able to assay clonogenic cells by counting the number of nodules formed in the lungs of recipient mice following the intravenous injection of tumour cell suspensions from a transplantable mouse sarcoma. Other cloning techniques have been developed for studying solid tissues *in vivo*. Kember (1965) presented data for the recovery of cartilage following irradiation, as did Withers (1967, 1968) for skin and for intestinal mucosa. A detailed review of many of these methods is given by Kallman (1968).

The application of these methods to human radiobiology is of considerable importance but for obvious reasons many of the methods are not practicable. Tumour heterogeneity makes work on biopsy samples difficult to interpret. Graft rejection makes the assay of cell viability in non-syngeneic recipient animals almost meaningless, except possibly in special systems such as the hamster cheek pouch where the immune response is depressed. Organ culture techniques provide a very synthetic environment remote from the *in vivo* situation. However, careful observation of tumour responses to irradiation, by the measurement of volume changes and of normal tissue reactions, can yield much information about the differences between the biological effects of varied methods of irradiation.

ACTION OF RADIATION AT A SUBCELLULAR LEVEL

Ionizing radiations produce their biological effect by the transfer of energy to target sites within the cells irradiated. The probability of a lethal event occurring will increase with the quantity of energy deposited in the tissue. The density of energy transfer is known as the linear energy transfer (L.E.T.) of the radiation measured in Kilo-electron-volts per micron (KeV/μ). Radiation with a high L.E.T. will be more effective biologically, rad per rad, than low L.E.T. radiations. X-rays generated at 250 K.V. and gamma rays produced by decay of ^{60}Co have a low L.E.T. When the biological effectiveness of a different radiation is compared with that of a specified standard type of radiation a ratio known as the relative biological effectiveness (R.B.E.) is obtained. This is characteristic for that radiation only at the specified conditions under which it is tested. High L.E.T. radiations have an R.B.E. of greater than one when compared with low L.E.T. radiation. Thus 6 MeV fast neutrons may have an R.B.E. of approximately 3 or more depending on the test conditions.

There is a considerable amount of evidence to suggest that a critical target for the radiation is the deoxyribonucleic acid (DNA) of the cell (Kaplan, 1966; Szybalski, 1967; Sawada and Okada, 1970). The effects of the irradiation may be due to a direct hit on the DNA molecule principally producing fission of the phosphate ester bonds between the sugars of one nucleotide and the next. There may be an indirect effect resulting from the production of highly reactive short-lived free radicals in the aqueous medium which then react with DNA molecules. Other effects of importance may be on the cell membrane, or the lysosomes inside the cell.

REPAIR OF RADIATION DAMAGE

The repair of sublethal damage is in some way dependent on the presence of oxygen. When cells are exposed to low L.E.T. radiation under conditions of low oxygen tension there is a reduction in the value of the extrapolation number (N). There is also a decreased recovery between doses of radiation which are separated by increasing time intervals (reviewed by Littbrand and Revesz, 1969; and Hall and Cavanagh, 1969). Indeed, absolute anoxia may reduce the extrapolation number to 1, implying an abolition of repair. These effects are observed when the oxygen tension falls below about 0·3 mm of mercury (the normal arterial oxygen tension is 100 mm Hg). The exact mechanism of this repair has not yet been elucidated. Studies with metabolic inhibitors and cooling to very low temperatures suggest that oxidative metabolic processes in part are involved but that some repair may occur in their absence (Dalrymple *et al.*, 1969). This oxygen effect is of considerable theoretical and practical importance, and is discussed more fully in a later section of this chapter and in chapter 9. At least part of the indirect effect mediated through free radical formation is oxygen dependent (Szybalski, 1967). With low L.E.T. radiation the inhibition of this mechanism of radiation damage in anoxic states results in a considerable diminution of the radiation effect. High L.E.T. radiations which are less dependent on this indirect method of cell killing are not so affected.

NORMAL TISSUE AND TUMOUR GROWTH

The events that have been described at a molecular and cellular level provide a framework for a more detailed analysis of the effects of radiation on solid tumours. Of ultimate interest to the radiotherapist is the achievement of a ratio of tumour to normal tissue damage greater than one. The radiation effects described demonstrate little quantitative or qualitative differences between normal and tumour cells. The successes of the past and the prospects for the future depend on exploiting whatever differences may be detected in the responses of these tissues. The response of normal tissue to irradiation is therefore of as fundamental importance to the successful radiotherapy of cancer as that of the cancer itself.

The morbid pathological response of various tissues has been well described by numerous authors over the years (reviewed by Rubin and Casarett, 1968). Recently there has been much more interest in the dynamic aspects of normal tissue and of tumour growth. The overall rate of growth of a tumour may be specified in terms of the time taken to double its volume, by measurement of the diameters of the primary cancer as in experimental animals (e.g. Laird, 1965). Similar measurements have been made in man (Spratt, 1965a and b), and also of secondary deposits as seen on chest X-rays (Collins *et al.*, 1956 and Breur, 1966a and b). The rate of growth is usually exponential in the early stages but later it slows down and the curve may fit a Gompertzian function. The doubling times range from about one day to many months.

The normal homeostatic mechanisms controlling the growth of non-malignant tissues do not exert the same control on tumour cells (see review by Burns, 1969). Continuous growth results from unlimited divisions until the tumour outgrows its vascular supply or kills the host. The detailed study of the kinetics of cell and tissue growth has followed the development of autoradiographic techniques. Phases of the cell division cycle have been defined and measured (reviewed by Baserga, 1965). The life cycle of the cell as illustrated in Fig. 3 may be divided into several stages related to the phase during which DNA is synthesized (S-phase). This phase is indicated by the incorporation of a specific radioactive labelled DNA precursor such as tritiated thymidine. This phase is followed by a premitotic stage (G_2) and then mitosis (M). The daughter cells which result from this division then pass into a part of early interphase known as G_1. They then proceed to S-phase and

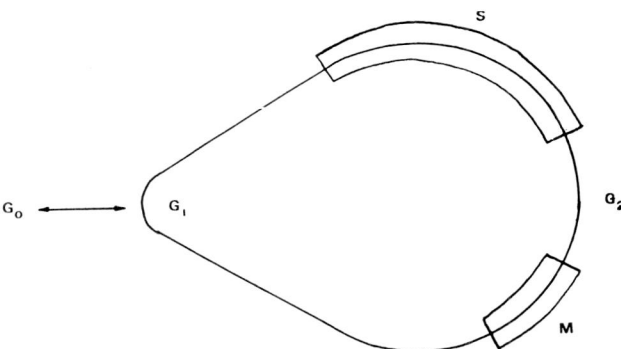

FIG. 8.3. Stages of the cell mitotic cycle as determined by autoradiography. Mitosis is represented by M and the synthetic stage by S. There may be considerable variations in the duration of G_1. Cells may enter the cycle from a non-dividing phase (G_0).

divide again or become differentiated and non-clonogenic. Some may pass into a resting phase (G_0) from which they may later be recalled into active division. The mean transit time for the cells to pass through one mitotic cycle is known as the generation time or cell cycle time (T_c). This may vary from approximately 0·5 days to several months. The greatest contribution to this variability is due to differences in the time spent in G_1. The M-phase usually takes between 0·5 and 2·5 hours; the S-phase is of the order of 8 hours (ranging from 4·5 to 36 hours) and the G_2 phase is $\frac{1}{2}$ to $1\frac{1}{2}$ hours (Baserga, 1965). These values are mean values for a group of cells in a culture, tissue or tumour; individual cells will have values ranging around this mean and may be modified following irradiation (e.g. Brown and Berry, 1969). The cell cycle time for normal tissues and tumours varies considerably over a range of a few hours to many days.

Considerable differences are observed when calculations are made of the expected volume doubling time of a tumour on the basis of all its cells dividing regularly with a mean T_c and then compared with the measured doubling time of the tumour (reviewed by Steel, 1968). Mendelsohn (1962), using continuous labelling of dividing cells with tritiated thymidine, showed that in a mouse mammary tumour only 40% of the tumour cells were actively participating in the mitotic cycle at any one time. These cells were termed the growth fraction. Growth fractions of other values have been found in the various tumours that have been investigated, both in man (e.g. Frindel *et al.*, 1968) and in animals (e.g. Tannock, 1968). Further investigations (reviewed by Steel, 1968) showed that it is still not possible to equate the measured doubling time with the estimated doubling time, as calculated from the product of the growth fraction and T_c of the cells in a tumour. A cell loss factor was therefore proposed. Thus Frindel and her co-workers (1968) in one of their patients with a basal cell carcinoma determined a T_c of 97 hours with a growth fraction of ⅓. This should indicate a potential doubling time of 10 days. The tumour was estimated to weigh between 2–3,000 G (i.e. approximately 3×10^{11} cells), which would suggest a clinical doubling time of approximately 10 months. A large proportion of the cells produced during successive divisions must have been lost from the tumour by a variety of methods such as necrosis, phagocytosis, metastasis and exfoliation. This cell loss factor, which may range from 0% to over 90%, has been estimated for a variety of animal tumours (see Steel, 1968) and in human tumours (Steel, 1967; Refsum and Berdal, 1967). The model so far developed of tumour growth, which may also be applied to that of normal tissues, is diagrammatically represented in Fig. 4. Tubiana (1971) has presented a comprehensive review.

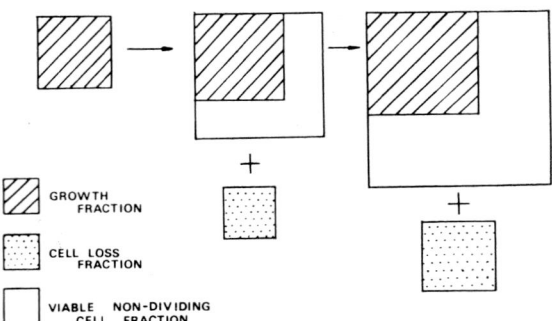

GROWTH FRACTION

CELL LOSS FRACTION

VIABLE NON-DIVIDING CELL FRACTION

FIG. 8.4. Diagrammatic representation of tumour growth showing the relative proportions of the growth, cell loss and viable non-dividing cell fractions with increase in size.

However, this does not give any indication of the dynamic changes that may occur in the distribution of the various cell compartments as growth proceeds or is perturbed by injury. It is an understanding of such changes which is of importance to the successful radiation treatment of tumours. The relationship of the tumour and of normal epithelial cells to the supporting stroma, and in particular to the vascular supply, has received much study recently. This has been of special interest, as it has been shown that the sensitivity of cells to radiation is partly dependent on their degree of oxygenation and that the late effects of radiation on normal tissues will depend on its effects on the vascular supply (reviewed by Rubin and Casarett, 1968). The growth pattern of tumours will also depend on their vascular supply. Thomlinson and Gray (1955) showed, by a study of histological sections of human lung cancers, that cords of viable cells surrounding capillaries may be separated by regions of necrotic cells at a relatively constant distance from the capillary. This distance was calculated to correspond with the distance over which sufficient oxygen might diffuse to maintain viability. The existence of a zone of viable hypoxic cells, between the well oxygenated cells near the capillaries and the necrotic cells at a distance, was postulated. Tannock (1968) has used an autoradiographic analysis to study a rather similar morphological situation in a mouse mammary tumour. He showed that although there was very little difference in the values of T_c for cells at varying distances from the central capillary, the growth fraction varied considerably from a value of 1 in the zone immediately next to the capillary to 0·5 in an outer zone adjacent to the necrotic cells. Similar observations have been reported by Bennington (1969) in tumours from two patients with carcinoma of the cervix where the growth fraction at the periphery of tumour nodules was 0·41 and 0·53 and in the interior of the nodules 0·17 and 0·20 respectively. In a later study, Tannock and Steele (1969) emphasized that the presence of a high vascular density with intact blood capillaries in the area may still be associated with necrosis. They showed that in that situation these vessels exhibit stasis of the blood flow, presumably resulting in a poor supply of oxygen and other nutrients to the cells.

We may now summarize the life history of a model tumour and its response to irradiation. Initially growth is likely to be at an exponential rate, whilst the cells are close to a good blood supply, with a growth fraction approximating to one. Later the growth fraction may progressively decline, cell loss occur and the volume increase depart from an exponential rate. Associated with this there is probably an increase in the proportion of poorly oxygenated cells. Radiation will destroy the reproductive viability of cells in a quantitative manner related to the dose. However, recovery from sublethal damage may occur. Tumour cure will depend on reducing the number of viable cells to below that likely to produce recurrence. This number may not need to be less than one, as host immunological factors (e.g. Maruyama, 1967), and effects on the stroma of the tumour bed (e.g. Hewitt and Blake, 1969), may produce growth restraint. Normal epithelial and connective tissues will similarly be damaged by radiation but the stimulus of injury produces responses which tend to minimize the effect. However, the tumour cells may show a shortened cell cycle time (Tubiana, 1971).

APPLICATION OF RADIOBIOLOGICAL OBSERVATIONS TO RADIOTHERAPY

One may now discuss in more detail the ways in which these varying responses to irradiation may be modified and exploited in the treatment of cancer. Since the early efforts at the cure of cancer with deep X-ray therapy or radium, there have been many attempts to improve the success rate. Variations in the conditions of irradiation have included changes in fractionation, dose-rate, quality of radiation, chemical sensitization and protection, and combinations with surgery and immunotherapy.

THE OXYGEN EFFECT

The earliest dose-modifying efforts were related to the fractionation and protraction of the irradiation administered. However, it is more convenient to discuss initially another phenomenon which has been found to have a profound dose-modifying effect on the biological action of ionizing radiations. This is the 'oxygen effect'. The importance of this in radiotherapy was recognized by Gray and his co-workers (1953) and has been subsequently confirmed in numerous experimental situations by them and by other workers (see Thomlinson, 1967, for general review). For the low L.E.T. radiations such as are used in conventional radiotherapy, there appears to be an approximately three-fold increase in sensitivity when the cells are changed from irradiation in a completely anoxic to a well oxygenated environment. This may be seen in the typical survival curves of cells plotted in Fig. 5. The ratio of the dose of radiation required to achieve a specified surviving fraction of cells when anoxic, as compared with the dose required after irradiation with complete oxygenation, is known as the oxygen enhancement ratio (O.E.R.) and is a measure of the relative radiosensitivity of the cells under the two conditions.

The work of Thomlinson and Gray (1956) with human lung tumours, suggested that the oxygen effect may be of clinical significance, and that recurrences following irradiation might be due to the protection

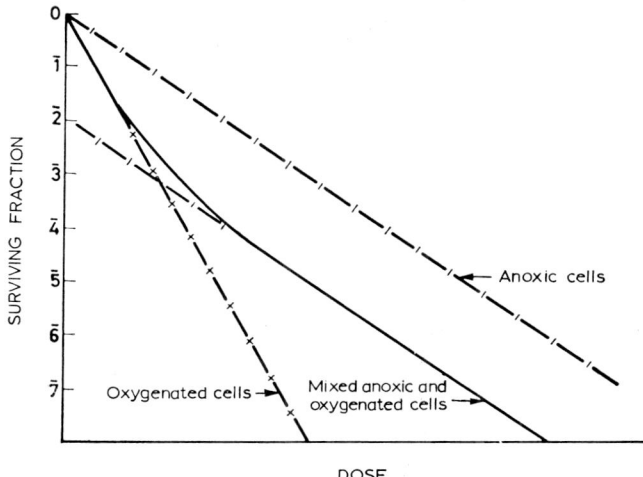

FIG. 8.5. Typical cell survival curves for cells under anoxic and oxygenated conditions and a composite curve for a mixed population of 1% anoxic cells in 99% oxygenated cells. (From Thomlinson, 1967.)

afforded to some cells by their hypoxic state. The presence of hypoxic cells relatively resistant to radiation has been demonstrated in tumour systems, as for example by Powers and Tolmach (1963) using a transplantable mouse lymphosarcoma. They demonstrated a biphasic response in the survival curve with increasing doses of irradiation. Survival curves for the *in vivo* irradiation in air or under anoxic conditions were compared with the *in vitro* responses of oxygenated and anoxic cells. At low radiation doses the proportion of cells killed was similar to that of well oxygenated cells *in vitro*, whilst at higher doses the response resembled that of the less sensitive anoxic cells. This is illustrated by the diagrammatic survival curve for a mixed tumour population of 99% oxygenated and 1% anoxic cells in Fig. 5. This response has been observed with other tumours (e.g. Van Putten and Kallman, 1968) and normal tissues such as skin (e.g. Withers, 1967). The proportions of hypoxic cells that have been estimated to be present in certain normal tissues and in solid tumours are frequently of the order of 15–20%. Hewitt and his co-workers (1967) have pointed out that this may be related to a critical intercapillary distance common to many tumours. Not only is this distance of importance, but the rate of flow of blood through the capillaries will be of significance. Churchill-Davidson, Sanger and Thomlinson (1957) have illustrated the very considerable changes in the oxygen tension across a capillary bed that may occur when blood flow through it is reduced. Tannock and Steele (1969) have discussed this phenomenon with regard to two experimental tumours. The mean distance of cells from the nearest capillary is greater in a large than in a small tumour, as was previously shown (Tannock, 1968), and there is a higher mitotic index in cells closer to the blood vessel than at a distance. In spite of areas of high vascularization there may be widespread areas of necrosis. These workers showed that such blood vessels exhibited stasis of flow, and commented that this pattern may be of considerable practical importance. It may be that tumours with necrosis between columns of viable cells, associated with a large intercapillary distance, would have more viable hypoxic cells than when there is necrosis associated with patchy stasis of flow. This was illustrated indirectly in two experimental tumours. In the one with a large intercapillary spacing, marked slowing of growth occurred when the animals breathed 10% oxygen; whereas in another tumour, with a smaller intercapillary distance, the growth rate was about the same in air and 10% oxygen. The intercapillary distances, and the pattern of blood flow, may change during the life history of a tumour receiving radiation, and the significance of this will be discussed later in this section.

The presence of a proportion of hypoxic cells makes it difficult to conceive how doses of radiation within the tolerance range of the host tissues will kill enough of the cells to reduce the probability of recurrence to a reasonable value. Factors other than those apparent in cell survival curves derived from single dose experiments, must be invoked. Suit (1968) make certain reasonable assumptions for values of D_0, N and the extent of repair from sublethal damage that may occur between fractionated doses of a course of radiation, in both well oxygenated and hypoxic cells. He calculated the dose required to cure 90% of the tumours irradiated (TCD_{90}) and he showed that for a small tumour of 10^7 cells all of which were viable and oxygenated, a dose of approximately 7,000 rads given over 30 fractions would be required. If the tumour contained from 1–10% hypoxic cells, the TCD_{90} might be from 11,000–15,000 rads, a dose which is considerably in excess of that successfully used in clinical radiotherapy for even larger tumours.

An explanation of this apparent paradox has been afforded by the recent work of Van Putten and Kallman (1968), Howes (1969) and others. The proportion of hypoxic cells in a tumour is not a static property of that tissue, but may vary during its growth, and be greatly altered by radiation treatment. It has been shown that following a large test dose of radiation there is an immediate increase in the proportion of hypoxic cells amongst the survivors. This approaches 100%. However, if the proportion of hypoxic cells is then assayed at intervals afterwards, there is a rapid reduction in this value over the next few days. Thus Van Putten and Kallman (1968), by varying the fractionation schedule, found that it was possible to reduce the proportion of hypoxic cells in a mouse fibrosarcoma from the pre-existing value of 14% down to 7% at 72 hours after the last dose of radiation. Other schedules resulted in higher values of residual hypoxic cells. The rapid time course of this re-oxygenation of cells was demonstrated following a single dose of irradiation (Kallman and Bleehen, 1968). Howes (1969), using a transplantable mammary tumour in C3H mice, has shown that as soon as 6 hours after a dose of 1,500 rads the percentage of hypoxic cells had started to fall towards a pre-irradiation value of 15% from an immediate post-irradiation value of 100%. By 4 days the percentage of hypoxic cells had fallen to a minimum which was significantly lower than the pre-irradiation value. This pattern of re-oxygenation will vary between tumours. Thus Van Putten (1968) showed that re-oxygenation was much slower and less complete in a mouse osteosarcoma. Thomlinson (1967) has summarized these effects in a useful model of the changing proportions of hypoxic cells in a tumour during growth and following irradiation (Fig. 6).

The explanation of this reoxygenation of cells is likely to be due to several factors. These will include a reduction of oxygen consumption by the tumour as a whole, as a result of the death of some of the cells; increased tumour necrosis and absorption of dead tissue resulting in a decreased intercapillary distance; an increased blood flow due to reduced tissue pressure; and possible vasodilator mechanisms. The investigation of these mechanisms is obviously of considerable interest and much work is in progress. Measurement of changes in oxygen tension following irradiation have been carried out in man (see Badib and Webster, 1969, for references) and in animals (e.g. Kruuv et al., 1967a, b and c) using a polarographic technique. Baker and his co-workers (1968) have shown that although these measurements are open to much criticism because of the disturbance caused by the electrodes, in fact the biological response to radiation matches the expected response from the oxygen tension measurements. Kolstad (1964) in a clinical study of carcinoma of the cervix showed that the radiocurability was related to the vascular pattern and oxygen tension of the tissue. Rubin and Casarett (1968) indicate some of the vascular changes to be observed following irradiation and demonstrate a state of 'super-vascularization' which may explain the change in proportion of hypoxic cells.

Various methods have been considered for overcoming the problem of the hypoxic cell fraction in a tumour. These have included attempts at improving the oxygenation by oxygen therapy, and reduction of the oxygen effect by anoxia, high L.E.T. irradiations, ultra-high dose-rate radiation and specific sensitizers. Of these hyperbaric oxygen therapy and neutron therapy have received the most study.

Oxygen therapy. Since the recognition of the importance of the

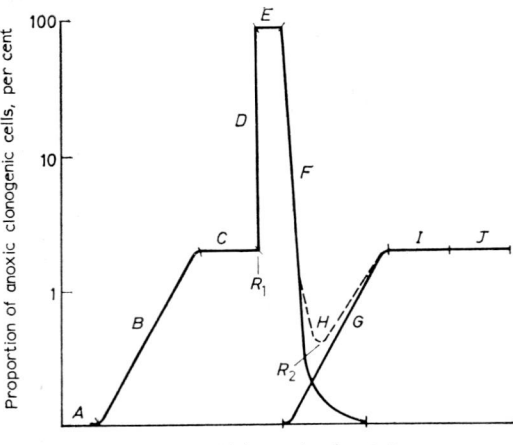

Life history of a tumour

Fig. 8.6. Diagram of changes in the proportion of anoxic clonogenic cells in a tumour. A, when a tumour is very small there are likely to be no anoxic cells: in some tumours they probably never occur. B, if any anoxic cells are produced they appear as the tumour grows. C, the proportion becomes limited to a level characteristic of the type of neoplasm, dependent on its growth rate, degree of differentiation and site. D, if a dose of radiation be given, R_1, the proportion of anoxic clonogenic cells amongst the survivors of radiation injury rises, perhaps to 100%. E, the proportion remains high until cells divide after irradiation. F, when cells divide irradiation injury leads to cell death, cessation of metabolism and relative increased availability of oxygen; the anoxic proportion therefore falls, at a rate dependent on the cell cycle time of the tumour and the number of injured cells. G, surviving clonogenic cells regrow the tumour at a rate dependent on cell-cycle time in the post-irradiation environment. H, the mean proportion of clonogenic cells reaches a minimum at a time dependent on the type of tumour and its growth rate; this time is optimal for a second dose, R_2. I, the characteristic level is restored. J, late irradiation ischaemia is not likely to alter the anoxic proportion greatly unless it were previously zero. (From Thomlinson, 1967.)

hypoxic fraction of cells in a tumour, much work has been carried out on attempts to improve the oxygenation, with a consequent reduction in the hypoxic fraction. These have included irradiation whilst breathing mixtures of 95% oxygen + 5% carbon dioxide. This may increase the blood flow and oxygen tension, as shown by Kruuv and co-workers (1967a) in a mouse mammary tumour, and of tumour cure rate as shown by du Sault (1963). Breathing pure oxygen at increased pressures of up to 4 atmospheres (Churchill-Davidson *et al.*, 1959) has been proposed. The hyperbaric oxygen method has attracted much attention and is the basis of numerous experimental and clinical trials which are beginning to indicate its possible clinical value (see Chapter 10).

Intra-arterial infusion of hydrogen peroxide (Mallams *et al.*, 1962) has been used to increase the oxygen tension of perfusing blood. This necessitates the catheterization of the arterial supply of the tumour with a possible morbidity. There may even be a reduction in oxygenation if there is a failure of catheterization followed by partial interruption of the blood supply by thrombosis or ligature. It therefore has not been the subject of more than random investigation with inconclusive results. Attempts to increase blood flow with chemical vasodilators in experimental tumours only decreased tumour blood flow and oxygen tension (Kruuv *et al.*, 1967b and c).

Anoxic therapy. An alternative approach to the problem of the poorly oxygenated cell fraction has been that used by Van den Brenk and his co-workers (1963) and Suit (1968). An attempt was made to reduce all the cells of the tissues to the same degree of hypoxia and then irradiate to a higher dose than usual, as suggested by the probable O.E.R. of 2 : 3. This anoxia may only be achieved clinically in peripheral tumours of limbs, such as bone and soft tissue sarcomas, by applying a tourniquet around the base of the limb. These tumours are known to be relatively insensitive to irradiation, and require a high dose under normal conditions to achieve growth restraint. Some satisfactory results and impressions have been obtained. However, there is no firm indication, from the very limited numbers reported, that the results are any better than those following conventional radiation techniques. They do provide an interesting clinical demonstration of the protective value of hypoxia on the normal tissues included in the radiation fields, when doses considerably higher than those usually tolerated in conventional schedules are given.

Other variations of anoxic therapy have been proposed. A period of complete anoxia of a duration still tolerated by the host might result in death of many of the hypoxic cells present. Then subsequent irradiation in the normal oxygenated state would result in the death of a higher proportion of remaining viable cells. However, it is not known for how long hypoxic cells can remain viable in an anoxic environment. Littbrand and Revesz (1968) have demonstrated survival of Chinese hamster cells in cultures held in extreme anoxia for periods of up to 72 hours, and Hall and Cavanagh (1969) maintained *Vicia faba* seedlings under extreme hypoxia for up to 9 hours without apparent damage. Therefore, it seems unlikely that such a method of treatment will be of value. An alternative interesting concept is that of the 'reciprocal oxygenated anoxic method' proposed by Wright and his co-workers (1966). They suggest that it may be possible to saturate the hypoxic cells with oxygen during the period of exposure to hyperbaric oxygen. If this is then followed by a rapid change to anoxia, the normal tissues will desaturate very rapidly. They will then be relatively protected against the effect of radiation whilst the previously hypoxic areas may still retain a higher oxygen tension. This method is obviously cumbersome, difficult to time and has not been tested practically.

High L.E.T. radiation. The use of high L.E.T. radiations has been proposed in an attempt to overcome the problem of the hypoxic fraction. Of the likely sources of high L.E.T. radiation available, to date the most suitable has been fast neutron beams obtained from a Cyclotron. Trials with fast neutron beams have been started (reviewed by Fowler, 1967a; Morgan, 1967; Duncan, 1969; and Chapter 9 of this book). The dependence of the oxygen enhancement ratio on the L.E.T. of radiation is illustrated in Fig. 7. The term 'anoxic gain factor' has been proposed by Alper; (1963). This is the ratio of the O.E.R. for X-rays to that for the high L.E.T. radiation and gives a measure of the advantage to be obtained in the treatment of mixed hypoxic and oxygenated cell populations by the high L.E.T. radiation. The increased relative biological effectiveness

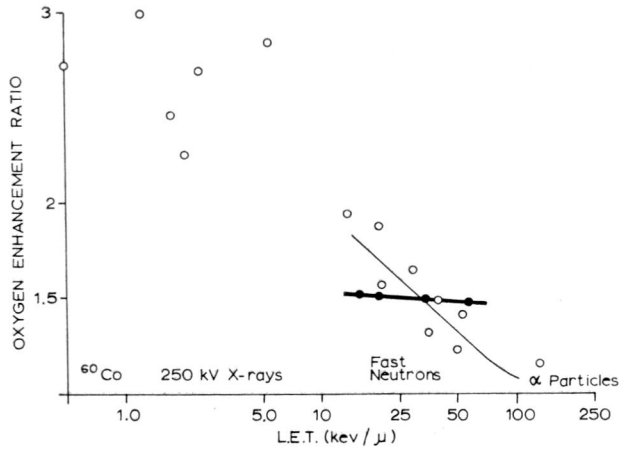

FIG. 8.7. The relationship of O.E.R. to different L.E.T. radiations. Fast neutron data (closed circles) from Barendsen and Broerse (1966), *Nature* **212**, 722. (From Duncan, 1969.)

and decreased O.E.R. associated with high L.E.T. radiation may be related to the formation of oxygen in the radiation path through an aqueous medium (Swallow and Velandia, 1962).

The practical problems involved in the use of fast neutrons in radiotherapy were illustrated by the early work of Stone and colleagues (Stone, 1948) who produced an unacceptably high complication rate in the patients treated on the Berkeley Cyclotron between 1937 and 1943. The increase in R.B.E. with fast neutrons was recognized but the nature of its variation with fractionation not appreciated. Current radiobiological work in experimental systems and man has been devoted to as exact a characterization of these variables as is possible. The practical interest in the value of fast neutrons in radiotherapy has been revived by the experiments and trials on the Hammersmith Cyclotron and the development of simpler D-T neutron generators (see Chapter 9). It is to be hoped that carefully designed clinical trials will provide answers to the similar questions that are being asked regarding hyperbaric oxygen treatment (see Chapter 10).

Neutron sources in a suitable needle form for implantation into tumours or surface applicators have become a possibility with the availability of Californium[252]. This is an isotope which produces neutrons of a suitable energy (Wright *et al.*, 1967). [252]Cf is not likely to be of much value as a neutron radiation source for teleradiotherapy because of the low dose-rate and the shielding problems involved (Lawson, 1969).

Fowler and Perkins (1961) suggested that another type of high L.E.T. radiation might be of use in radiotherapy. Negative π mesons generated by a high energy particle accelerator at 50–75 MeV will have an anoxic gain factor in excess of 2·5 in the region of maximum dose in the irradiated tissue. Over the first part of its path the radiation is only sparsely ionizing and will not deposit much energy in the tissue. The depth dose distribution and anoxic gain factor are therefore theoretically of more value than fast neutrons. Preliminary radiobiological studies have been carried out by Richman and his colleagues (e.g. Raju *et al.*, 1970) and other workers with access to the highly sophisticated machines required. As yet no practical form of π meson generator suitable for routine radiotherapy has been produced, although the new generation of cryogenic accelerators have promise for the future.

Ultra-high dose rate. Of theoretical interest is the possibility of the use of low L.E.T. radiation at a very high dose-rate to change the proportion of hypoxic cells. Town (1967) demonstrated a change in the shape of the survival curve of the HeLa cells in culture at doses above approximately 900 rads, given as very short (1·3 microsecond) single pulses. A comparison with the survival curves obtained at conventional dose-rates of the order of 100 rads/minute showed that at higher doses the ultra-high dose-rate survival curve changed from the slope of oxygenated cells to that resembling the survival curve of anoxic cells. It was postulated that severe oxygen depletion, as a result of the rapid energy transfer, had taken place during the radiation which was of too short a duration to permit re-oxygenation by diffusion. Other workers (Kannon *et al.*, 1968; and Phillips and Worsnop, 1968) have confirmed these results with microsecond pulses. However, Nias and his co-workers (1969) were unable to do so with pulses down to 100 nanoseconds duration using HeLa and Chinese hamster cells. Berry and his co-workers (1969), using two generators of very short pulses in the range of 7–35 nanoseconds and instantaneous dose rates in excess of 7×10^{10} rads/sec., confirmed these effects for different sublines of HeLa and

Chinese hamster cells in culture. Slightly larger pulse durations of 50 nanoseconds gave survival curves of the conventional pattern. Oliver (1969) has pointed out that the survival curves are not in fact correctly drawn, as varying the dose within a uniform pulse size will give further alterations of the dose-rate and has suggested that the curves should be redrawn. This criticism, however, does not remove the general validity of the observations. Berry and his colleagues (1969) have suggested that the effect on survival is more likely to be the result of secondary interactions between the free radicals at high concentrations, thus reducing their availability for reaction with sensitive biological sites in the presence of oxygen. In the absence of oxygen this effect should be minimal as the radicals are destroyed without producing a permanent biological effect.

This effect has obvious implications for radiotherapy if confirmed in other systems. Apart from the practical difficulties involved with a new generation of radiation sources, there remains the problem represented by the first part of the survival curve in which there is no anoxic protection of the cells. The high initial fraction of over 900 rads which is required before the deviation in the curve is seen (Town, 1967) could be a considerable disadvantage in the usual fractionation schemes for radiation. However, Berry and his colleagues (1969) showed that a progressive reduction in duration of the radiation pulse from 35 to 7 nanoseconds was accompanied by a progressive decrease from 2,400 rads down to 500 rads of the dose which was required to produce the deviation in the survival curve. This suggests that it might be possible with even higher dose-rates to produce this phenomenon sooner. Advantage of the effect might then be taken with fractionated doses which are more likely to be tolerated by the patient. Further work on this subject is required as suitable generators would probably cost no more than many of the neutron generators and accelerators being considered at present (Berry et al., 1969), although later work by Berry and Stedeford (1971) is discouraging.

Chemical sensitization. The use of chemical substances other than oxygen to increase the radiosensitivity of cells is discussed in a later section. Of particular interest in the present context would be sensitizers acting specifically on the hypoxic fraction of cells, or protectors which could specifically act on the oxygenated fraction. Adams (1963) suggested that high electron-affinity compounds might sensitize hypoxic cells. Unfortunately no such agents of practical value are known, although sensitizers acting preferentially on hypoxic cells *in vitro* have been described.

Compounds that have aroused interest recently include indanetrione hydrate (ninhydrin), N-ethylmaleimide (NEM) and triacetoneamine N-oxyl (TAN). Hornsey and her colleagues (1967) have reviewed some of the results with indanetrione and also presented their own results suggesting some preferential sensitization of hypoxic cells in the gastro-intestinal tract of mice. However, with the dosage used, the gain factor of 1·3 was much smaller than the factor of 2·6 obtained with oxygen. Higher concentrations of the drug were too toxic.

Moroson and colleagues (1968) have studied the effect of NEM on bacteria and shown that in four strains of *E. coli*, it will only sensitize anoxic cells to radiation. However, Moroson and Frinlan (1967) using the P388 leukaemia ascites tumour showed that NEM was a moderate radiosensitizer for both oxygenated and hypoxic cells. Higher doses of the drug were too toxic for the mice.

Emmerson (1968) has shown that in one mutant of *E. coli*, TAN will increase the radiosensitivity of anoxic cells by a factor of 3·9 whilst oxygen only gave a factor of 1·9. However, with another mutant it was only half as effective as oxygen. TAN had no sensitizing effect on oxygenated cells. He suggested that the effect was due to an action similar to that of oxygen in reacting with the free radicals induced by irradiation of vital molecules such as DNA. Reduced repair following sublethal damage may explain the result in the mutant with a response greater than that found in oxygen. Hewitt and Blake (1970) studied the value of TAN *in vivo* with a transplantable leukaemia of CBA mice. They were unable to demonstrate any sensitization of anoxic cells. This may have been due to the inadequate concentration of drug reaching the leukaemic cells in the sublethal doses administered.

It is to be hoped that radiosensitizers preferentially acting on hypoxic cells *in vivo*, without excessive general toxicity, may be developed. It is to be expected that much more work will be carried out on this very promising aspect of radiation sensitization.

FRACTIONATION

The early work on radiotherapy was almost solely concerned with variations in time-dose relationships. Numerous treatment schedules were developed which exploited the possibility of sparing normal tissues whilst obtaining the desired effect on the tumour as a result of splitting the total dose of radiation into smaller individual fractions spread over several days. The experiments of Regaud (1923) were extended by Coutard (1932) in the treatment of cancer of the upper respiratory and digestive tracts. A decrease in skin reaction for a comparable tumour effect was achieved by spreading the dose over 2–4 weeks. Baclesse (1964) spread the radiation dose over an even longer period of time, that is 9–10 weeks, calling the technique hyperfractionation. Massive tumours could be treated this way without untoward normal tissue reaction. A further modification of these methods is the split dose technique introduced by Scanlon (1960) and Sambrook (1962) and reviewed by Levitt (1969). One or more radiation-free intervals of 2–3 weeks are interspersed between the fractionated course to allow time for normal tissue recovery.

The splitting of a total dose of radiation into several fractions is now known to be associated with several effects. It will allow time for intracellular recovery from sublethal damage, reoxygenation of hypoxic cells, cell division with repopulation and possibly some synchronization of these cells when they subsequently divide. These effects will vary for different tumours and normal tissues. It is the exploitation of these variables, and in particular the difference between the repopulation of tumour and normal tissues, that may explain the value of some fractionation schedules.

All these techniques were developed when the principal radiation sources were orthovoltage X-ray machines with a generating voltage of the order of 200 KV. The maximum reaction was at the skin surface, making analyses of reactions easy. Newer machines, producing X or γ rays, with energies of the order of megavolts have resulted in a reduction of the skin dose for equivalent tumour dose and removed some of the immediately apparent necessity for these more complicated fractionation procedures.

Comparative analyses of the effect of various time-dose schedules on normal skin and squamous cell carcinomas have been made by several workers since the classical comparison by Strandqvist (1944). These have been reviewed by Ellis (1967). Iso-effect curves of dose and time expressed logarithmically for cure of squamous carcinoma, skin tolerance and erythema were constructed, as collated by Cohen (1960) in Fig. 8. An expression of the advantageous effect of prolonged fractionation may be observed in the different slopes of the curves for skin tolerance and cure of carcinoma. Until recently most analyses were more concerned with the total duration of the treatment in days, than the number of individual fractions. Theoretical consideration of cell survival curves show that for each dose of irradiation given more than 12 hours apart, there must be a portion of the dose from which the cells will have completely recovered (Elkind, 1959). Thus the greater the number of fractions into which the radiation is split, the greater the final total dose likely to be required to achieve the same effect. There have been several mathematical attempts to relate the individual contributions of the overall time and number of fractions to the effectiveness of the total dose. The earlier work has been reviewed by Ellis (1967). In a later paper (Ellis, 1969) he summarizes his concept of the Nominal Standard Dose (N.S.D.) which is a parameter representing a specific biological effect, that is a normal tissue tolerance dose. This dose is not meant to represent a dose given in a single treatment but is a basis of comparison between differing schedules. The normal tissue represented is skin and its supportive stromal elements. Analysing previous data he obtains a unitary expression relating the parameters of total dose (D), number of fractions (N) and total duration (T) of treatment in days. He derives the equation: $D = NSD \times N^{0.24} \times T^{0.11}$.

The exponents for the time and fraction corrections are derived from consideration of the regression coefficients of the data of Cohen (1960) in Fig. 8. The effect due to the number of fractions is considered to be the same for normal tissue and carcinoma but the difference in regressions of the slopes will give a measure of the normal tissue recovery time. Ellis has calculated a N.S.D. of 1,800 for the normal tissue tolerance. This dose is expressed in a new unit proposed for this purpose

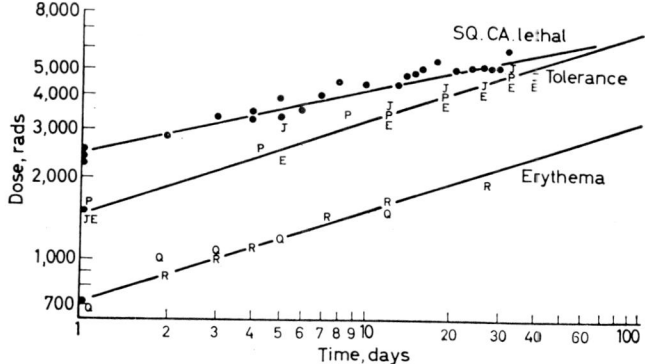

Fig. 8.8. Graphs relating the lethal dose for squamous cell carcinoma, the dose tolerated by normal skin and the dose producing erythema of skin, to the total time over which the dose was delivered in one or more fractions. The initials refer to the authors responsible for the various points. (From Cohen, 1960.)

called the ret (rad equivalent therapy). Ellis and his colleagues (Winston et al., 1969) have produced a slide rule from which equivalent dose schedules may be calculated. Cohen (1968a and b) has attempted a more detailed analysis involving constants representing the radiosensitivity parameters of a single target component, multitarget component and a regeneration or growth constant. These constants will have differing values for different tissues and tumours. The introduction of a computer program based on his proposals, with estimates of the various constants for the tumour and normal tissues involved, provides the possibility of optimizing dose fractionation schedules to achieve the maximum therapeutic ratio.

Theoretical objections to analyses such as these of Ellis and Cohen are that arbitrary values for constants are used which are often derived from inadequate data and that allowance is not made for volume treated. The more detailed analysis by Cohen still does not directly allow for changes in the radiosensitivity of component cells during fractionated irradiation due to reoxygenation of hypoxic cells or semi-synchronization. However, these analyses are of value in providing methods by which fractionation schedules may be designed and tested experimentally in animals and man. Prospective fractionation trials are being established (e.g. British Institute of Radiology Trial 1970) to compare the efficacy of various schedules in the control of disease in patients. More work is needed on comparable experimental work in animals. A valuable illustration of the desirability of such analyses is shown by some recent work on carcinoma of the breast. Bates, Fleming and Wiernik (1969) reported the results of a retrospective survey comparing radiation dose schedules in carcinoma of the breast. They showed a significantly better survival response in patients receiving radiotherapy three times per week than in those treated five times per week. Cohen (1970) has used his kinetics analysis to calculate the theoretical advantage to be gained by a change from a five to a three times a week treatment schedule. He found an increase of the order of 10 fold in the ratio of tumour to normal cells killed. Montague (1968) reported an increase in complications associated with three times per week treatment of carcinoma of the breast when compared with five times per week. However, Ellis, Winston, Fowler and De Ginder (1969) have pointed out that by irradiating only one of the two radiation fields on each treatment day, a very inhomogeneous dose distribution was obtained. When analysed in terms of NSD by the Ellis formula (Ellis, 1969), ret doses in excess of tolerance were demonstrated at the near edge of the fields. This would be enough to explain the increased complication rate. Such analyses will become even more valuable when the various parameters for different tissues can be defined with more precision.

A further theoretical and mathematical approach is being developed in Glasgow, defining a new function termed 'Cumulative Radiation Effect' (Kirk, Gray and Watson, 1971).

SYNCHRONY

Changes in the radiosensitivity of partially synchronized cultures of mammalian cells as they pass through successive stages of the mitotic cycle were demonstrated by Terasima and Tolmach (1961), and many later workers, as reviewed by Elkind and Whitmore (1967) and Sinclair (1968). A varying response has been observed, but in general mitosis and G_2 are the most sensitive stages of the cycle. Cells with a long G_1 stage may, in addition, have a sensitive part at the end of G_1. After a dose of radiation a variable delay in mitosis is observed. There may be a tendency for all the cells to accumulate in G_2 from which they may then be released in partial synchrony. Kallman (1963) has reviewed the data from *in vitro* studies and proposed that such a mechanism might also achieve synchronization *in vivo*.

Recent work on mice has shown that some significant cyclic variation in radiation sensitivity following a first dose of radiation can be observed in bone marrow (Kallman, Silini and Taylor, 1966), a transplantable sarcoma (Kallman and Bleehen, 1968) and the skin (Denekamp, Ball and Fowler, 1969). It has been inferred that these variations are due to semi-synchronization of mitosis or metabolic processes, although this has not been demonstrated directly. The periodicity of the systems

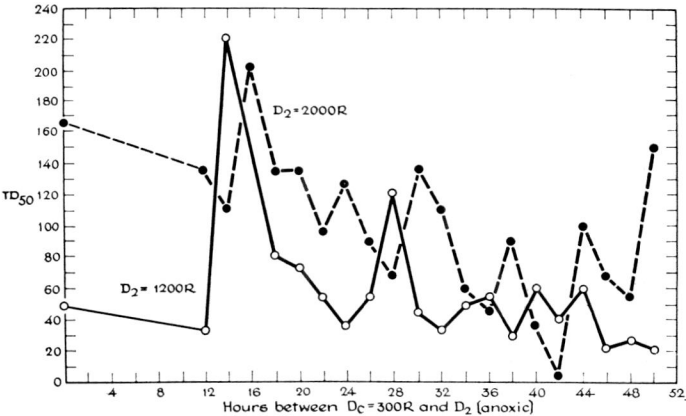

FIG. 8.9. TD_{50} of a transplantable sarcoma in C3H mice assayed following an initial. dose of 300 rads and a second dose (D_2) of either 1200 R or 2000 R given at a time of between 12 and 50 hours later. The second dose was administered under anoxic conditions. An increase in TD_{50} represents a reduction in radio-sensitivity of the tumour at that time. (From Kallman and Bleehen, 1968.)

varied. Kallman and his co-workers (1966) found a periodicity for the marrow response of C57 BL mice of approximately 8 hours, over the 50 hours following a preliminary dose of radiation. Similar cyclical fluctuations in the DNA synthesis of bone marrow stem cells following irradiation *in vivo* has been demonstrated by Frindel and her co-workers (Frindel *et al.*, 1966).

Fluctuations in the radiosensitivity of a transplantable fibrosarcoma of C3H mice following a first dose radiation have been observed by Kallman and Bleehen (1968) as seen in Fig. 9. Analysis of the data revealed significant peaks of radiosensitivity with a frequency of about 7 hours and lower peaks with a mean frequency of about 14 hours. Thus there was a 3 to 7-fold decrease of the surviving fractions of sarcoma cells when exposure to a second dose of radiation was applied at the maximum of radiosensitivity as compared with the same dose at minimum radiosensitivity.

A similar phenomenon has been observed in mouse skin by Denekamp, Ball and Fowler (1969). Over a period of 15 to 74 hours variations with a periodicity of 12 to 17 hours were seen. These times are consistent with the known cell cycle times for cells of the basal layer of the mouse hair follicle. Young and Fowler (1969) have constructed a mathematical model to incorporate the available data from the two-dose cell survival experiments on Chinese hamster cells by Sinclair (1968). Making some reasonable assumptions they observed that the data can in large part be explained by the progression of partially synchronized cells through mitosis with variations in the radiosensitivity of those cells at different stages. Hahn (1968a) with a different model system has shown that it is possible to calculate the optimum fractionation schedule for the selective killing of one cell line in the presence of cells of another type.

Attempts have been made to use other parameters to determine periodic fluctuations of radiosensitivity. Hale and his colleagues (Bullen et al., 1963) have developed an in vivo method of measuring fluctuations in the radioactive phosphorus (^{32}P) concentration of tumours in patients to whom a dose of the agent had previously been administered systemically. They have suggested that the periodic fluctuations they observed may be used as an indication of possible changes in radiosensitivity. This technique has been used by other workers and extended to animal tumours without any firm conclusion being reached (Bleehen and Bryant, 1968; Woolley-Hart et al., 1968). A similar technique using a more reliable indicator of synchrony could be of considerable value but no such radioactive tracer is yet available.

Methods other than radiation to achieve synchronization are also feasible. Kaplan (1965) has suggested the possibility of augmenting the radiation induced block in G_2 by using colchicine in small doses to achieve a secondary bunching in mitosis, and Hale and his co-workers have used methotrexate in their clinical investigations (Bullen et al., 1963).

The variations in radiosensitivity associated with synchronization would only be of clinical value if the following criteria could be satisfied. A reasonable proportion of dividing cells must be synchronized. The synchrony should be maintained for a sufficient duration so that advantage may be taken in a practical fractionation schedule. The periodicity of the radiosensitivity changes must be easily predicted or measured concurrently. There should be a sufficient difference between the maximum and minimum of radiosensitivity to make the procedure worthwhile. Finally, if all these criteria can be met, it is of importance that the periodicities of the cells of the tumour and normal tissue bed are sufficiently different to achieve a useful therapeutic ratio. It is not possible to fulfil these conditions in other than very limited experimental circumstances at the present time.

DOSE-RATE

Little emphasis was made in the past on the rate at which radiation was given (i.e. rads/min), as the early studies had shown only minor differences within the clinical range used (e.g. McWhirter, 1936). There were, however, some indications that dose-rate effects might perhaps be of importance as instanced by the different doses tolerated when radiation is given continuously over approximately 1 week by interstitial implant, or by fractionated external regimes.

A wide range of dose-rates are now available for radiation therapy. Ultra high dose-rates in the range of 10^{10} rads per second are as yet only of experimental interest (see previous section). High dose-rates in the range of 100 rads per minute are used in conventional external beam therapy. These have recently been used in intracavitary therapy for uterine cancer and some surface applicator treatments with an after-loading radioactive source dispenser such as the Cathetron (Joslin et al., 1967). Alternatively, low dose-rate therapy in the range of 100 rads per hour has been used for conventional intracavitary and interstitial radium therapy and has been proposed for external beam therapy by Pierquin and Baillet (1970).

Recent work on the recovery from sublethal intra-cellular damage has provided a basis for some understanding of dose-rate effects. In general, radiation at a low dose-rate will produce less cell killing than at a high dose-rate because of recovery and repopulation during the radiation exposure (reviewed in the Symposium on 'Dose-Rate in Mammalian Radiation Biology', 1968). Liversage (1966) has discussed the theoretical changes in dosage schedule likely to be necessary when intracavitary radiations are given at a high dose-rate instead of the more usual low dose-rate radium techniques. An increased use of fractionation becomes important to allow for recovery of normal tissue damage. A preliminary clinical report of its application to the Cathetron has been given by Joslin and his colleagues (Joslin et al., 1967) (see Chapter 12).

Apart from the changes of dose and fractionation required by alterations in dose-rate, the possible reduction in oxygen enhancement ratio with low dose-rates must be considered. Hall, Bedford and Oliver (1966) demonstrated this effect with HeLa cells in vitro. However, Berry (1968a) showed only a slight reduction in O.E.R. with ascites tumour cells irradiated in vivo at low dose-rates. This latter system is more akin to the solid tumour systems of interest in clinical radiotherapy. It may be that much of the success of low dose-rate radium treatments has been due to the low O.E.R. of such therapy with consequent greater effect on the hypoxic portion of the tumours irradiated.

CHEMICAL SENSITIZATION AND PROTECTION

Considerable effort has been devoted to the search for chemical agents which will sensitize cells to the effects of radiation. Recent reviews of the subject by Doggett, Bagshaw and Kaplan (1967) and several authors in Moroson and Quintiliani (1970) list many of the agents used. These include halogenated pyrimidines, purine analogues, certain antibiotics and miscellaneous other agents. There does not appear to be a selective sensitization of tumour cells, and normal tissues will also demonstrate the same phenomenon, thus maintaining the same therapeutic ratio. Brown and Ellis (1969) have suggested that it might be possible to incorporate more sensitizer into tumour cells than normal tissues, assuming a longer cell cycle time for the latter. If the sensitizer is only given for a period shorter than the average tumour cell-cycle time, then a greater proportion of tumour cells than normal cells passing through S phase will be exposed to the sensitizer.

The alternative attempts selectively to sensitize the hypoxic cell fraction have been discussed in an earlier section of this chapter. Berry (1968b), working with HeLa cells in culture, found a potentiation of the X-ray dose response by methotrexate. This was the result of both an increased D_0 and an abolition of the 'shoulder' on the dose-response curve. Of interest was the increased O.E.R. resulting from a greater potentiation seen with anoxic cells. One explanation of this effect may have been partial synchronization of the cell culture by the methotrexate with a varying O.E.R. for the different stages of the cell cycle. However, Kruuv and Sinclair (1968) with synchronous cultures of Chinese hamster cells, were unable to detect any difference in O.E.R. during the different states of the cell cycle. The reduced recovery and increased O.E.R. observed by Berry (1968b) may explain the excellent clinical results sometimes seen with combinations of radiotherapy and methotrexate (Friedman and Daly, 1963).

Attempts at the practical use of radioprotective agents have been even more disappointing. The majority of these contain –SH groups which act as 'radical scavengers' or promote repair. Although protective *in vitro*, they are often toxic *in vivo* when given in effective doses. Other pharmacological protectors such as 5-hydroxy-tryptamine and adrenaline may produce a large part of their effect by alterations in tissue blood flow and consequent hypoxia.

In spite of the present lack of therapeutic promise of known radio-protective agents, more work on the subject is needed. Combinations of protective agents may be more effective than single agents (Maisin *et al.*, 1968). It is perhaps possible that agents with certain diffusion characteristics may selectively protect well-oxygenated cells close to the vascular supply leaving the remoter hypoxic cells unprotected, when these agents are injected a short time before the radiation exposure.

CONCLUSIONS

The radiobiological basis of radiotherapy has advanced considerably over the past few years. This review has not attempted to be comprehensive in its scope and only selected references to individual topics have been discussed. Other developments which may be no less significant have been omitted. Such important topics as combinations of irradiation and surgery (e.g. Rush and Greenlaw, 1968), heavy particle irradiation effects (e.g. Chang, Linfoot and Lawrence, 1969), tumour immunology and response to irradiation (e.g. James, 1969) have received scant or no attention.

Developments in cancer therapy by radiation in the near future are likely to come from a better understanding of normal and tumour cell kinetics and the responses of these tissues to radiation. More fundamental knowledge is required to improve our interpretation of present data. For example, there has been considerable emphasis on the 'oxygen effect', its significance and the measures taken to overcome the problem presented by the hypoxic fraction of cells. This is the most extensively defined radiation dose-modifying phenomenon. However, the biological significance of even this effect remains in some doubt. It has usually been assumed that cells which are completely anoxic in a tumour are of no further biological interest as they will eventually die. However, Littbrand and Revesz (1968) have shown with monolayer cell cultures grown under conditions of anoxia, that a significant proportion of cells may survive up to 72 hours. They point out that the anoxic cells may be of importance, as following a first dose of irradiation they might pass into the hypoxic state as part of a general re-oxygenation phenomenon. They (Littbrand and Revesz, 1969) have demonstrated impairment of repair mechanisms in Chinese hamster cells cultured under extreme anoxia, as have Phillips and Hanks (1968) with mouse bone marrow colony-forming cells *in vivo*. Suit and Urano (1969) defined two compartments of hypoxic cells in mouse mammary carcinoma. Those which were acutely hypoxic showed rapid repair; the chronically hypoxic cells, remaining after irradiation under hyperbaric oxygen conditions, did not repair so well. It may be that some of the cells which are chronically hypoxic in tumours will be more sensitive to the effects of irradiation, as a result of this lack of repair, than general consideration of the survival statistics for a mixed hypoxic population would suggest. As is pointed out by Phillips and Hanks (1968) a reduction of the extrapolation number from 2 to 1 could almost completely cancel out the effect of hypoxia on cell survival in fractionated dose regimes.

Another modification to our general evaluation of the oxygen effect has been introduced by the work of Hahn (1968b) who showed that Chinese hamster cells after prolonged growth in culture with overcrowding, passed into a stationary phase with no further increase in the total number of cells. In these circumstances the D_0 of the survival curve became steeper, the 'shoulder' disappeared and the cells tended to accumulate in G_1. Split dose experiments confirmed a failure of repair processes. Berry, Hall and Cavanagh (1970) showed that stationary phase HeLa cells were more sensitive to radiation than cells in the log phase of growth. It would seem possible that some cells in tumours might be in an equivalent stationary phase as evidenced by the small growth fraction seen in cells remote from capillaries. If the hypoxic cells of a tissue become arrested in one of the more radiosensitive stages of the mitotic cycle, then methods to improve oxygenation may not be of any advantage. This concept has been discussed in more detail by Kruuv and Sinclair (1968).

It can be seen that although radiobiological studies have produced much valuable information to help and explain the radiotherapeutic management of malignant disease, they have also posed many new questions. It is from the solution of these problems and the further questions raised that improvements in radiotherapy will come.

REFERENCES

ADAMS, G. E., & DEWEY, D. L. (1963). *Hydrated Electrons and Radiobiological Sensitisation.* Biochemistry and Biophysics Research Commission, **12**, 473.

ALPER, T. (1963). Comparison between oxygen enhancement ratio for neutrons and X-rays as observed in *Escherichia coli* B. *Br. J. Radiol.*, **36**, 97.

ANDREWS, J. R. (1968). *The Radiobiology of Human Cancer Radiotherapy.* Philadelphia: Saunders.

BACLESSE, F. (1964). Hyperfractionation. *Am. J. Roentg.*, **91**, 32.

BADIB, A. O., & WEBSTER, J. H. (1969). Changes in tumor oxygen tension during radiation therapy. *Acta radiol. scand.*, **8**, 247.

BAKER, D. J., LINDOP, P. J., & HEWITT, H. B. (1968). The effect of breathing oxygen at high pressure on the oxygenation of a sarcoma in CBA mice. *Br. J. Radiol.*, **41**, 318.

BASERGA, R. (1965). The relationship of the cell cycle to tumour growth and control of cell division: a review. *Cancer Res.*, **25**, 581.

BATES, T., FLEMING, J. A. C., & WIERNIK, G. (1969). Carcinoma of the breast. The effect of dose fractionation and radiotherapeutic technique on survival. *Clin. Radiol.*, **20**, 278.

BENNINGTON, J. L. (1969). Cellular kinetics of invasive squamous carcinoma of the human cervix. *Cancer Res.*, **29**, 1082.

BERRY, R. J. (1968a). Hypoxic protection and recovery in tumor cells irradiated at low dose-rates and assessed *in vivo. Br. J. Radiol.*, **41**, 921.

BERRY, R. J. (1968b). Some observations on the combined effects of X-rays and methotrexate on human tumour cells *in vitro* with possible relevance to their most useful combination in radiotherapy. *Am. J. Roentg.*, **102**, 509.

BERRY, R. J., HALL, E. J., & CAVANAGH, J. (1970). Radiosensitivity and the oxygen effect for mammalian cells cultured *in vitro* in stationary phase. *Br. J. Radiol.*, **43**, 81.

BERRY, R. J., HALL, E. J., FORSTER, D. W., STORR, T. M., & GOODMAN, M. J. (1969). Survival of mammalian cells exposed to X-rays at ultra-high dose rates. *Br. J. Radiol.*, **42**, 102.

BERRY, R. J., & STEDEFORD, J. B. H. (1971). Reproductive survival of mammalian cells after irradiation at ultra-high dose-rates: further observations and their importance for radiotherapy. *Br. J. Radiol.*, in press.

British Institute of Radiology Working Party on dose fractionation (1970). Third Progress Report. *Br. J. Radiol.*, **43**, 558.

BLEEHEN, N. M., & BRYANT, T. H. E. (1967). *In vivo* studies of radioactive phosphorus in malignant tumours. *Clin. Radiol.*, **18**, 237.

BREUR, K. (1966a). Growth rate and radiosensitivity of human tumours. 1. Growth rate of human tumours. *Eur. J. Cancer*, **2**, 157.

BREUR, K. (1966b). Growth rate and radiosensitivity of human tumours. *Eur. J. Cancer*, **2**, 173.

BROWN, J. M., & BERRY, R. J. (1969). The effects of X-irradiation on the cell population kinetics in a model tumour and normal tissue system. Implications for the treatment of human malignancies. *Br. J. Radiol.*, **49**, 372.

BROWN, J. M., & ELLIS, F. (1969). The use of pyrimidine analogues in radiotherapy. *Br. J. Radiol.*, **42**, 155.

BULLEN, M. A., FREUNDLICH, H. F., HALE, B. T., MARSHALL, D. H., & TUDWAY, R. C. (1963). The activity of malignant tumours and response to therapeutic agents, studied by continuous records of radioactive phosphorus uptake. *Postgrad. med. J.*, **39**, 265.

BURNS, E. R. (1969). On the failure of self-inhibition of growth in tumours. *Growth*, **33**, 25.

CHANG, C. Y. L., LINFOOT, J. A., & LAWRENCE, J. H. (1969). High energy heavy charged particles in medicine. *Radiologic Clins N. Am.*, **7**, 319.

CHURCHILL-DAVIDSON, I., SANGER, C., & THOMLINSON, R. H. (1957). Oxygenation in radiotherapy. *Br. J. Radiol.*, **30**, 406.

COHEN, L. (1960). Ph.D. thesis, University of Witwatersrand, quoted by Ellis, F. (1967).

COHEN, L. (1968a). Theoretical 'iso-survival' formulae for fractionated radiation therapy. *Br. J. Radiol.*, **41**, 522.

COHEN, L. (1970). Three or five fractions per week for breast cancer. *Br. J. Radiol.*, **43**, 74.

COHEN, L., & SCOTT, M. J. (1968b). Fractionation procedures in radiation therapy: a computerised approach to evaluation. *Br. J. Radiol.*, **41**, 529.

COLLINS, V. P., LOEFFLER, R. K., & TIVEY, H. (1956). Observations on growth rates of human tumours. *Am. J. Roentg.*, **76**, 988.

COUTARD, H. (1932). Roentgen therapy of epitheliomas of the tonsillar region, hypopharynx and larynx from 1920–1926. *Am. J. Roentg.*, **28**, 313.

DALRYMPLE, G. V., SANDERS, J. L., BAKER, M. L., & WILKINSON, K. P. (1969). The effect of 2:4 dinitrophenol on the repair of radiation injury by L-cells. *Radiat. Res.*, **37**, 90.

DEELEY, T. J., & WOOD, C. A. P. (1967). (Eds.) *Modern Trends in Radiotherapy.* London: Butterworths.

DENEKAMP, J., BALL, M. M., & FOWLER, J. F. (1969). Recovery and repopulation in mouse skin as a function of time after x-irradiation. *Radiat. Res.*, **37**, 361.

DOGGETT, R. L. S., BAGSHAW, M. A., & KAPLAN, H. S. (1967). Combined Therapy Using Chemotherapeutic Agents and Radiotherapy. *Modern Trends in Radiotherapy*, p. 107. Deeley, T. J. and Wood, C. A. P. (Eds.). London: Butterworths.

Dose Rate in Mammalian Radiation Biology (1968). *A Symposium.* U.S. Atomic Energy Commission. CONF-680410.

DUNCAN, W. (1969). Fast-neutron radiotherapy. *Br. J. Hosp. Med.*, **2**, 1486.

ELKIND, M. M., & SUTTON, H. (1959). X-ray damage and recovery in mammalian cells in culture. *Nature, Lond.*, **184**, 1293.

ELKIND, M. M., & WHITMORE, G. F. (1967). The Radiobiology of Cultured Mammalian Cells. New York: Gordon and Breach.

ELLIS, F. (1967). Fractionation in Radiotherapy. *Modern Trends in Radiotherapy*, p. 34. Deeley, T. J. and Wood, C. A. P. (Eds.). London: Butterworths.

ELLIS, F. (1969). Dose, time and fractionation. A clinical hypothesis. *Clin. Radiol.*, **20**, 1.

ELLIS, F., WINSTON, B. M., FOWLER, J. F., & DE GINDER, W. L. (1969). Three or five fractions per week: treated on alternate treatment days. *Br. J. Radiol.*, **42**, 715.

EMERSON, P. T. (1968). Sensitisation of anoxic recombination-deficient mutants of *Escherichia coli* K12 to X-rays by triacetoneamine N-oxyl. *Radiat. Res.*, **36**, 410.

FRIEDMAN, M., & DALY, J. F. (1963). Combined irradiation and chemotherapy in the treatment of squamous cell carcinoma of the head and neck. *Am. J. Roentg.*, **90**, 246.

FRINDEL, E., CHARRUYER, F., TUBIANA, M., KAPLAN, H. S., & ALPEN, E. L. (1966). Radiation effects in DNA synthesis and cell division in the bone-marrow of the mouse. *Int. J. Radiat. Biol.*, **11**, 435.

FRINDEL, E., MALAISE, E., & TUBIANA, M. (1968). Cell proliferation kinetics in five human solid tumours. *Cancer*, **22**, 611.

FOWLER, J. F. (1967a). Fast Neutron Therapy—Physical and Biological Considerations. *Modern Trends in Radiotherapy*, p. 145. Deeley, T. J. and Wood, C.A.P. (Eds.). London: Butterworths.

FOWLER, J. F. (1967b). Kinetics of injury and repair to mammalian tissue by high L.E.T. radiation. *Radiat. Res.*, **7**, 276.

FOWLER, P. H., & PERKINS, D. H. (1961). The possibility of therapeutic applications of beams of negative π-mesons. *Nature, Lond.*, **189**, 524.

GRAY, L. H., CONGER, A. D., EBERT, M., HORNSEY, S., & SCOTT, O. C. A. (1953). The concentration of oxygen dissolved in tissues at the time of irradiation as a factor in radiotherapy. *Brit. J. Radiol.*, **26**, 638.

HAHN, G. M. (1968a). Possible improvement in differential cell killing by cell cycle modulation. *Br. J. Radiol.*, **41**, 239.

HAHN, G. M. (1968b). Failure of Chinese hamster cells to repair sublethal damage when x-irradiated in the plateau phase of growth. *Nature, Lond.*, **217**, 741.

HALL, E. J., BEDFORD, J. S., & OLIVER, R. (1966). Extreme hypoxia. Its effect on the survival of mammalian cells irradiated at high and low dose-rates. *Br. J. Radiol.*, **32**, 302.

HALL, E. J., & CAVANAGH, J. (1969). The effect of hypoxia on recovery of sublethal radiation damage in *Vicia* seedlings. *Br. J. Radiol.*, **42**, 270.

HEWITT, H. B., & BLAKE, E. R. (1969). The growth of transplanted murine tumours in pre-irradiated sites. *Br. J. Cancer*, **22**, 808.

HEWITT, H. B., & BLAKE, E. R. (1970). Studies of the toxicity and radiosensitising activity of triacetoneamine-N-oxyl in mice. *Br. J. Radiol.*, **43**, 91.

HEWITT, H. B., CHAN, D. P. S., & BLAKE, E. R. (1967). Survival curves for clonogenic cells of a murine keratinising squamous carcinoma irradiated *in vivo* or under hypoxic conditions. *Int. J. Radiat. Biol.*, **12**, 535.

HEWITT, H. B., & WILSON, C. W. (1959). A survival curve of mammalian cells irradiated *in vivo. Nature, Lond.*, **183**, 1060.

HILL, R. P., & BUSH, R. S. (1969). A lung-colony assay to determine the radiosensitivity of the cells of a solid tumour. *Int. J. Radiat. Biol.*, **15**, 435.

HORNSEY, S. J., HEDGES, M. J., & BRYANT, P. E. (1967). The sensitisation of the hypoxic gastro-intestinal tract, *in vivo*, to radiation damage by indanetriane hydrate. *Int. J. Radiat. Biol.*, **13**, 581.

HOWES, A. E. (1969). An estimation of changes in the proportion and absolute numbers of hypoxic cells after irradiation of transplanted C3H mouse mammary tumours. *Br. J. Radiol.*, **42**, 441.

JAMES, K. W. (1969). Tumour immunology and response to radiation therapy. *Radiologic Clins N.A.*, **7**, 353.

JOSLIN, C. A. F., O'CONNELL, D., & HOWARD, N. (1967). The treatment of uterine carcinoma using the Cathetron. *Br. J. Radiol.*, **40**, 895.

KALLMAN, R. F. (1963). Recovery from radiation injury. A proposed mechanism. *Nature, Lond.*, **197**, 557.

KALLMAN, R. F. (1968). Methods for Study of Radiation Effects on Cancer Cells. *Methods in Cancer Research*, Vol. 4. Busch (Ed.). Academic Press.

KALLMAN, R. F., & BLEEHEN, N. M. (1968). Post-irradiation cyclic radiosensitivity changes in tumours and normal tissues. Dose-rate in mammalian radiation biology, U.S. Atomic Energy Commission, CONF-680410, 20.1.

KALLMAN, R. F., SILINI, G., & TAYLOR, H. M. (1966). Recuperation from lethal injury by whole body irradiation. *Radiat. Res.*, **29**, 362.

KANNON, W. (1968). Abstract Fc8. Sixteenth Annual Meeting of the Radiation Research Society, Houston, April 1968.

KAPLAN, H. S. (1965). Clinical Potentialities of Recent Advances in Cellular Radiobiology, p. 584. Baltimore: Williams and Wilkins Company.

KAPLAN, H. S. (1966). DNA strand scission and loss of viability after x-irradiation of normal and sensitised bacterial cells. *Proc. natn Acad. Sci., U.S.A.*, **55**, 1442.

KEMBER, N. F. (1965). An *in vivo* cell survival system based on the recovery of rat growth cartilage from radiation injury. *Nature, Lond.*, **207**, 501.

KIRK, J., GRAY, W. M., & WATSON, E. R. (1971). Cumulative Radiation Effect. Part 1: Fractionated Treatment Regimes. *Clin. Radiol.*, **22**, 145.

KOLSTAD, P. (1964). Vascularisation, oxygen tension and radiocurability in cancer of the cervix. Universitetsforlaget, Oslo. *Acta obst. gynec. scand.*, **43** (suppl. 7), 100.

KRUUV, J. A., INCH, W. R., & McCREDIE, J. A. (1967). Blood flow and oxygenation of tumours in mice. *Cancer*, **20**, 51 (1967a); *Cancer*, **20**, 60 (1967b); *Cancer*, **20**, 66 (1967c).

KRUUV, J., & SINCLAIR, W. K. (1968). X-ray sensitivity of synchronised Chinese hamster cells irradiated during hypoxia. *Radiat. Res.*, **36**, 45.

LAIRD, A. K. (1965). Dynamics of tumour growth. Comparison of growth rates and extrapolation of growth curve to one cell. *Br. J. Cancer*, **19**, 278.

LAWSON, R. C. (1969). Californium 252 as an external source of neutrons for radiotherapy treatment. *Br. J. Radiol.*, **42**, 714.

LEVITT, S. H. (1969). The split-dose approach in radiation therapy. *Radiologic Clin. N. Am.*, **7**, 293.

LITTBRAND, B., & REVESZ, L. (1968). Survival of cells in anoxia. *Br. J. Radiol.*, **41**, 479.

LITTBRAND, B., & REVESZ, L. (1969). The effect of oxygen on cellular survival and recovery after radiation. *Br. J. Radiol.*, **42**, 914.

LIVERSAGE, W. E. (1966). The application of cell survival theory to high dose-rate intracavitary therapy. *Br. J. Radiol.*, **39**, 338.

MAISIN, J. R., MATTELIN, G., FRIDMAN-MANDUZIO, A., & VAN DER PARREN, J. (1968). Reduction of short- and long-term radiation lethality by mixtures of chemical protectors. *Radiat. Res.*, **35**, 26.

MALLAMS, J. F., FINNEY, J. W., & BALLA, G. A. (1962). Use of hydrogen peroxide as a source of oxygen in a regional intra-arterial infusion system. *Sth. med. J.*, **55**, 230.

MARUYAMA, Y. (1967). Contribution of host resistance to radiosensitivity of an isologous murine lymphoma *in vivo*. *Int. J. Radiat. Biol.*, **12**, 277.

McWHIRTER, R. (1936). Radiosensitivity in relation to the time intensity factor. *Br. J. Radiol.*, **9**, 287.

MENDELSOHN, M. L. (1962). Autoradiographic analysis of cell proliferation in spontaneous breast cancer of C3H mouse. III. The growth fraction. *J. natn. Cancer Inst.*, **28**, 1015.

MONTAGUE, E. D. (1968). Experience with altered fractionation in radiation therapy of breast cancer. *Radiology*, **90**, 962.

MORGAN, R. L. (1967). Fast Neutron Therapy—Clinical Applications. *Modern Trends in Radiotherapy*, p. 171. Deeley, T. J. and Wood, C. A. P. (Eds.). London: Butterworths.

MOROSON, H., & FURLAN, M. (1967). Can N-ethylmaleimide preferentially radiosensitise hypoxic tumour cells *in vivo*? *Int. J. Radiat. Biol.*, **13**, 585.

MOROSON, H. L., & QUINTILIANI, M. (1970). *Radiation Protection and Sensitisation.* London: Taylor and Francis.

MOROSON, H., & TENNEY, D. N. (1968). Radiation sensitisation by thiol binding agents of radioresistant and radiosensitive *Escherichia coli* and the oxygen effect. *Radiat. Res.*, **36**, 418.

NIAS, A. H. W., SWALLOW, A. J., KEENE, J. P., & HODGSON, B. W. (1969). Effects of pulses of radiation on the survival of mammalian cells. *Br. J. Radiol.*, **42**, 553.

OLIVER, R. (1969). The effect of irradiation at extremely high dose-rates. *Br. J. Radiol.*, **42**, 231.

PHILLIPS, T. L., & HANKS, G. E. (1968). Apparent absence of recovery in endogenous colony-forming cells after irradiation under hypoxic conditions. *Radiat. Res.*, **33**, 517.

PHILLIPS, T. L., & WORSNOP, R. B. (1968). Abstract Fc8, Sixteenth Annual Meeting of the Radiation Research Society, Houston, April, 1968.

PIERQUIN, B., & BAILLET, F. (1970). Communication to the Annual Congress of the BIR.

PIZZARELLO, D. J., & WITCOFSKI, R. L. (1967). *Basic Radiation Biology.* London: Henry Kimpton.

POWERS, W. E., & TOLMACH, L. J. (1963). A multicomponent X-ray survival curve for mouse lymphosarcoma cells irradiated *in vivo*. *Nature, Lond.*, **197**, 710.

PUCK, T. T., & MARCUS, R. I. (1956). Action of X-rays on mammalian cells. *J. exp. Med.*, **103**, 653.

RAJU, M. R., AMER, N. M., GRIANAPIVANI, M., & RICHMAN, C. (1970). The oxygen effect on π-mesons in *Vicia faba*. *Radiat. Res.*, **41**, 135.

REFSUM, S. B., & BERDAL, P. (1967). Cell loss in malignant tumours in man. *Eur. J. Cancer*, **3**, 235.

REGAUD, C. (1923). The latent period of the biologic effect of X-rays, etc. as an explanation of the histophysiology. *Bull. Acad. natn. Méd.*, **91**, 375.

REINHOLD, H. S. (1965). A cell dispersion technique for use in quantitative transplantation studies with solid tumours. *Eur. J. Cancer*, **1**, 67.

RUBIN, P., & CASARETT, G. W. (1968). *Clinical Radiation Pathology*. Philadelphia: Saunders.

RUSH, B. F., & GREENLAW, R. H. (1968). *Symposium on Cancer Therapy by Integrated Irradiation and Operation*. Springfield, Illinois: Charles C. Thomas.

SAMBROOK, D. K. (1962). Clinical trial of a modified (split-course) technique of X-ray therapy in malignant tumours. *Clin. Radiol.*, **13**, 1.

DU SAULT, L. A. (1963). The effect of oxygen on the response of spontaneous tumours in mice to radiotherapy. *Br. J. Radiol.*, **36**, 749.

SAWADA, S., & OKADA, S. (1970). Rejoining of single-strand breaks of DNA in cultured mammalian cells. *Radiat. Res.*, **41**, 145.

SCANLON, P. W. (1960). Initial experience with 'split-dose' periodic radiation therapy. *Am. J. Roentg.*, **84**, 632.

SINCLAIR, W. K. (1968). Cyclic X-ray responses in mammalian cells *in vitro*. *Radiat. Res.*, **33**, 620.

SPRATT, J. S. (1965a). The rates and patterns of growth of neoplasms of the large intestine and rectum. *Surg. Clins N. Am.*, **45**, 1103.

SPRATT, J. S. (1965b). The rates of growth of skeletal sarcomas. *Cancer*, **18**, 14.

STEEL, G. G. (1967). Cell loss as a factor in the growth rate of human tumours. *Eur. J. Cancer*, **3**, 381.

STEEL, G. G. (1968). Cell loss from experimental tumours. *Cell Tissue Kinetics*, **1**, 193.

STONE, R. S. (1948). Neutron therapy and specific ionisation. *Am. J. Roentg.*, **59**, 771.

STRANDQVIST, M. (1944). Studien über die kumulativ Wirkung der Röntgenstrahlen bei Fraktionierung. *Acta radiol.* (suppl. 55), 1.

SUIT, H. D. (1968). Application of radiobiologic principles to radiation therapy. *Cancer*, **22**, 809.

SUIT, H. D., & SHALEK, R. J. (1963). Response of anoxic C3H mouse mammary carcinoma isotransplants (1–25 mm³) to x-irradiation. *J. natn. Cancer Inst.*, **31**, 479.

SUIT, H., & URANO, M. (1969). Repair of sublethal radiation injury in hypoxic cells of a C3H mouse mammary carcinoma. *Radiat. Res.*, **37**, 423.

SWALLOW, A. J., & VELANDIA, J. A. (1962). Oxygen effect as an explanation of differences between the action of α-particles and X- or γ-rays in aqueous solutions of amino acids and proteins. *Nature, Lond.*, **195**, 798.

SZYBALSKI, W. (1967). Molecular events resulting in radiation injury, repair and sensitisation of DNA. *Radiat. Res.*, Suppl. 7, 147.

TANNOCK, I. F. (1968). The relation between cell proliferation and the vascular system in a transplanted mouse mammary tumour. *Br. J. Cancer*, **99**, 258.

TANNOCK, I. F., & STEEL, G. G. (1969). Quantitative techniques for study of the anatomy and function of small blood vessels in tumours. *J. natn. Cancer Inst.*, **42**, 771.

TERASIMA, T., & TOLMACH, L. J. (1961). Changes in X-ray sensitivity of HeLa cells during the division cycle. *Nature, Lond.*, **190**, 1210.

THOMLINSON, R. H. (1960). An experimental method in comparing treatments of intact malignant tumours in animals and its application to the use of oxygen in radiotherapy. *Br. J. Cancer*, **14**, 555.

THOMLINSON, R. H. (1967). Oxygen Therapy—Biological Considerations. *Modern Trends in Radiotherapy*, p. 52. Deeley, T. J. and Wood, C. A. P. (Eds.). London: Butterworths.

THOMLINSON, R. F., & GRAY, L. H. (1955). The histological structure of some human lung cancers and the possible implications for radiotherapy. *Br. J. Cancer*, **9**, 539.

TILL, J. E., & McCULLOCH, E. A. (1961). A direct measurement of the radiation sensitivity of normal mouse bone marrow cells. *Radiat. Res.*, **14**, 213.

TOWN, C. D. (1967). Effect of high dose rates on survival of mammalian cells. *Nature, Lond.*, **215**, 847.

TUBIANA, M. (1971). The kinetics of tumour cell proliferation and radiotherapy. *Br. J. Radiol.*, **44**, 325.

VAN DEN BRENK, H. A. S., MADIGAN, J. P., KERR, R. C., & RICHTER, W. (1963). Treatment of malignant disease of the extremities by megavoltage irradiation under tissue anoxia. *J. Coll. Radiol. Australasia*, **7**, 142.

VAN PUTTEN, L. M. (1968). Tumour reoxygenation during fractionated radiotherapy; studies with a transplantable mouse osteosarcoma. *Eur. J. Cancer*, **4**, 173.

VAN PUTTEN, L. M., & KALLMAN, R. F. (1968). Oxygenation status of a transplantable tumour during fractionated radiation therapy. *J. natn. Cancer Inst.*, **40**, 441.

WINSTON, B., ELLIS, F., & HALL, E. J. (1969). The Oxford N.S.D. calculator for clinical use. *Clin. Radiol.*, **20**, 8.

WITHERS, H. R. (1967). The dose-survival relationship for irradiation of epithelioma cells of mouse skin. *Br. J. Radiol.*, **40**, 187.

WITHERS, H. R., & ELKIND, M. M. (1968). Dose-survival characteristics for irradiation of cells of the mouse intestinal mucosa. *Radiology*, **91**, 998.

WRIGHT, C. N., BOULOGNE, A. R., REINIG, W. C., & EVANS, A. G. (1967). Implantable californium-252 neutron sources for radiotherapy. *Radiology*, **89**, 337.

WRIGHT, E. A., HAHN, G. M., & STEELE, R. E. (1966). Towards the ideal use of the 'oxygen effect' in radiotherapy; the reciprocal oxygenated anoxic method. *Am. J. Roentg.*, **96**, 749.

WOOLLEY-HART, A., TWENTYMAN, P., CORFIELD, J., JOSLIN, C., MORRISON, R., & FOWLER, J. F. (1968). Changes in ^{32}P counting-rate in human and animal tumours. *Br. J. Radiol.*, **41**, 440.

YOUNG, J. M., & FOWLER, J. F. (1969). The effect of X-ray induced synchrony on two dose cell survival experiments. *Cell Tissue Kinetics*, **2**, 95.

9 Fast Neutrons in Radiotherapy

WILLIAM DUNCAN

NEUTRON RADIOTHERAPY

Neutron radiation has been considered for clinical use in two quite distinct ways which depend essentially on whether high energy 'fast' neutrons or low energy 'slow' neutrons are employed.

Fast neutrons are arbitrarily defined as having an energy over 10 KeV, but for radiotherapy only neutrons of energy over 1 MeV are of significant interest, for at this energy penetration in tissues begins to be sufficiently good to treat deep-seated tumours. All neutrons, when attenuated in tissues, release densely ionizing particles and their biological effect is much less influenced by availability of oxygen at the time of irradiation than is that of X-rays. Many malignant tumours contain hypoxic cells which retain their capacity to proliferate and fast neutrons will kill a much greater number of these cells than X-rays with no greater damage to normal tissues. (Fowler *et al.*, 1963).

Slow neutrons are used for neutron capture therapy. This treatment requires selective localization within the tumour of a chemical, such as boron, with a high affinity for slow neutrons. If this is achieved, irradiation with slow neutrons produces nuclear reactions in the localized chemical which will emit secondary radiation of very limited range (within a cell) and so destroy only tumour cells. This application holds much less promise of therapeutic advantage generally and is not the subject of this review (see Brownell *et al.*, 1967).

THE OXYGEN EFFECT AND FAST NEUTRONS

Oxygen is one of the most powerful dose-modifying agents known and the effect of X-rays is increased by a factor of about three when irradiation is performed in well oxygenated conditions rather than in an atmosphere of nitrogen (Gray *et al.*, 1953). By comparison, the effect of fast neutrons is only modified by a factor of about 1·6. This general phenomenon in radiobiology is called the 'oxygen effect'. The magnitude of the oxygen effect is measured by the oxygen enhancement ratio (OER) and is usually derived from the ratio of the slopes (D_0 values) of cell survival curves (Fig. 1). HeLa cells *in vitro* have been found to have an OER of 2·4 when irradiated with 250 KeV X-rays and an OER of 1·5

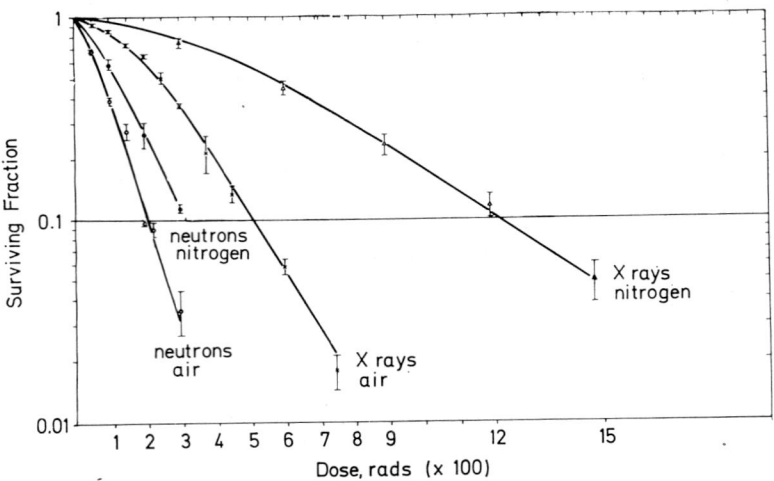

Fig. 9.1. HeLa cell survival curves following irradiation, in air and in nitrogen, with 14 MeV neutrons and 250 KV X-rays (Nias *et al.*, 1967). (Reproduced by courtesy Editors *International Journal, Radiation Biology*.)

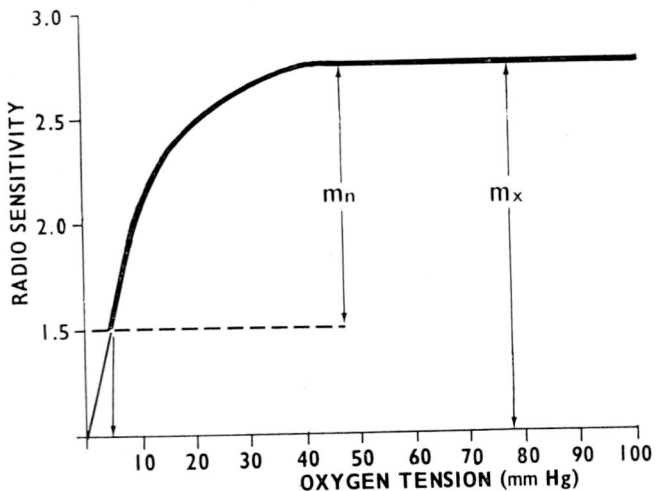

Fig. 9.2. The relationship of cellular radiosensitivity to the oxygen concentration in tissues at the time of irradiation. (After Alper and Moore, 1967.)

with fast neutrons (Nias *et al.*, 1967). The ratio of the OER for X-rays compared with fast neutrons has been called the 'Gain Factor' (Alper 1963) and is the measure of the relative effectiveness of fast neutrons in killing hypoxic cells.

Under normal conditions in the well oxygenated capillary bed of tissues, the relative radiosensitivity is near its maximum (Fig. 2). When the oxygen concentration falls below 40 micromoles per litre, radio-sensitivity rapidly diminishes. The shape of the response curve is the same for X-rays and fast neutrons although the OER is much less with fast neutrons. The explanation for this difference, first demonstrated by Giles *et al.* (1952), is not yet established. Alper and Moore (1967) produced evidence suggesting that the neutron curve is raised to a level dependent on the amount of increased oxygen formation occurring in the tracks of the high LET particles. If this is so, then the relationship of the OER for X-rays and the OER for fast neutrons must be inter-dependent. The largest 'Gain Factor' will be obtained for mammalian cells with high OER values with X-rays, a fact of some importance in choosing suitable tumours for therapeutic trials with fast neutrons.

However, the gain factor is irrelevant unless it be demonstrated that there are significant proportions of hypoxic and anoxic cells in tumours. This has indeed been shown, very comprehensively for animal tumours, and more than a *prima facie* case has been stated for most human tumours (see Chapter 8). The evidence thus strongly suggests that most experimental and human tumours contain a proportion of hypoxic cells which retain their ability to proliferate. Some degree of re-oxy-genation of these cells may take place during a fractionated course of X-ray treatment, but this is often suboptimal, and the presence of a very small proportion of anoxic cells in a tumour at the last treatment greatly reduces the chance of cure (Munro, 1967).

Fast neutrons, having a low OER, should be much more effective in the treatment of hypoxic tumours. Neutron generators are now being developed, and their properties evaluated, for possible application in radiotherapy.

CRITERIA OF FAST NEUTRON SOURCES FOR BEAM THERAPY

The first essential property of fast neutron beams for radiotherapy is that the OER is advantageously low compared with that of X and γ radiation. In addition, the penetrating properties of the beam must be great enough to allow the treatment of deep seated tumours, and this is best achieved with high energy neutrons. It is also necessary for the fast neutron beam to be sufficiently intense to provide dose-rates which would allow reasonable treatment times at distances of at least 75 cm, the minimum thickness of material required for adequate shielding and collimation.

At present there are four types of neutron generator which may be considered as possible sources for clinical use: Nuclear Reactors, Compact Cyclotrons, Large Cyclotrons and Deuterium-Tritium Generators. Their important physical and biological parameters are detailed in Table I.

Nuclear reactors produce a beam of neutrons with a mean energy of about 1 MeV, with penetration in tissues too poor for general use in radiotherapy and suitable for treating only the most superficial tumours. It is possible to use only fixed beams of fast neutrons and this restriction would be unacceptable to most radiotherapists.

Compact cyclotrons have been built using a new principle in design. Although much smaller than conventional cyclotrons, it was expected that high beam currents and high outputs of neutrons could be attained (Fleischer, 1968). When actual measurements were made (Broerse and Barendsen, 1967; Brennan, 1969), using the reaction of 20 MeV tritons on beryllium, the intensity of neutrons was disappointingly low and the penetration of the beam was also poor.

Large cyclotrons, on the other hand, are reliable and versatile machines. Intense beams of neutrons are produced by accelerating positive ions at very high energies on to targets of low atomic number (Bewley, 1970). The Medical Research Council 30 in cyclotron at the Hammersmith Hospital (Fig. 3) accelerates 16 MeV deuterons on to a beryllium target giving a beam of neutrons with a mean energy of 7 MeV, and depth doses very similar to those provided by orthovoltage X-ray machines. The 70 in TAMVEC cyclotron accelerates 30 MeV deuterons on to beryllium and produces a beam of 15 MeV neutrons. This beam is much more penetrating than 7 MeV neutrons and the dose-rate is high enough for radiotherapy. The staff of the M.D. Anderson Hospital in Houston, Texas, have decided to use this 70 in cyclotron to undertake clinical trials. Elaborate plans have been made to give a steerable beam of neutrons and also to have a moving floor and couch assembly so that a wide range of treatment axes can be provided (Almond, 1970).

Cyclotrons are too large and complex to be used in most radiotherapy clinics but may be suitable for university departments where facilities and responsibility for operation can be shared with others. The initial cost of a large cyclotron is perhaps about £500,000 and the services of many highly skilled staff are needed for its maintenance and reliable performance.

The deuterium-tritium generators accelerate deuterium ions at relatively low voltage on to a tritium target. The resulting fusion reaction produces 14 MeV mono-energetic neutrons which are emitted isotropically from the target. An output of 10^{12} neutrons per second

TABLE I

POSSIBLE SOURCES FOR FAST NEUTRON BEAM THERAPY

Group	Actual source	Reaction	Average Neutron energy	Field size = 10 × 10 cm SSD = 75 cm		Gain factor mx/mn	
				Dose rate rads/min	50% dose (cm) $(n + \gamma)$	Berry (1969)	Barendsen (1966)
1. Nuclear reactors	TRIGA Reactor Bethesda, Maryland	235 uranium fission	1	60	5	2·7	1·7
2. Compact cyclotrons	CS–15 cyclotron Berkeley, California	^{9}Be (d,n) ^{10}B	4	3	5	—	—
		^{9}Be $(^3$He,n$)$ ^{11}C	5	6	7	—	—
	A.V.F. cyclotron Eindhoven, Holland	^{9}Be $(^3$He,n$)$ ^{11}C	5	21	7	—	1·6
3. Large cyclotrons	30 in cyclotron Hammersmith Hospital, London	^{9}Be (d,n) ^{10}B	6	100	8	1·9	1·6
	70 in cyclotron TAMVEC Texas, A. & M	^{9}Be (d,n) ^{10}B	15	40	10	2·0	—
4. D.T. generators	D.T. (rotating target) generator Livermore, California	^{3}H (d,n) ^{4}He	14	6	10	1·8	—
	D.T. (sealed tube) generator Christie Hospital, Manchester	^{3}H (d,n) ^{4}He	14	10	10	—	1·6*

* This value was obtained by Nias et al. (1967). Barendsen et al. (1966) obtained the same result using the D.T. generator at Rijswijk.

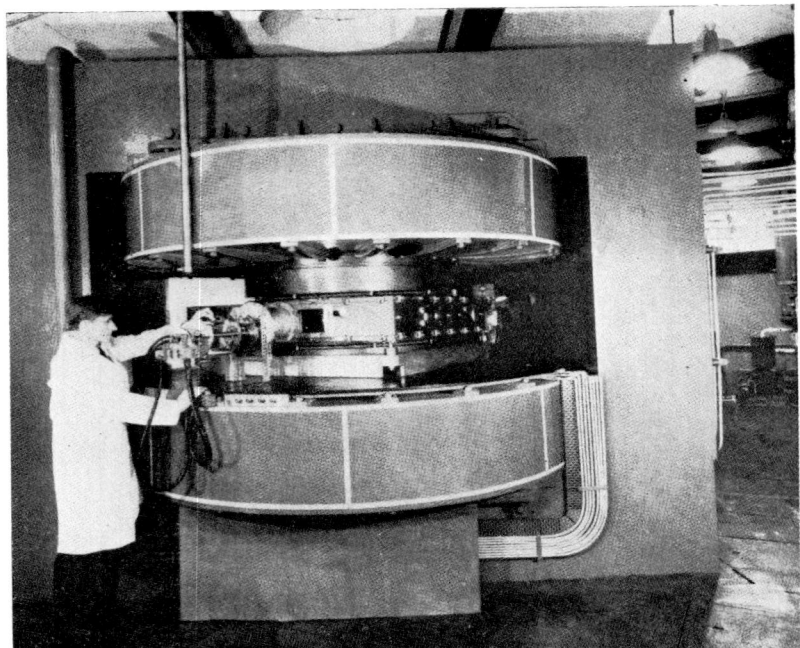

FIG. 9.3. The M.R.C. cyclotron at Hammersmith Hospital. (Reproduced by courtesy of Editors, *British Journal of Radiology*).

gives a dose-rate of about five rads per minute at 75 cm from the target and this is considered the minimum requirement for radiotherapeutic trials. The other limitation of D.T. generators has been the short life of the target. When these generators are used at high power, the great heat produced in the target drives off the bound tritium leading to reduced neutron output within a few hours. Several independent research groups are now working to develop D.T. generators with an output of at least 1×10^{12} neutrons per second combined with a long target life.

The most favourable approach is to use a 'mixed' beam system in which both deuterium and tritium ions are accelerated on to the target. The tritium from the beam replenishes tritium lost from the target. In the U.S.A., work has centred on continuously pumped generators—a system which carries some disadvantages from the point of view of radiotherapeutic application. The potential hazards of operation are considerable because of the high activity of tritium gas in the tube and the ancillary apparatus required is cumbersome. Brennan (1969) of Philadelphia has initiated the design of an accelerator using a mixed beam of deuterons and tritons which is directed on to a special copper target. Here the tritium is driven in and lodged in the lattice of the metal by the incident beam and, in this way, long target lives may be attained. It is hoped to achieve an output of 4×10^{12} neutrons per second from this type of generator.

Another research group in Madison, U.S.A., is considering the design of a mixed beam—gas target generator which should in principle give an unlimited target life but this system is a long way from practical testing. (Kelsey *et al.*, 1971.)

The alternative approach to a continuously pumped apparatus is a sealed tube device. Sealed generators are much more attractive from the standpoint of tritium safety and should also provide long operational lifetimes. In England, the Services Electronics Research Laboratories (S.E.R.L.) (Downton *et al.*, 1968) and Philips Research Laboratories in the Netherlands (Reifenschweiler, 1968) have produced high output neutron generators of this type. Since 1963, research has been conducted by S.E.R.L. to develop a compact sealed tube neutron generator especially for radiotherapy (Lomer and Greene, 1963).

THE SEALED TUBE NEUTRON GENERATOR

In principle, the generator (Fig. 4) consists of two sections—an ion source and an accelerating zone. A mixture of deuterium and tritium gas is ionized by a powerful radio-frequency coil and the ions, both tritons and deuterons, are extracted through an aperture and accelerated on to a tritium loaded rare earth target (Paris *et al.*, 1968). The generator developed for clinical use has special features in design and in particular the target is at earth potential (Hillier *et al.*, 1971). The neutron output

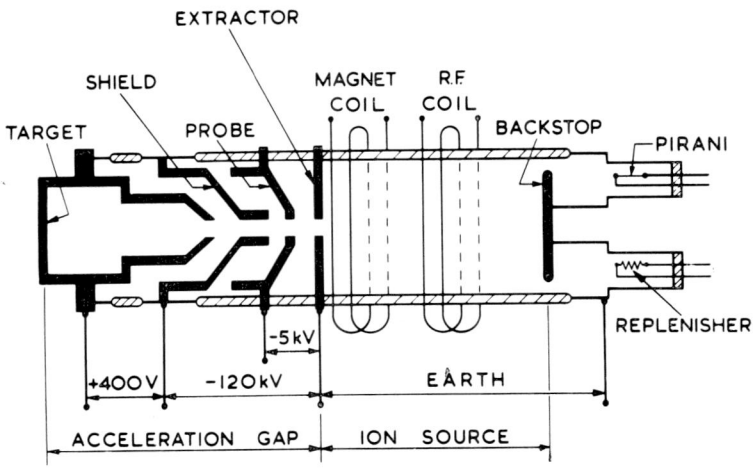

FIG. 9.4. Diagram of a sealed tube neutron generator, and its supplies. (Paris, 1968.)

is improved considerably by increasing the accelerating voltage to 250 kV (30 mA) and an emission of over 1×10^{12} neutrons per second has been obtained. The life of these tubes is greater than 100 hours and this may be extended with further tube development (Bounden *et al.*, 1967). Their operation is simple and reliable, essential features for apparatus designed for routine clinical use.

This compact unit (Fig. 5) may be suitably insulated in a steel container which can easily be inserted and removed from a specially designed radiotherapy machine. The English Department of Health and Social Security, in co-operation with the National Research and Development Corporation, has sponsored the development of the S.E.R.L. neutron generator and the manufacture of a Neutron Therapy machine. Elliott Automation Radar Systems Ltd. are responsible for the development of this equipment, which has been called the 'Hiletron'.

THE HILETRON

This is the first machine designed exclusively for fast neutron therapy with facilities comparable with modern megavoltage equipment (Lundberg 1971) (Fig. 6). The sealed tube neutron generator, enclosed in its oil-filled insulating container, is mounted in the treatment head (Fig. 7). The neutron shield consists of layers of steel, polythene and lead, which reduce the transmitted radiation around the treatment head to a level of 1% of that in the main beam. The beam will be collimated by a series of interchangeable applicators handled by a mechanical trolley. The limits of each field are to be illuminated and light sources will also indicate the correct source to skin distance. A fixed S.S.D. of either 80 cm or 85 cm may be obtained. Mechanical front and back pointers are also provided. Field sizes will range from 5×5 cm to a 30 cm circular field.

The treatment head is mounted isocentrically, mechanized for rotational therapy and can be angled to 110° from the vertical position on both sides.

The treatment couch has the usual freedom of movements and its vertical movement is motorized. Special features in design have been used to minimize the induced radioactivity which will occur in the couch assembly. The S.E.R.L. neutron generator tube will initially give an output of about 1×10^{12} neutrons per second and a dose-rate of about 5 rads per minute at 80 cm.

The power supply is mounted on the annulus counterbalancing the treatment head and the 250 kV cable pierces a dividing partition which separates the treatment room from the service area.

The machine is operated from a simple console by radiographers and controlled by a single ON-OFF button. The dose to be delivered will be

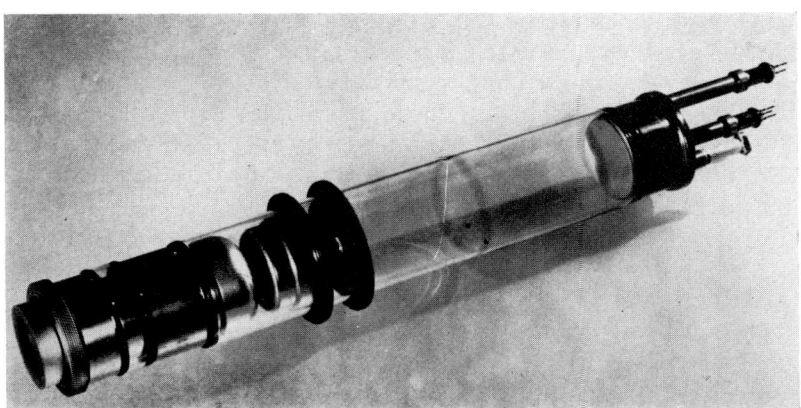

FIG. 9.5. A sealed tube neutron generator designed for the production of 14 MeV neutrons at a rate of 1×10^{11} neutrons/sec. The tube is about 45 cm long (Paris, 1968).

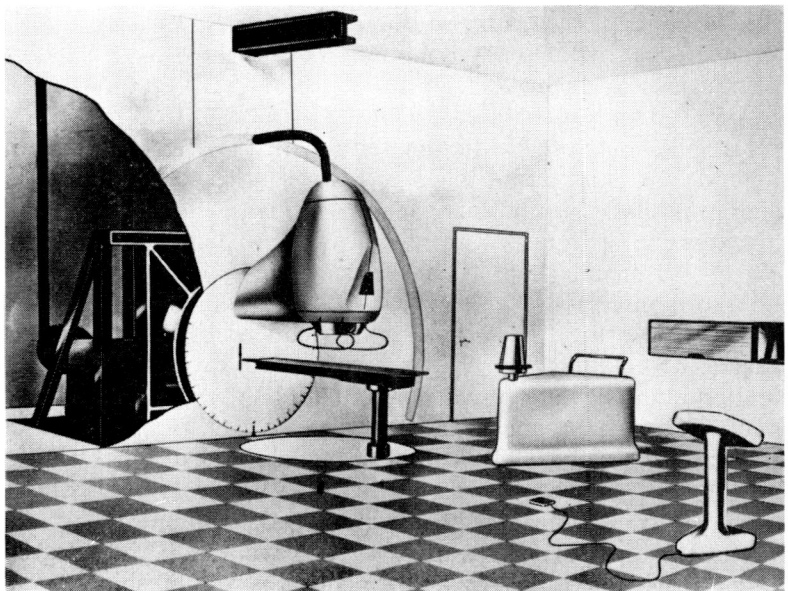

FIG. 9.6. An artist's impression of the 'Hiletron'.

pre-set and the machine will switch off automatically. Double dose meters are incorporated in the treatment head and in addition the console has a clock mechanism which will also, if necessary, switch off the neutron generator. Meters registering dose rate and integrated dose are provided in the control console.

The first of the machines is to be installed at the Christie Hospital and Holt Radium Institute in Manchester in July 1971, and the second Hiletron will be delivered to the Glasgow Institute of Radiotherapeutics at Belvidere Hospital about 6 months later.

PHYSICAL PROPERTIES OF FAST NEUTRON BEAMS

SHIELDING AND COLLIMATION

Normal clinical radiotherapy will require collimation of the beam of neutrons and shielding of the remainder of the patient as much as possible from stray radiation. The design of a suitable shield for 14 MeV neutrons has to be undertaken within the limitations of space determined by the neutron output of the generator. Reasonable treatment times can only be obtained if the source to skin distance (S.S.D.) is kept as short as possible. The shielding and collimation of neutrons from a cyclotron is much easier to achieve (Bewley 1970) than from 14 MeV D.T. generators (Greene and Major, 1970).

It is the thickness of shielding material which is of prime importance with 14 MeV neutrons and whereas hydrogenous materials are more efficient in terms of weight, Greene (1964) showed that steel is the most suitable material with respect to thickness. More detailed studies on the design of the shield have been conducted by Greene and Thomas (1969) and Greene and Major (1970). They have shown that the transmitted radiation through steel is further reduced by adding a layer of polythene, which effectively absorbs the slowed-down neutrons arising from attenuation of the neutron beam in steel. Attenuation in this layer produces gamma rays and these may be absorbed in another layer of high density material such as lead. The treatment head for the Hiletron (Fig. 7) is built on the principle of a composite shield of this type. In this way the transmitted radiation is reduced to about 1%; it seems impractical with D.T. generators to achieve the higher degree of shielding provided with X-ray and telecurie therapy machines.

The design of a collimation system presents many technical problems. Beam collimators made largely of steel are far from ideal, not only because of their great weight but also because of the hazard of induced radioactivity in the metal. Greene and Major (1970) have compared

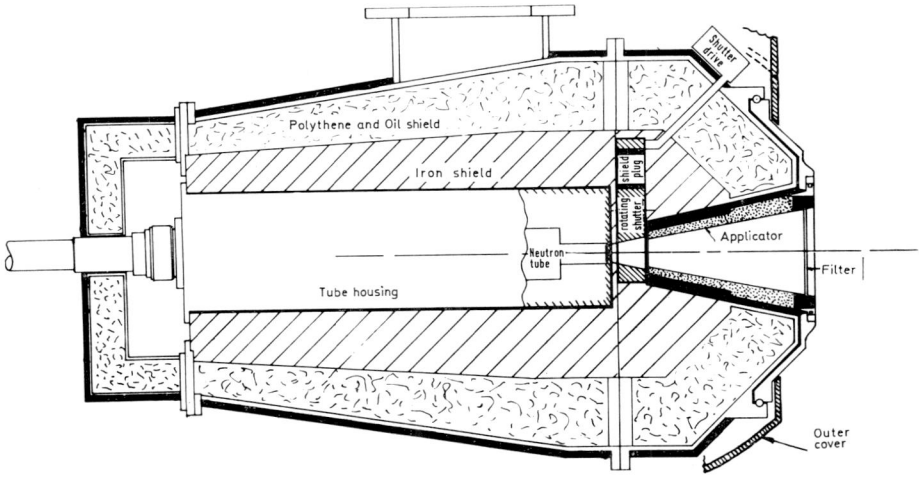

FIG. 9.7. The design of the treatment head of the Hiletron showing the shielding materials. (Reproduced by courtesy of Elliott Automation Ltd.)

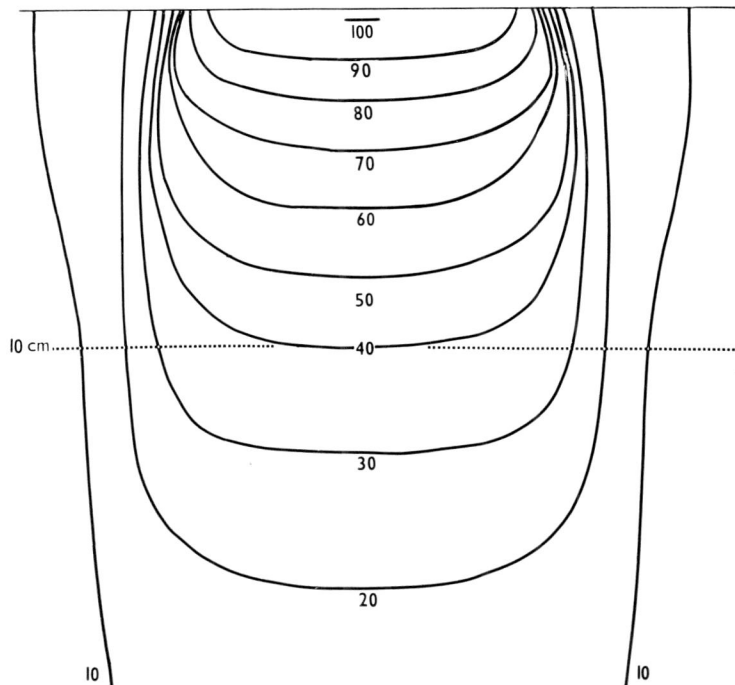

FIG. 9.8. Isodose chart for a 10 × 10 cm field 14 MeV neutrons at 55 cm source to skin distance (Greene and Major, 1970).

collimators made mostly of polythene with those made mainly of steel, and around the edge of the beam there is no significant difference in definition. However, beyond this region the level of stray radiation is significantly higher with the polythene collimator. It is important that the level of whole body radiation be kept as low as is practicable and the optimum design of collimator is being actively pursued. The dose distribution measured across the axis of a beam of 14 MeV neutrons using a composite steel, polythene steel collimator shows good flatness and definition (Fig. 8).

The high intensity of the neutron beam from the M.R.C. cyclotron at Hammersmith Hospital eases the problem of its collimation (Bewley and Parnell, 1969). The main shield material is a mixture of iron pellets and of boric acid in paraffin wax around a thick steel collimator. Into this can be placed a series of borated wooden applicators to define the treatment field (Fig. 9).

STRAY WHOLE BODY RADIATION FROM NEUTRON BEAMS

The levels of stray radiation outside a collimated beam of neutrons may be much greater than with photon radiation. The relative dose levels measured to 35 cm from the central axis of the beam for megavoltage X-rays, cobalt gamma rays and fast neutrons are shown in Fig. 10. The fast neutron data include the estimation of gamma ray contribution to dose (except for the 14 MeV neutron curve) measured using a 75 cm experimental collimator and a nuclear emulsion film technique (Marshall, 1970). The quality of this stray radiation is of great importance and has not been fully investigated. Preliminary measurement in a water phantom with 14 MeV neutrons (Greene and Major, 1970) shows that at about 8 cm from the central axis of the beam, gamma rays contribute about 50% of the total dose increasing to almost 100% at 50 cm from the central axis. Similar measurements have been made with the 7 MeV neutron beam at Hammersmith (Bewley and Parnell, 1969) with which the gamma radiation dose exceeded the neutron dose at 10 cm from the central axis but quickly became negligible beyond this. The large gamma ray component reduces considerably the biological effectiveness of stray radiation from neutron beams. It has been estimated that the dose levels outside the 14 MeV neutron beam using a 50 cm collimator are derived about two thirds from stray radiation transmitted through the shield and about one third from scattered radiation from the primary beam. An attempt has been made to assess the clinical significance of this stray radiation contribution to the whole body dose, and although higher than desirable, these dose levels are considered to be tolerable (Duncan, Greene and Major, 1970).

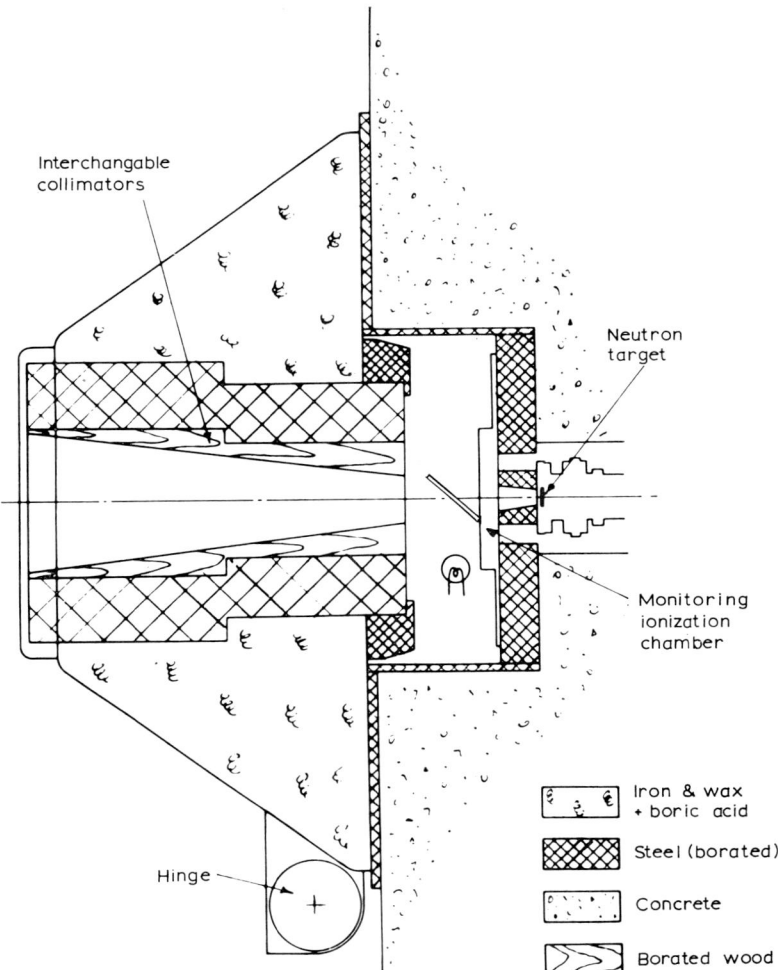

Interchangable
collimators

Neutron
target

Monitoring
ionization
chamber

Hinge

	Iron & wax + boric acid
	Steel (borated)
	Concrete
	Borated wood

FIG. 9.9. Diagram of the shielding and collimation of the neutron target of the M.R.C. cyclotron at the Hammersmith Hospital (Bewley and Parnell, 1969). (Reproduced by courtesy of the Editors, *British Journal of Radiology*.)

BEAM PENETRATION AND NEUTRON QUALITY AT DEPTH

It is essential for the treatment of deep-seated tumours that good penetration of the neutron beam is obtained. The depth dose characteristics have been studied theoretically by Snyder and Neufield (1955) and by Auxier *et al.* (1968) and it has been shown that penetration improves with increasing energy of the beam. For radiotherapy it is necessary that

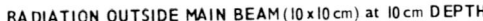

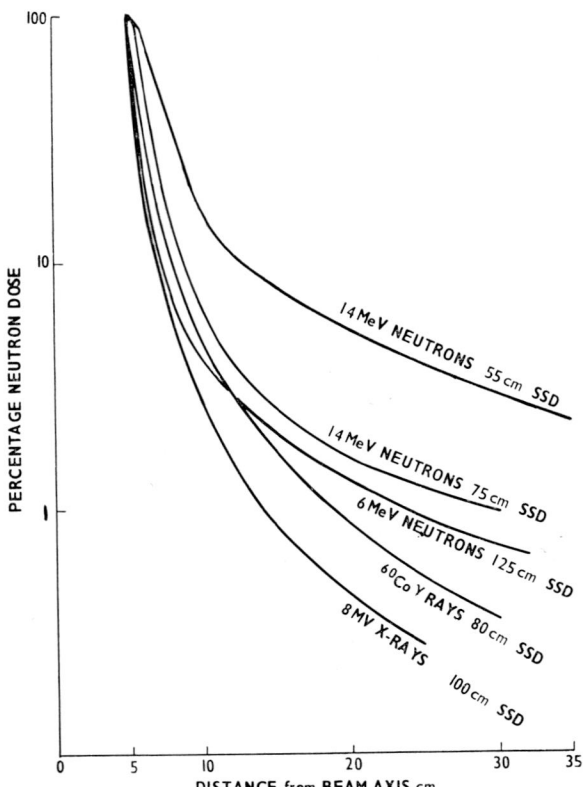

FIG. 9.10. Stray radiation from 10 × 10 cm collimated beams of X-rays and fast neutrons at 10 cm deep in phantom.

the 50% dose should be at a depth in tissue of at least 10 cm, and only large cyclotrons and D.T. generators can at present produce such a penetrating beam.

A collimated beam of 14 MeV neutrons gives depth doses very similar to those of telecobalt therapy beams (Fig. 11), and if the output of D.T. generators can be increased depth doses will be improved by using greater source to skin distances (Fig. 12). A beam of 7 MeV neutrons has appreciably less penetrating power than 14 MeV neutrons but this can be offset to some extent by using a much greater S.S.D. because of the higher neutron output from a cyclotron.

The percentage depth doses for fast neutrons, like those of ortho-voltage X-rays, are dependent on field size, (Fig.13).

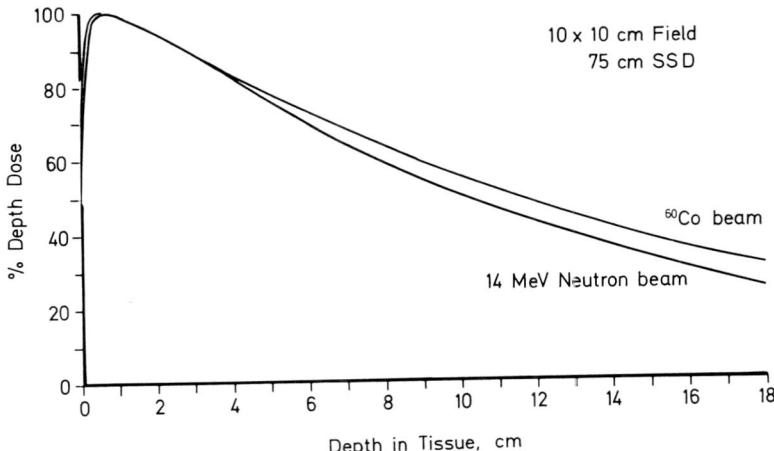

FIG. 9.11. Depth dose curves of 14 MeV neutrons compared with telecobalt gamma radiation.

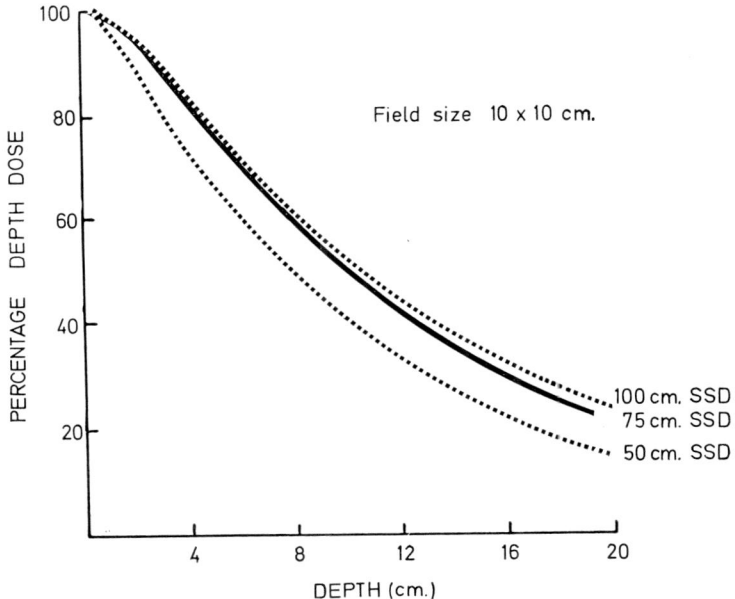

FIG. 9.12. Variation of depth dose curve of 14 MeV neutrons with change in source to skin distance. (Data from Greene and Thomas, 1968.)

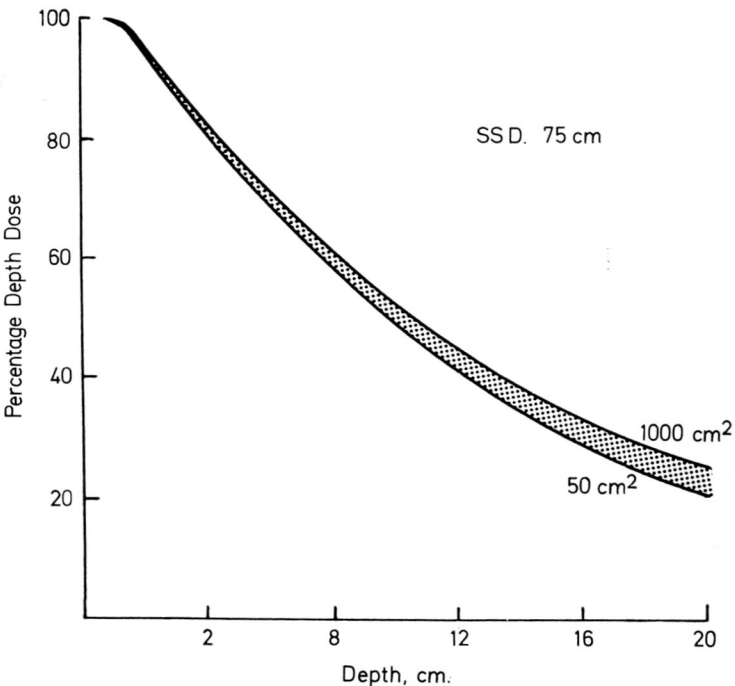

FIG. 9.13. Variation in depth dose curve of 14 MeV neutrons with change in field size. (Data from Greene and Thomas, 1968.)

NEUTRON BEAM QUALITY

The beam of fast neutrons is contaminated by slowed-down neutrons and gamma rays produced by attenuation in the shield and collimator. Greene and Thomas (1968), using an experimental 14 MeV generator with a 50 cm steel collimator, have shown that the gamma ray dose in the beam is about 8% and the slow neutron fluence about 2%. The gamma ray contamination of the M.R.C. cyclotron beam is about 4% (McNally and Bewley, 1969).

In the same way, the quality of the neutron beam will change as it penetrates tissues and it is important to determine the nature and extent of this alteration and its biological significance.

The gamma ray contribution to the total depth dose is never greater than 10% and with 14 MeV neutrons the gamma ray contribution to the local dose at depth in tissues may not significantly exceed this level (Greene and Thomas, 1968). With the 7 MeV neutron beam from the M.R.C. cyclotron the gamma ray contribution to the local dose rises to about 25% at 20 cm depth (Bewley, 1970). The biological significance of the gamma ray dose is reduced by an R.B.E. factor of perhaps 2·5 so that the effective gamma ray dose from 14 MeV neutrons is not greater than 4%.

It is also of practical importance to know how the spectrum of neutron energies changes with attenuation in tissues, for changes in the linear energy transfer (L.E.T.) may greatly alter the biological properties of the neutron beam at different depths. Much more detailed study is necessary on this aspect of fast neutron beams, although some measurements have been made using threshold detectors and sensitive biological models. With mono-energetic 14 MeV neutrons progressive scattering in tissues reduces the neutron energy with a slight increase in mean L.E.T. at depth (Lawson and Watt, 1967). By comparison, the 7 MeV neutron beam produced by the M.R.C. cyclotron includes a wide spectrum of neutron energies. In this case, it is found that filtration by tissues of the lower energy neutrons results in a slight 'hardening' of the beam (Field and Parnell, 1965) and this effect is greater than the reduction in mean neutron energy produced by scattering processes. Lawson and Watt (1968) found a slight increase in L.E.T. at depth in the 7 MeV neutron beam but this has not been confirmed by Wilson and Field (1969). Scattering effects produce a considerable increase in thermal and epithermal neutrons in the beam but they still make only a small contribution to the total dose (Bewley and Parnell, 1969). When comparing experimental results from different neutron sources it should be noted that differences in geometry may account for large changes in the values of the physical and biological parameters of the beam (Broerse et al., 1971).

BIOLOGICALLY EFFECTIVE DEPTH DOSES

R.B.E. at depth. Changes in the biological parameters for mammalian cells have been studied in relation to their position in scattering medium irradiated with fast neutrons. Ehrlich ascites tumour cells have been irradiated at four different depths (2, 10, 16 and 24 cm) in a tissue equivalent phantom (McNally and Bewley, 1969). The relative sensitivity of the tumour cells to the neutron beam at these depths was found to compare well with the relative doses measured by an ionization chamber and by activation of sulphur pellets (Fig. 14). This demonstrated that no change in RBE had occurred at depth. Berry et al. (1965) had previously shown no difference in the biological efficiency of 7 MeV neutrons measured in air and at 10 cm deep in phantom by *in vivo* assay of P-388 lymphoma cells. A similar experiment using 14 MeV neutrons also showed no alteration in the biological effectiveness at depth (Berry and Ellis, 1966). Preliminary experimental results (Nias and Greene, 1971) using HeLa cells in culture have shown a slight decrease

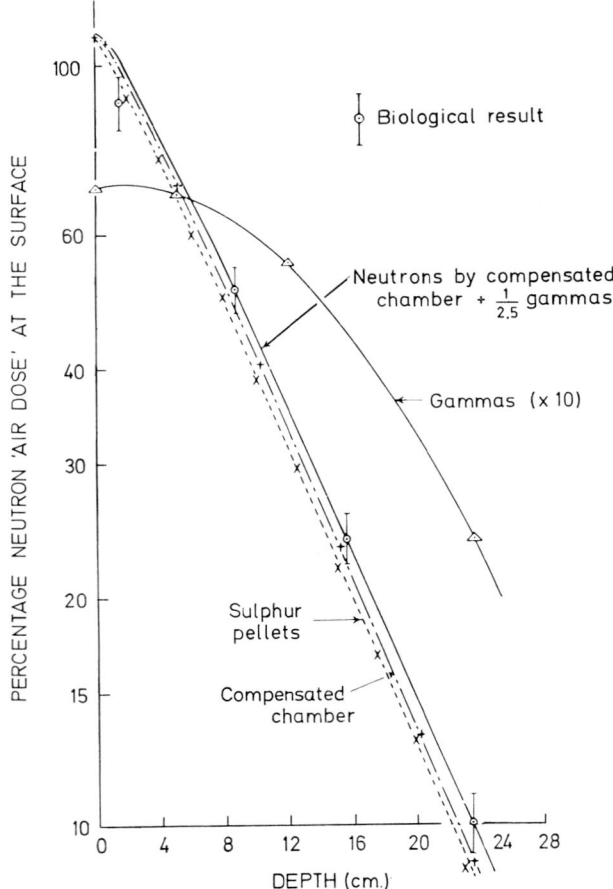

Fɪɢ. 9.14. A comparison of central axis depth doses in tissue equivalent phantom,
measured by physical and biological methods (McNally and Bewley, 1969).
(Reproduced by courtesy of Editors, *British Journal of Radiotherapy.*)

in the R.B.E. values for cells irradiated with 14 MeV neutrons at 10 cm
depth in a water phantom and in the penumbra in air. Evans *et al.*
(1970) have recently reported decreasing effectiveness of an uncollimated 6 MeV neutron beam with depth. They measured the survival of
HeLa cells irradiated at 2·4 cm, 8 cm and 16 cm deep in a tissue equivalent phantom and for 37% survival obtained R.B.E. values of 3·2,
2·7 and 2·2. Further experimental work of this kind is required.

O.E.R. at depth. Berry (1969) has examined the oxygen enhancement
ratio of several different collimated beams of fast neutrons in air and
at 10 cm depth in a phantom filled with tissue equivalent fluid. The
biological system used was the P-388 lymphoma, in which the anoxic

response was obtained by *in vivo* irradiation, and the well oxygenated response measured by irradiation *in vitro*, and in both cell survival was assayed in normal recipient mice of the same strain. The results (Table II) show a reduction in O.E.R. at depth for the three neutron beams of therapeutic interest and could be of great importance. However, Berry *et al.* (1965) had earlier found no significant change in O.E.R. of the 7 MeV neutron beam from the M.R.C. cyclotron when irradiation of P-388 cells was performed 8·7 cm deep in a tissue equivalent phantom compared to measurements in air. Similarly no alteration in O.E.R. of the 7 MeV neutron beam at depth was found when Ehrlich ascites tumour cells were examined (McNally and Bewley, 1969). Other experiments with 14 MeV neutrons also produce evidence conflicting with Berry's results. Hall (1969) has shown no difference in O.E.R. in air and at 10 cm deep in a water phantom when Vicia seedlings were exposed to an uncollimated beam of 14 MeV neutrons. Nias and Greene (1971) also found no significant difference in O.E.R. for a collimated 14 MeV neutron beam when the response of HeLa cells was measured in air and at 10 cm depth in phantom.

It is obviously essential that further measurements be made of R.B.E. and O.E.R. values of collimated beams of fast neutrons at depth in phantoms. It is of the greatest practical importance that it be confirmed that the biological advantages of fast neutrons are maintained at depth in spite of attenuation of the beam in tissues.

TABLE II

Oxygen enhancement ratios measured by R. J. Berry (1969) for various fast neutron beams on the surface and at 10 cm deep in a tissue equivalent phantom.
The biological model is the P.388 lymphoma cell irradiated *in vivo* for anoxic conditions and *in vitro* for well-oxygenated conditions and both assayed *in vivo*.

Source	Neutron beam average energy	O.E.R. Surface	O.E.R. 10 cm depth
Fission reactor	1 MeV	1·12 (0·92–1·36)	1·24 (1·15–1·33)
Hammersmith cyclotron	7 MeV	1·63 (1·44–1·84)	1·28 (1·22–1·34)
D.T. generator Livermore	14 MeV	1·75 (1·58–1·96)	1·27 (1·08–1·49)
TAMVEC cyclotron Texas	15 MeV	1·50 (1·15–2·24)	1·11 (0·94–1·32)

ATTENUATION OF FAST NEUTRON BEAMS IN TISSUES

The deposition of energy in tissues depends on the release of charged particles from atomic nuclei following their interaction with fast neutrons.

The principal reaction is known as 'elastic' scattering in that the kinetic energy of the particles is changed, as in billiard ball collisions. Fast neutrons are most likely to collide in this way with hydrogen nuclei, ejecting a recoil proton and transferring on average half their energy. This reaction accounts for about 80% of the dose absorbed in wet tissues and the relative absorption in other tissues is roughly proportional to the hydrogen content. Fatty tissue, which is rich in hydrogen, will absorb 20% more dose than skin. Bone, by comparison contains relatively little hydrogen and absorbs about 15% less dose than skin. Elastic collisions also occur with other atomic nuclei such as oxygen, carbon and nitrogen, which produce densely ionizing heavy recoil particles and may be responsible for about 10% of the transfer of energy to tissue. The doses of neutron radiation received by different tissues have been calculated by Bewley (1963) taking into account elastic interactions only (Fig. 15).

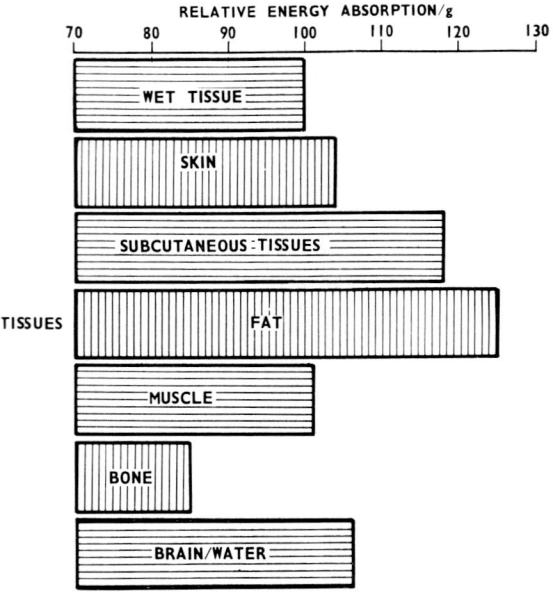

FIG. 9.15. The relative absorption of fast neutrons in tissues. (Data from Bewley, 1963.)

Other processes of attenuation also take place, some of which produce densely ionizing secondary particles of great biological importance. Nuclear disintegrations may take place following the absorption of neutrons in nuclei, which become so excited and unstable that they explode, giving rise to alpha particles, deuterons, protons and other neutrons. Such reactions may contribute almost 30% of the absorbed dose from 14 MeV neutrons (Randolph, 1957) and may account for their low oxygen enhancement ratio.

Neutron capture may take place in hydrogen and in nitrogen, producing their radio-isotopes and the emission of gamma rays and low energy protons respectively. Inelastic scattering of fast neutrons by the heavier atomic nuclei in tissues also results in a very small contribution of gamma rays to the absorbed dose.

AIR SOFT TISSUE INTERFACES—SKIN SPARING

A great advantage of megavoltage X and γ radiation is the skin sparing effect produced by the build-up of secondary electrons below the incident skin surface. With fast neutrons secondary protons are emitted similarly in a forward direction, and a build-up of dose occurs just below the surface. With 14 MeV neutrons the maximum dose is reached at 2·0 mm depth (Greene and Thomas, 1968) and at about 1·0 mm with a 7 MeV neutron beam (Bewley and Parnell, 1969). If the end of a collimator contains a hydrogenous filter to remove slow neutrons in the beam, the build-up effect would be lost unless a thin layer of aluminium is placed over it. In the same way, the surface of the oral mucosa may be protected by coating a wax bite block in the mouth with a very thin layer of lead (Catterall, 1971).

BONE—SOFT TISSUE INTERFACES

The dose of fast neutrons absorbed in wet bone free from bone marrow is only about half that received by soft tissue (Bewley, 1970). The effects of perturbations around bone marrow have been studied in detail by Broerse (1965) and he has found that the dose received by the bone marrow stem cells is about 10% less than the soft tissue dose. He has taken into consideration the large contribution to dose of heavy recoil particles which could have a higher R.B.E. than recoil protons. However, when mammalian cells were irradiated with 14 MeV neutrons adjacent to bone equivalent plastic, they received about 12% less dose. Indeed, when the number of recoil protons was greatly reduced by irradiating the cells on a carbon plaque, so that the energy deposition occurred mainly by recoil nuclei with L.E.T. values over 100 KeV/μ, the sensitivity of the cells was reduced by almost 50%.

BIOLOGICAL PROPERTIES OF FAST NEUTRONS

CELLULAR RADIOBIOLOGY

It is primarily by examining the experimental results of cellular radiobiology that the fundamental differences between the biological effect of low L.E.T. radiations and of fast neutrons may be seen. Cell survival curves have demonstrated three important differences in the response to fast neutrons compared with X or γ radiations. First, all mammalian cells show a greater sensitivity to fast neutrons than to low L.E.T. radiations, demonstrated (Fig. 17) by smaller D_0 values. Secondly, following irradiation with fast neutrons, the shoulder region of the survival curve is always smaller (or absent) than after X-rays, indicating a reduced capacity to repair sublethal radiation damage. Thirdly, the dose-modifying influence of the presence of oxygen at the time of irradiation is much less with fast neutrons and other high L.E.T. radiations than with X-rays.

OXYGEN ENHANCEMENT RATIO AND GAIN FACTOR

O.E.R. measurements are usually made *in vitro* with a cell culture being irradiated in air and in nitrogen (Fig. 1). The ratio of the slopes (D_0 values) of the survival curves gives the O.E.R. and is independent of dose. HeLa cells (Nias *et al.*, 1967) have shown an O.E.R. of 2·4 with 250 KeV X-rays and an O.E.R. of 1·5 with 14 MeV neutrons. The ratio of the O.E.R. for X-rays and the O.E.R. for neutrons has been called the 'Gain Factor' (Alper, 1963) and is a measure of the increased effectiveness of neutrons in killing anoxic cells. There appears to be little difference in the gain factor of 7 MeV and 14 MeV neutron beams and the mammalian cell systems used give a value of about 1·6 (Tables III and IV). The small differences in results may depend on the cell

TABLE III

Gain Factors Measured for 7 MeV Cyclotron Neutrons

Mammalian cell system	Gain factor Mx/Mn.	Reference
Ehrlich mouse ascites tumour cells	1·7 1·6	Bewley and Hornsey (1964) McNally and Bewley (1969)
Mouse leukaemia (P.388) cells	1·5 1·9	Berry *et al.* (1965) Berry (1969)
Mouse thymus	1·6	Wright *et al.* (1966)
Human kidney cells	1·6	Broerse and Barendsen (1967)
Rat cartilage	1·3	Kember (1969)

TABLE IV
GAIN FACTORS MEASURED FOR 14 MeV D. T. NEUTRONS

Mammalian cell system	Gain factor Mx/Mn.	Reference
Human kidney cells (TI)	1·6	Broerse and Barendsen (1967)
HeLa cells	1·6	Nias et al. (1967)
	1·6	Masuda (1968)
Rat rhabdomyosarcoma	1·6	Barendsen (1968)
Chinese hamster (CHL–F) cells	1·8	Hall (1969)
Mouse leukaemia (P 388) cells	1·8	Berry (1969)

system used and on the experimental conditions at the time of irradiation. The gain factor is the comparative difference in response of a wholly anoxic population of cells and that of a well-oxygenated population of cells to X-rays and neutrons and represents the greatest possible advantage in this respect of fast neutrons over X-rays. If an increased effectiveness of this order were applicable in the clinical situation, fast neutrons could possibly produce permanent regression in a very much greater number of anoxic tumours than could be cured by X-rays. However, in most malignant tumours only a small proportion of the cells are anoxic. The gain factor is accordingly reduced and is expected from other evidence to be about 1·2 (Fowler, 1967a).

O.E.R. AND FRACTIONATION

The response of a tumour containing 1% anoxic cells following irradiation with fast neutrons and X-rays is represented in Fig. 16 (Hornsey and Silini, 1963). The positions of the initial slopes of the survival curves have been superimposed by applying a single R.B.E. factor observed for well-oxygenated cells. For these cells the O.E.R. for X-rays and for 7 MeV neutrons is 3·1 and 1·8 respectively, giving a gain factor of 1·7. With doses of fast neutrons greater than 500 rads the response of the anoxic cells predominates and the maximum gain factor is obtained. However, with doses under this 'threshold' value the gain factor quickly falls to unity. In general the greater the proportion of anoxic cells in a tumour cell population the lower is the 'threshold' dose below which the practical gain factor is lost. It is possible that the improvement in tumour response which might be obtained with fast neutron therapy could be lost if too small dose fractions were given.

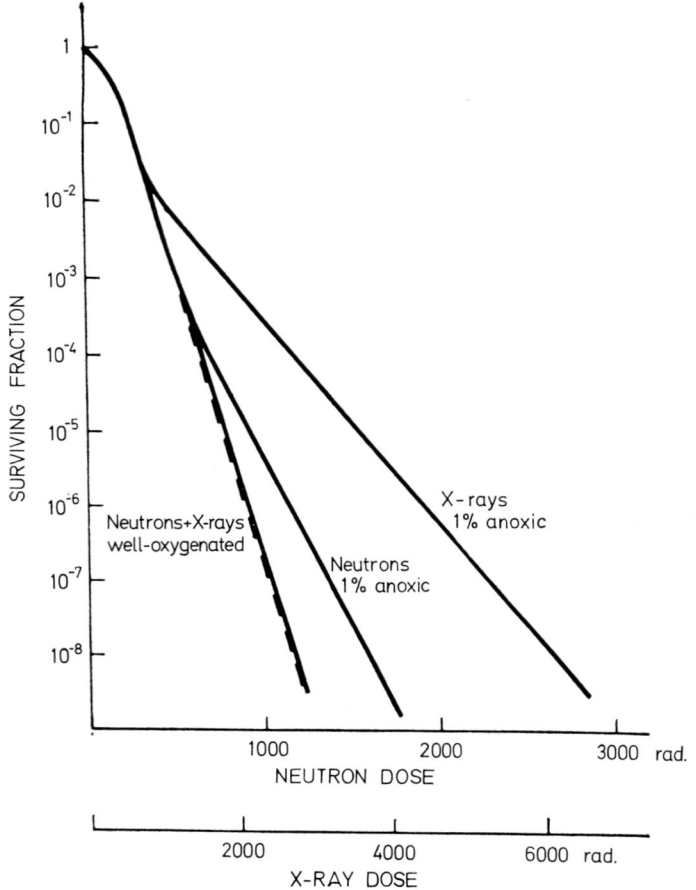

Fɪɢ. 9.16. Survival curves for well oxygenated tumour cells and for a population of cells with 1% anoxic, irradiated with fast neutrons or X-rays. The curves for well oxygenated cells have been superimposed by application of an R.B.E. of 2·2 (Hornsey and Silini, 1963).

R.B.E. AND FRACTIONATION OF FAST NEUTRONS

It has been pointed out that fast neutrons are more effective than low L.E.T. radiations in cell killing. The shape of cell survival curves for the two radiations is different because of the reduction of the size of the shoulder region with fast neutrons (Fig. 17). It is impossible therefore in these circumstances to give a single value for the effectiveness of neutrons compared to X-rays. With small doses the rate of change is much greater than with large doses. Table V shows the dependence of R.B.E. values on 14 MeV neutron dose as calculated from the survival curves

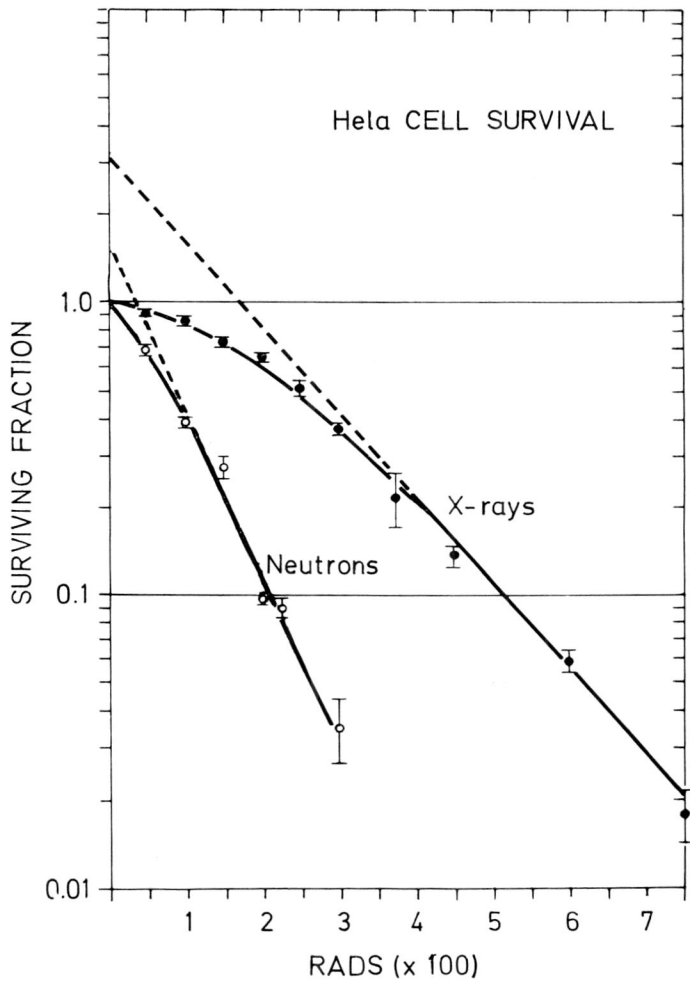

Fig. 9.17. Survival curves for HeLa cells irradiated with 250 KV X-rays and 14 MeV neutrons (Nias *et al.*, 1967). (Reproduced by courtesy of Editors, *International Journal of Radiation Biology*.)

of HeLa cells (Fig. 18) (Nias *et al.*, 1967). This is the explanation for the increase in R.B.E. noted by Stone (1948) when small fractionated doses of 6 MeV neutrons were given, compared to the single erythema doses from which he estimated R.B.E. Indeed, with very small doses of fast neutrons the R.B.E. compared to low L.E.T. radiation increases very rapidly (Fig. 22). An extremely sensitive model is required to demonstrate effects following very small doses, but this is possible with the murine lens and a value of 70 has been recorded (Bateman *et al.*, 1970).

TABLE V

R.B.E. values of 14 MeV neutrons compared to 250 KV X-rays as a function of dose.
Values taken from survival curves of HeLa cells (Fig. 17) (Nias *et al.*, 1967).

Survival level %	Neutron dose (rad)	X-ray dose (rad)	R.B.E.
90	15	65	4·3
80	30	115	3·8
70	45	160	3·6
60	60	200	3·3
50	80	240	3·0
40	100	280	2·8
30	125	335	2·7
20	160	400	2·5
10	210	515	2·4
3	305	695	2·3

'RECOVERY' FROM FAST NEUTRON RADIATION AND FRACTIONATION

Fractionation has traditionally been used in X-ray therapy in the belief that it gives a greater sparing effect to normal tissues than tumour and in this way increases the therapeutic ratio. The total dose of X-radiation has to be increased with larger number of fractions and this is because of the ability of all mammalian cells to repair sublethal damage (Elkind and Sutton, 1960). The relatively smaller recovery after fast neutron radiation, measured by the decreased size of the shoulder on cell survival curves, implies that the increase in total dose to be given with increasing number of fractions must be less than with X or γ rays. This will be illustrated when the experimental studies of skin reactions to fast neutrons are reviewed later.

SOMATIC RADIOBIOLOGY

It is important to confirm that the principles deduced from fundamental research using single cell systems do correspond with changes occurring in organized tissues. The few experimental studies so far made with normal tissues and tumours do indeed demonstrate that gross response may be related to cell survival data (Barendson, 1968; Van den Brenk, 1969).

SKIN

One of the initial biological investigations carried out on the M.R.C. cyclotron at Hammersmith was a study of the reactions of skin and of subcutaneous tissue to fast neutron radiation. Pig skin was chosen because it closely resembles human skin, particularly in the relation to the layer of subcutaneous fat. It was felt that the increased absorption of fast neutron beams in this subcutaneous layer of fat might have been an important factor in the development of the severe skin damage experienced by Stone (1948) in the first trial of neutron therapy.

Early skin reactions. The original experiments reported by Bewley *et al.* (1963) found the R.B.E. for single doses of 7 MeV fast neutrons relative to 8 MeV X-rays was 2·5, and for 6 fractions given over 18 days the R.B.E. increased to 3·3. Reactions were assessed up to a period of about 3 months after treatment. A further series of experiments (Bewley *et al.*, 1967) with various fractionated treatments, ranging from 2 fractions given in 1 day to 15 fractions in 3 weeks, have provided more detailed information on the change of R.B.E. measured by the early response of pig skin. The relationship of the increase in total dose required with 8 MeV X-rays and with 7 MeV fast neutrons to increasing numbers of fractions producing the same level of early skin reaction is shown in Fig. 18. The treatments with 6, 9 and 15 fractions were all given in the same overall time of 3 weeks. The increase in neutron dose for various fractionated regimes expressed as the ratio of the equivalent

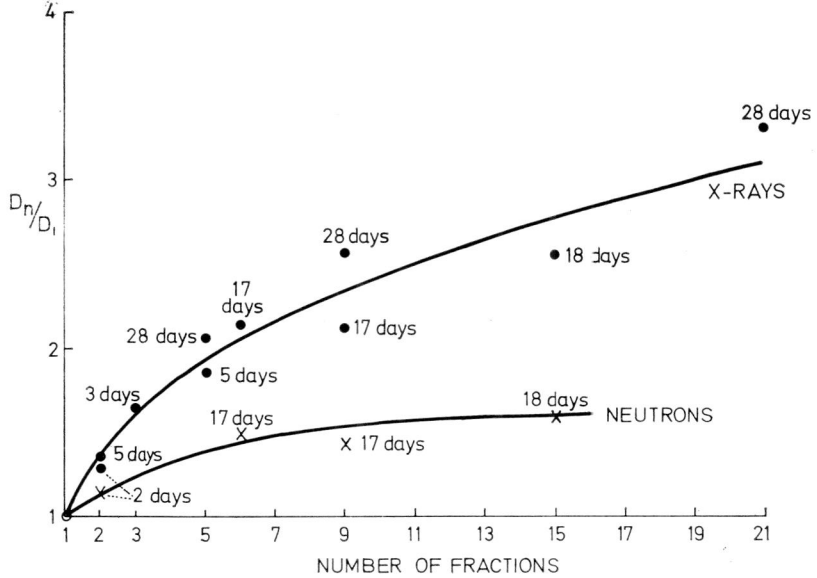

FIG. 9.18. The increase in total dose of 7 MeV neutrons and 8 MV X-rays required to produce the same level of skin reaction with different numbers of fractions (Bewley *et al.*, 1967). (Reproduced by courtesy Editors, *British Journal of Radiology*.)

TABLE VI

Number of fractions	Overall time (days)	Ratio of fractionated dose to single dose for early skin reactions in various species				
		Mouse	Rat	Pig	Man	
		(Fowler 1966)	(Field et al. 1968)	(Bewley et al. 1967)	(Morgan 1967)	(Stone 1948)
2	2	1·15	1·25	1·2	—	—
5	5		1·47	1·4		
6	20			1·5	1·5	
9	20			1·5		
12	40				1·7	
15	20			1·6		
18	35					1·7

single dose for skin reaction in mice, rat, pig and man is shown in Table VI.

The much smaller increment of dose required with neutrons is obvious, and an attempt has been made to establish to what extent this difference is due to a reduction in short term recovery, or to changes in repopulation, in pig skin. A series of split dose experiments up to 24 hours was carried out and the results from X-rays and neutrons compared (Fig. 19). The recovery following neutron radiation was found to be about two-thirds that measured after X-rays. A similar estimate of short term recovery was found in mouse skin (Denekamp et al., 1966) and it was deduced that the rate of cellular repopulation was similar after high and low L.E.T. radiation.

Late reactions. Many of the irradiated skin areas on the experimental pigs have been assessed at periods of up to 2 years following exposure to fast neutrons (Bewley et al., 1967). The signs of radiation damage, slight induration and atrophy and sometimes epilation, were similar to those found after X-ray treatment and there was no evidence of any increase in R.B.E. for late damage to skin and subcutaneous tissues.

The pathological changes which occur in the skin, subcutaneous tissues and underlying muscle following heavy overdosage of goats' skin with fast neutrons have been described by Edmondson (1968).

Field (1969a) has studied the relationship of different levels of early reactions to late skin reaction and also to progressive deformity of the hind limbs of rats following X-rays and fast neutrons. He demonstrated

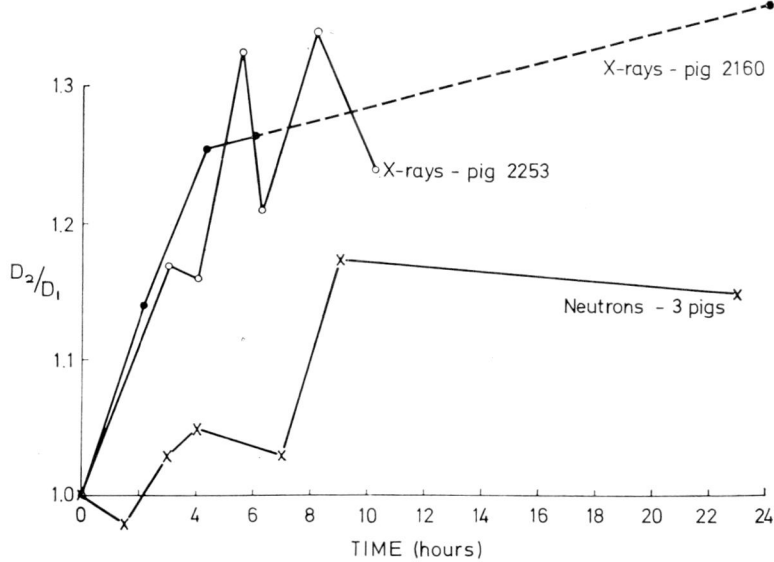

FIG. 9.19. Recovery in pig skin after X-rays and 7 MeV neutrons illustrated by split dose experiments up to 24 hours (Bewley *et al.*, 1967). (Reproduced by courtesy of Editors, *British Institute of Radiology*.)

that the relationship of early and late changes was the same for X-rays and for fast neutrons for single and fractionated treatments. After a certain degree of early skin reaction the severity of late reactions increased sharply with increasing dose but this relationship was still the same for X-rays and for fast neutrons (Fig. 20). It seems that early skin reactions following fast neutron therapy are a poor index of late morbidity, and, as with X-rays, tolerance levels of dose will have to be found by careful clinical trials and based on the incidence of late necrosis of normal tissues.

HAEMOPOIETIC SYSTEM

The response of the bone marrow to fast neutrons is particularly important because of the possible hazards of the high levels of whole body dose which may have to be tolerated during fast neutron therapy (Duncan, Greene and Major, 1970).

The early effects of 14 Mev neutrons on the peripheral blood count in mice are similar to those found after X-radiation (Darden *et al.*, 1967). There is a rapid dose dependent fall in the total white blood count after acute doses of fast neutrons. The neutrophil count usually had returned to normal values within 3 weeks and the lymphocyte count in 1–2

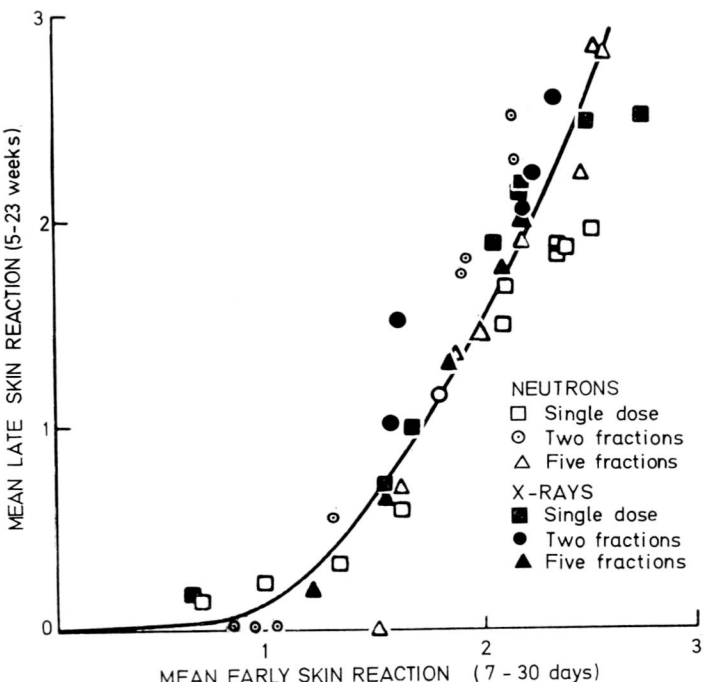

Fig. 9.20. The relationship of early and late skin reactions after various treatments with 250 KV X-rays and 7 MeV fast neutrons (Field, 1969). (Reproduced by courtesy Editors, *Radiology*.)

months. There is no significant quantitative or qualitative difference in the response of the peripheral blood count to neutrons and to X-rays (Davies *et al.*, 1965).

The sensitivity of mouse haemopoietic stem cells to fast neutrons and to X-rays has been estimated by assay of thirty-day mortality doses and by measuring the number of spleen colonies formed by irradiated haemopoietic cells injected into syngeneic mice.

After exposure to the lowest lethal doses of fission spectrum neutrons, it is found that many animals die in the first week after exposure as a result of intestinal injury (Bond, 1964; Gambino *et al.*, 1968). It has, however, also been shown that the characteristic bone marrow death occurs at doses only slightly lower than those producing the gastro-intestinal syndrome not only in mice (Davies, 1965) but also in Rhesus monkeys (Broerse and Van Bekkum, 1969).

Sawada and Yoshinaga (1963) using 14 MeV neutrons (compared with orthovoltage X-rays) found an R.B.E. of 1·14 for thirty-day mortality in mice and Broerse (1969) found a value of 1·1.

Recently the response of mouse haemopoietic stem cells to 14 MeV neutrons has been studied in Manchester (Duncan *et al.*, 1969) and in Rijswijk (Broerse *et al.*, 1969) using the spleen colony-forming unit technique. Again, low values of R.B.E. were obtained and Broerse's results were consistent with his value of 1·1 for haemopoetic death in mice. The Manchester results were found to be about 25% higher but a later collaborative study (Broerse, Duncan *et al.*, 1971) has indicated that this difference can be attributed to differences in neutron dosimetry and in neutron beam quality. The Manchester experiments, unlike those performed at Rijswijk, used a collimated beam of neutrons and scattering phenomena may have increased the numbers of lower energy neutrons and biological effectiveness of the beam. However, even with collimated beams of fast neutrons and at low doses and dose-rates, the R.B.E. was about 1·8, significantly lower than found with similar energy fast neutrons and other mammalian cells (Fig. 21) (Field, 1969b). Broerse (1966a and 1969) has suggested that the explanation probably depends on differences of intrinsic radiosensitivity; inhomogeneity of dose in the bone marrow cavities would not seem to be responsible.

GASTRO-INTESTINAL TRACT

The sensitivity of the intestinal stem cells are commonly assessed by determining the acute lethality of irradiated mice. Hornsey *et al.* (1965) found that the L.D.50/5 was reduced by a factor of 2·3 for the 7 MeV

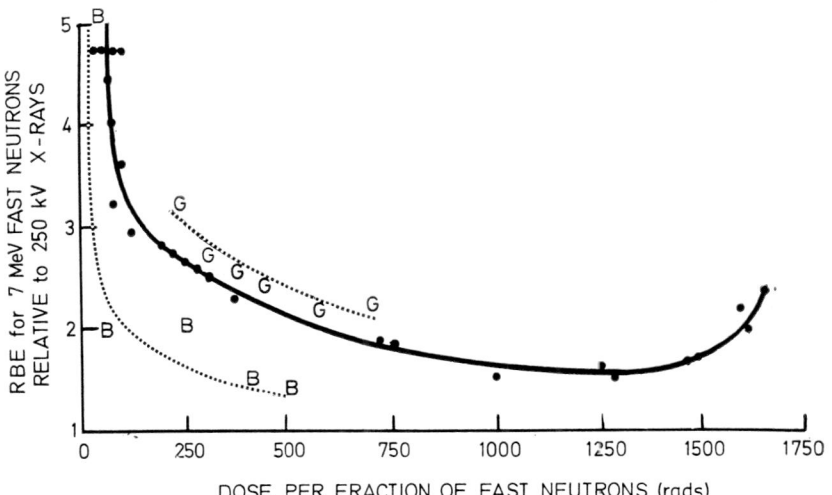

FIG. 9.21. The relationship of R.B.E. to dose of 7 MeV neutrons for skin reactions (continuous line), haemopoietic stem cells (B) and intestinal crypt cells (G) (Field, 1969).

neutron beam from the M.R.C. cyclotron, compared to orthovoltage radiation. This high R.B.E. was associated with a failure to demonstrate any recovery from sublethal damage after neutron irradiation, no sparing effect having been seen in the intestinal crypts when the neutron dose was divided over less than 12 hours. Intestinal stem cells have been shown to have a large capacity for repair of sublethal damage after low L.E.T. radiation (Hornsey, 1970) and this is not seen in haemopoietic stem cells.

However, R.B.E. values for intestinal deaths (L.D.50/5) using 14 MeV neutrons have been found to be much lower; Broerse (1966b) has given a value of 1·4, Yamomoto (1967) 1·6 and Withers et al. (1970) 1·4. Withers and colleagues used a technique measuring the survival of clonogenic cells in the intestinal mucosa to demonstrate only a small difference in the intrinsic radiosensitivity (D_0 values) of intestinal crypt cells to 14 MeV neutrons and to 250 KV X-rays (Fig. 22). Recovery after 14 MeV neutrons was reduced by about half that following 250 KV X-rays but was still appreciable.

It would seem that mono-energetic 14 MeV neutrons may have some advantage over 7 MeV cyclotron neutrons in producing less damage to the gastro-intestinal tract and particularly in relation to the sparing effect during fractionated treatments. The morphological changes in the intestinal mucosa to be seen after exposure to 14 MeV neutrons have been described by Hirose (1968) and Vogel and Jordan (1967) and have been found to be qualitatively similar to changes seen after exposure to X-rays.

The leakage of P.V.P. (polyvinylpyrrolidine) into the gut is a useful functional test of damage to the intestinal tract and has been used to compare the effect of 7 MeV neutrons and of orthovoltage X-rays (Hornsey and Vatistas, 1968). An R.B.E. of 3·0 was found for fast neutrons, higher than that for intestinal death. The time relationship also indicated that protein leakage from the gut could not be correlated with the morphological damage which is found soon after irradiation.

THE LENS

The lens is known to be highly sensitive to neutron radiation and very high R.B.E. values for cataract formation have been reported (Upton et al., 1956). It seems that the murine lens is particularly sensitive to the cataractogenic effects of radiation whereas in dogs, monkeys and goats the dose of fast neutrons required to induce cataract formation sufficiently severe to impair vision is in the lethal range (Edmondson, Batchelor and Lloyd, 1967). It is also important to note that 14 MeV neutrons are much less efficient in producing cataracts in mice than are fission spectrum neutrons (Darden et al., 1967; Bateman et al., 1970).

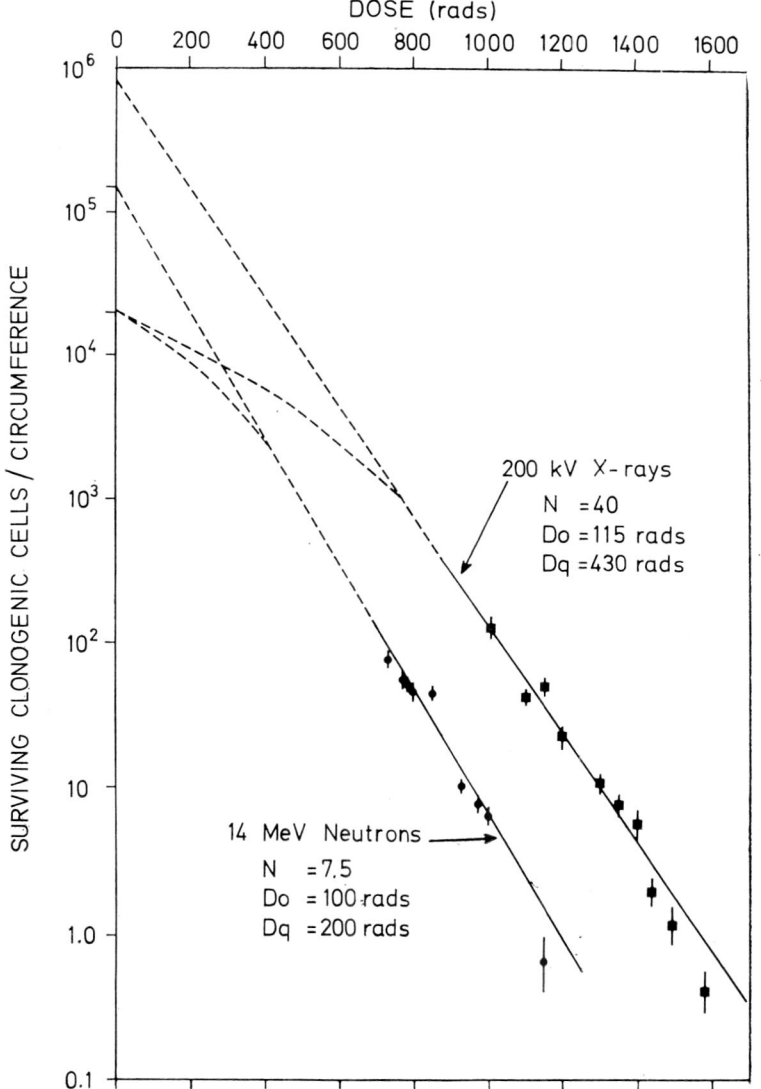

FIG. 9.22. Survival curves from intestinal crypt cells after single dose irradiation with 14 MeV neutrons or 250 KV X-rays (Withers *et al.*, 1970). (Reproduced by courtesy Editors, *British Journal of Radiology.*)

Information concerning cataract formation in man is unreliable because of the uncertainties of dose calculation and of retrospective estimation of the quality of a mixed beam of radiation in studies of both radiation accidents (Kraus and Bond, 1961; Ham, 1960) and in the assessment of atomic bomb casualties (Cogan *et al.*, 1949). Opacities in the human lens have been reported with doses of 200 rads (Poppe, 1957) but these were non-progressive, and for significant opacification the R.B.E. for 7 and 14 MeV neutrons may be no greater than that for other mammalian cells (Field, 1969b). In controlled studies with monkeys (Pickering *et al.*, 1960; Brown, 1960) it was found that only minimal changes in the lens were detected after a whole body dose of 150 rads of fast neutrons.

Thus the mouse lens is one of the most sensitive tissues for the measurement of the R.B.E. of fast neutrons. Using 0·43 MeV neutrons Bateman *et al.* (1970) showed a gradual rise of R.B.E. from 10 to about 30 with a decrease of neutron dose from 40 rads to about 5 rads and then a rapid rise to a value of 65 at a dose level of 0·5 rads. These results are of great radiobiological significance even though the lens changes are only just detectable at the lowest dose levels and cannot be related to the opacities which may occur in the human lens.

EXPERIMENTAL RADIOTHERAPY

The therapeutic advantage of fast neutrons has been demonstrated experimentally by comparing the regression of both tumours and normal tissues in animals after various regimes of treatment.

A transplantable fibrosarcoma in rats has been treated with single doses of 7 MeV fast neutrons and 250 KV X-rays (Field *et al.*, 1967) when about 8–10 mm in size. The delay in regrowth (to an arbitrary size of 25 mm) after irradiation was compared with degrees of early skin reaction, and fast neutrons were seen to be much more effective than X-rays (Fig. 23). The experiments were later extended to investigate the effect of two and five daily fractions and the results are shown in Fig. 24 (Field *et al.*, 1968). It can be seen that although two and five fractions of X-rays are more effective than single doses, five fractions of neutrons appear to have no therapeutic advantage over a single exposure. All three neutron treatments however are superior to the X-ray treatments. Two fractions of fast neutrons given 24 hours apart are the most effective of the regimes tested and with this particular tumour 'cure' may be expected at a dose level which would produce only an erythema reaction, much less than with any of the other regimes. The explanation given for these results is that a large proportion of cells surviving each fraction of radiation is hypoxic but that this proportion reduces in time.

Similar experiments have been carried out by Barendsen and Broerse (1969, 1970). The 90% tumour cure dose for a rhabdomyosarcoma in rats was measured for 300 KV X-rays and for 14 MeV neutrons. The R.B.E. of fast neutrons was found to be 2·8 for single doses. When

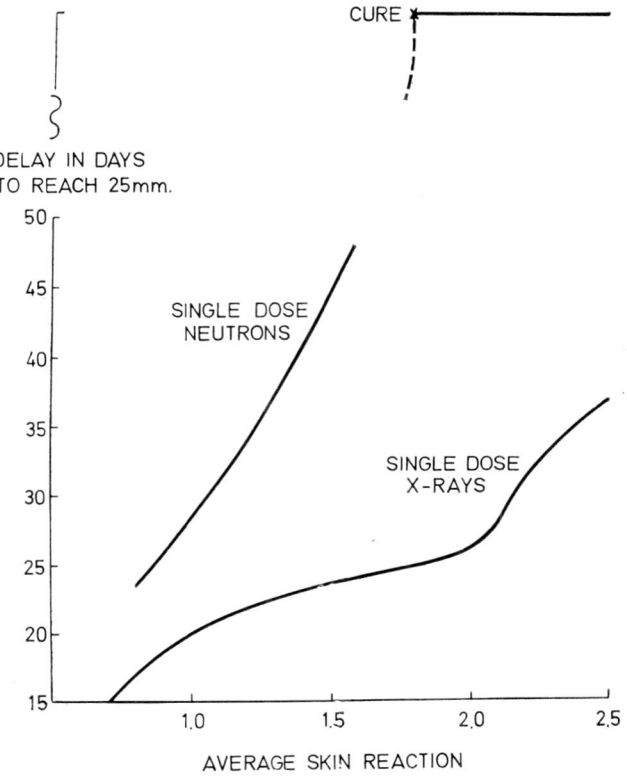

FIG. 9.23. Tumour injury (measured by the delay in growing to an arbitrary 25 mm diameter compared with controls) as a function of skin reaction after single exposure of 7 MeV fast neutrons and 250 MV X-rays (Field *et al.*, 1967). (Reproduced by courtesy Editors, *British Journal of Radiology*.)

delay in growth was measured, the fast neutrons, over a wide range of doses, were shown to be 3·3 times more effective than the X-rays. In another series of experiments daily fractions of X-rays or fast neutrons were given 5 days per week for 3 weeks. Doses of 50, 70 and 100 rads of fast neutrons were given and compared with 200, 300 and 400 rads X-rays. The R.B.E. for tumour growth delay varies greatly, depending on the dose schedule used (Table VII), and is considered to be due to differences in the effects of re-oxygenation and repopulation in the tumour.

This tumour may be dispersed into a cell suspension and cultured *in vitro*, and in this way the relative numbers of clonogenic cells surviving after each treatment may be found. An R.B.E. of 2·9 is obtained for

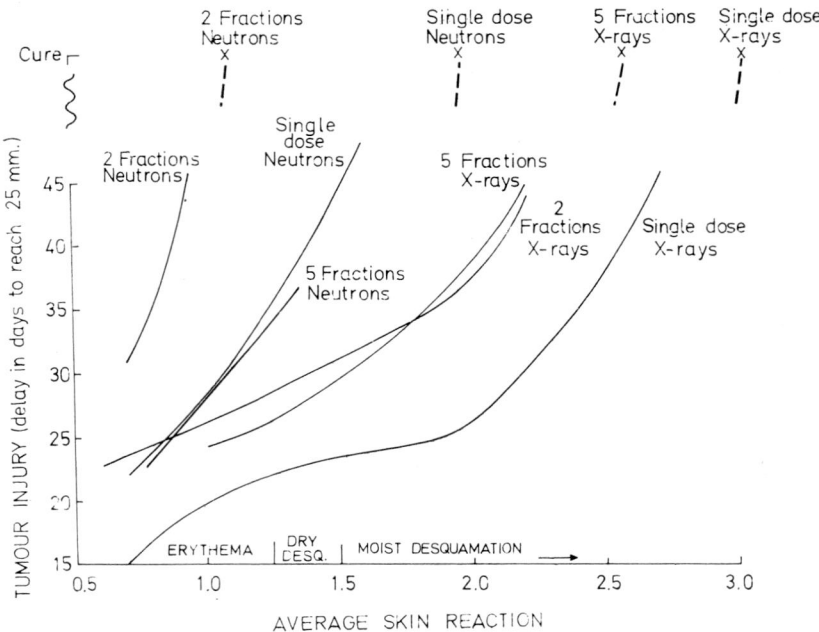

Fig. 9.24. Tumour injury as a function of skin reaction after various treatments with 7 MeV fast neutrons and 250 KV X-rays (Field *et al.*, 1968). (Reproduced by courtesy of Editors, *British Journal of Radiology*.)

single doses, a value determined by the presence of a large proportion of anoxic cells in the tumour. At low levels of survival following fractionated treatments the R.B.E. is as high as 3·0 because of the reduced capacity of the tumour cells to repair sublethal damage after neutron radiation. The therapeutic implications of these R.B.E. values for this tumour will of course depend on the relative damage sustained by normal tissues treated similarly (Broerse, Barendsen *et al.*, 1971).

Fractionated treatments with 14 MeV fast neutrons have also been given to a transplantable osteosarcoma in mice (Van Putten *et al.*, 1971). This tumour is known to contain a large proportion of hypoxic cells and also has been shown to re-oxygenate only poorly between fractions of X-rays (Van Putten, 1968). In these respects, this tumour would seem to be an excellent biological model for neutron therapy. It has been found, however, in experiments with this osteosarcoma, unlike the rat rhabdomyosarcoma, that after large dose fractions of over 400 rads the R.B.E. for tumour regression does not increase as would be expected and a surprisingly small therapeutic gain factor for neutrons is obtained.

Lindop (1970) has reported the measurement of the therapeutic gain factors for large single doses of 6 MeV neutrons compared with

TABLE VII

R.B.E. values of 15 MeV neutrons compared to 300 KV X-rays for single and fractionated exposures of R.1 rhabdomyosarcomas in the rat.
Barendsen and Broerse (1970) (Reproduced by courtesy Editors, *European Journal of Cancer*).

A. Reduction of numbers of clonogenic cells

Treatments compared	at 10%	RBE at 1%	at 0·1%
1. Single doses	2·4	2·7	2·9
2. 5 fractions in 5 days	2·9	3·4	—
3. 10 fractions in 12 days	3·4	3·0	3·0
4. 15 fractions in 19 days	3·3	3·0	2·9

B. Growth delay of 20 days

Treatments compared	RBE
1. Single doses	3·3
2. 200 rads/day of 300 kV X-rays and 50 rads/day of 15 McV neutrons	2·3
3. 200 rads/day of 300 kV X-rays and 70 rads/day of 15 MeV neutrons	2·2
4. 300 rads/day of 300 kV X-rays and 100 rads/day of 15 MeV neutrons	3·4
5. 400 rads/day of 300 kV X-rays and 100 rads/day of 15 MeV neutrons	4·3

14 MeV electrons, measuring the response of spontaneous mammary carcinoma in C3H mice in comparison with the early radiation reaction of the skin overlying the tumour. A gain factor of 1·5 was obtained at an equivalent electron dose of 2,000 rads but then diminished as the dose increased and above 4,000 rads became negative as the relative damage to skin rapidly increased.

More experimental data of this kind is required using animal tumours, particularly with fractionated treatments, in the hope of providing evidence which may be of some relevance to clinical radiotherapy. It would appear from the evidence of the response of experimental tumours that the therapeutic gain factor with fast neutrons may be about 1·3, and this could predict large improvements in the local control of many human tumours.

CLINICAL EXPERIENCE WITH FAST NEUTRONS

INITIAL TRIALS AT BERKELEY, CALIFORNIA

In Berkeley, California in 1932, shortly after the discovery of the neutron, Livingstone and Lawrence were developing the cyclotron. Within a year or two, they had adapted the machine to accelerate 16 MeV deuterons on to a beryllium target, producing neutrons with a mean energy of about 6 MeV.

The possible medical application of this new radiation was soon realized and early radiobiological studies seemed to confirm the hope that fast neutrons might have a place in the treatment of human cancer (Lawrence *et al.*, 1936). By 1938, shielding of the cyclotron and collimation of the neutron beams had been achieved and it was decided to embark on a clinical trial of patients with advanced malignant disease (Stone *et al.*, 1940).

The clinical trial was begun by determining the skin erythema dose in a group of 24 patients. An R.B.E. of 2·5 was estimated for single doses and this figure was applied to fractionated treatments with much smaller increments of dose (Stone and Larkin, 1942). Most patients were treated three times weekly for 6 weeks, because there was no reason to expect that the R.B.E. would vary with the size of dose fraction. Stone (1948) estimated that the R.B.E. for fractionated treatments had increased by a factor of 1·6 but did not realize the significance of this.

A group of 225 patients with advanced incurable cancers were treated on the 60 in medical cyclotron. Some of these patients had been treated previously with X-rays and this must explain to some extent at least the severe normal tissue reactions which followed neutron therapy. One patient who had an early carcinoma of the larynx chose to have neutron therapy and was alive and well, with severe stigmata in the treated area, 6 years later, presumably the first patient to be cured by this form of treatment.

It is impossible to judge the relative effectiveness of fast neutron therapy in terms of tumour resolution from this trial. A heterogeneous group of tumours was treated and none received comparative treatment with conventional radiation, but impressive resolution of advanced tumours was seen at times, particularly in secondary deposits in lymph nodes. The outstanding clinical impression gained by Stone was that fast neutrons produced unusually severe reactions with a particularly high incidence of late skin and soft tissue necrosis. It was thought this was due to some intrinsic difference between the action of neutrons and of X-rays, but it is clear in a retrospective analysis that the severity of reactions was due to overdosage. Stone reported that among a group of 16 patients treated for advanced cancer of the larynx, 7 (44%) died of necrosis with no evidence of recurrent tumour at autopsy. In a group of

24 patients treated for carcinoma of the prostate gland, 6 patients had persistent ulceration of the skin in one or more of the treated areas. Eleven patients with pharyngeal tumours were treated and immediate necrosis was a major factor in their short survival, the best result in this group was obtained by a patient who failed to attend to complete treatment. These results do indicate that too high a dosage of neutron radiation was given leading to unduly severe reactions.

Recently, Stone's records have been critically reviewed (Sheline et al., 1971) and the prescribed doses analysed in relation to an equivalent single dose of X-rays using the Ellis formula (Ellis, 1967). All but one of the records, many of which included photographs, were available for examination. Four patients who were treated in this trial are still alive and are being seen at follow-up. In 27 records, the observations were not considered adequate for any assessment to be made. The records of another 51 patients showed that they had received previous X-ray therapy in the neutron-irradiated fields. The treatment of several patients was irregular because of the uncertain operation of the cyclotron and in one patient treatment was so often interrupted that the record was not included in the analysis. These exclusions left 144 patient records suitable for critical assessment of the observations of skin reactions at 274 different sites. It has been conclusively demonstrated that the neutron doses delivered were mostly extremely high and that the severe late reactions produced were due in most patients to overdosage. The reason for these untoward effects has been called the 'fractionation trap', namely that the relative effectiveness of fast neutrons increases as the size of dose fractions diminishes.

CLINICAL TRIALS AT THE HAMMERSMITH HOSPITAL, LONDON

Clinical trials were started at the M.R.C. Cyclotron Unit in 1964 after a careful programme of pre-therapeutic assessment (Fowler et al., 1963). The beam of fast neutrons is of the same quality as used by Stone. The fixed horizontal beam is collimated to the required treatment field size by a series of boronated wood applicators and alignment of the beam is achieved by moving the patient who is treated lying, sitting or in the knee-chest position. A dose-rate of about 50 rads per minute is obtained at 125 cm source to skin distance.

At first, a number of experimental studies were undertaken on volunteer patients (Morgan, 1967). Adjacent areas of skin (5 × 4 cm) on the lateral aspect of the thigh were treated with either 6 MeV neutrons or 8 MeV X-rays. The doses of fast neutrons given were always less than two-thirds those used in the earlier pig skin experiments (Bewley et al., 1967). The erythema reactions produced were similar following both types of radiation and the R.B.E. increased in a predictable way when smaller dose fractions were given. Some patients have been observed for many months after treatment and no evidence of progressive damage after fast neutron treatment has been found.

More detailed assessment of skin reactions has continued (Catterall, 1971) and an R.B.E. of 3·0 has been determined for the usual course of 12 fractions given in 26 days. At present, the neutron dosage schedule is 1440 rads given in fractions three times weekly for 4 weeks and is found to be equivalent to 4300 rads orthovoltage radiation. It has also been confirmed that skin sparing is obtained with this energy of fast neutron radiation.

About 80 patients have now been treated at the Hammersmith Hospital. The qualitative response of tumours has been similar to that seen after X-ray therapy. All the patients treated have had advanced malignant disease and no comparative assessment can be made yet of the effectiveness of fast neutrons. Clinical trials with patients with locally advanced accessible tumours are now being undertaken. (Catterall *et al.*, 1971).

CLINICAL APPLICATION OF FAST NEUTRONS IN MANCHESTER

For some months now, the experimental facility at the Christie Hospital (Greene and Thomas, 1968) has provided a fixed horizontal beam of 14 MeV neutrons of sufficient intensity to allow clinical research to begin. The neutron generator has an output of about 3 rads per minute at 55 cm from the target and the beam is collimated by composite steel and polythene applicators. The patient is positioned in relation to applicator which has a 2 mm polythene facing to ensure full build-up of dose on the skin surface. In this way, the R.B.E. of skin is being determined by treating one skin area on the thigh with neutrons as part of a palliative course of radiotherapy, while other fields are treated with telecobalt gamma rays. Few patients have as yet been treated and it can only be confirmed that there is no qualitative difference in the immediate reaction following neutrons and gamma rays.

RADIO-ISOTOPE AND RADIO-CHEMICAL SOURCES OF FAST NEUTRONS

Sources of fast neutrons which may be suitable for interstitial and intracavitary treatments are now being developed. These are Californium-252, made in the United States, and a Curium 242—beryllium mixture, made by the Radio-Chemical Centre in England.

Such sources are unsuitable for telecurie therapy units not only because the energies of the neutrons emitted are too low to give sufficiently good depth doses but also because of other problems such as the large amount of radioactive material required, its extremely high cost and the great difficulties of shielding such a source and collimating the beam (Lawson, 1969).

Californium-252 is a transplutonic radioisotope produced by the United States Atomic Energy Commission in special high flux reactors at the Oak Ridge National Laboratory and at the Savanah River Plant. Its interest for radiotherapists lies in the fact that it spontaneously emits fast neutrons ($2 \cdot 34 \times 10^{12}$ neutrons per second per gram) and its use for interstitial and intracavitary therapy was first suggested by Schlea and Stoddard (1965). Decay of Californium-252 is by alpha particle emission and spontaneous fission with a half life of $2 \cdot 6$ years. The neutrons have a mean energy of about 2 MeV and are accompanied by gamma rays, fission fragments and alpha particles.

The Savanah River Laboratory sources are made by the electro-deposition of Californium hydroxide on to a platinum-iridium rod which is then oxidized by heating. This form is then relatively insoluble in saline (Boulogne and Evans, 1969). Sources are placed in sealed platinum-iridium cells and ensheathed in platinum iridium needles (Fig. 25) (Wright et al., 1967). The dose-rates from the sources are determined largely by the inverse square law and a 1 µg Californium needle gives similar dose distribution to a 1 mg radium needle (Fig. 26). In addition to fast neutrons, gamma rays account for about 37% of the total dose, assuming a relative biological effectiveness of five.

Californium-252 is at present available only in very small quantities and is expensive, but its price has just been reduced to $10 per microgram.

Three medical research centres in the United States, Brookhaven National Laboratory in New York, the M.D. Anderson Hospital in Houston and the Hospital of the University of Pennsylvania in Philadelphia, have been investigating the biological effects of Californium-252 and its application in radiotherapy.

CELLULAR RADIOBIOLOGY

THE O.E.R. OF CALIFORNIUM-252

Great technical difficulties exist in measuring the O.E.R. at low dose rates and few results have been reported. The available data are tabulated (Table VIII) and suggest that the gain factor with Californium-252 is much smaller than following irradiation at high dose-rates.

Fairchild et al. (1970) have found an O.E.R. of $1 \cdot 3$ for HeLa cells in culture irradiated with Californium-252 at a dose-rate of 16 rads per hour. They did not evaluate the O.E.R. with radium at the same dose-rate but reference may be made to earlier work (Hall et al., 1966) which

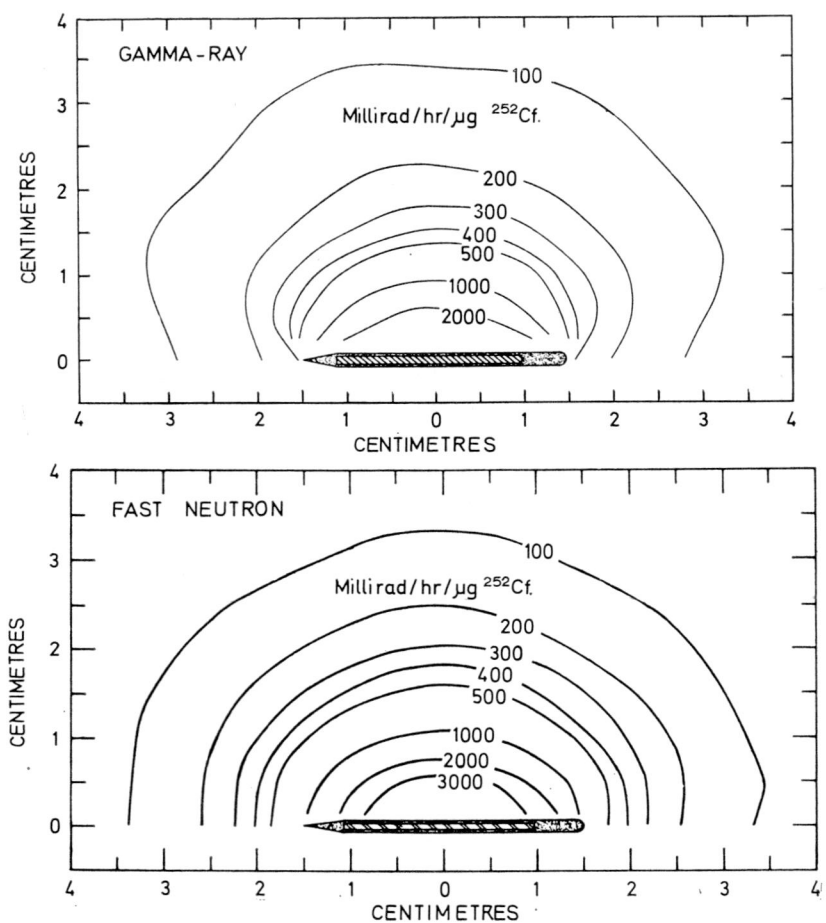

Fig. 9.25. The fast neutron and gamma ray isodose charts for a Californium 252 needle in a tissue equivalent solution (units in rad/hr per μg) (Oliver and Wright, 1969). (Reproduced by courtesy Editors, *Radiology*.)

gave an O.E.R. of 1·5 with the same HeLa cell line using 60 cobalt gamma rays at a dose-rate of 32 rads per hour. The irradiation of *Vicia faba* seedlings is technically much easier and an O.E.R. of 1·66 was determined for Californium-252 (Hall and Fairchild, 1970) and this may be a more reliable measurement than that obtained using HeLa cells. When low dose-rate radium treatment was given, the O.E.R. was 2·02 and the gain factor is only 1·2.

Bushong *et al.* (1970) have measured the number of chromosome aberrations occurring in Chinese hamster ovarian cells obtaining O.E.R. values of 1·75 and 2·5 for Cr-252 neutrons and radium gamma rays respectively.

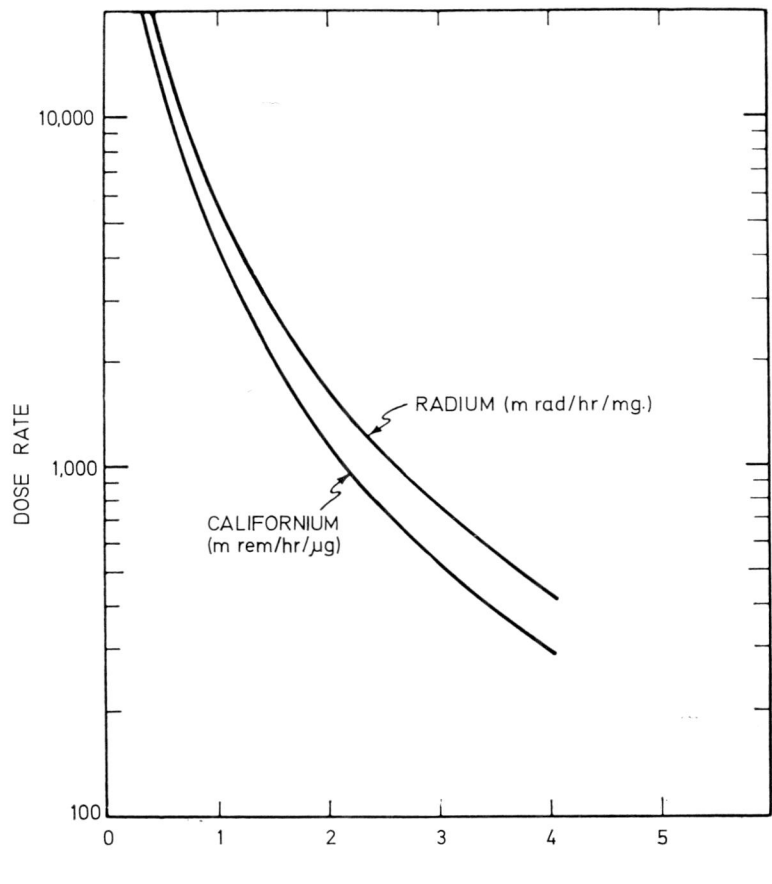

FIG. 9.26. Comparison of dose-rates from Californium 252 and from radium. (Oliver and Wright, 1969). (Reproduced by courtesy Editors, *Radiology*.)

This scanty evidence suggests that, Californium-252 may have only a small therapeutic advantage over radium. It had already been suggested that continuous low dose-rate gamma radiation may be as effective as neutrons in situations of extreme hypoxia (Hall *et al.*, 1966).

THE R.B.E. OF CALIFORNIUM-252

Fairchild *et al.* (1969) have irradiated HeLa S3 cells *in vitro* with Californium-252 at 16 rads per hour, radium at 31 rads per hour and acute exposure to 250 KV X-rays. The survival curves had the same shape and extrapolation number and so the R.B.E. could be expressed

TABLE VIII

COMPARATIVE O.E.R. VALUES FOR RADIUM AND CALIFORNIUM-252

Reference	Biological model	Irradiation *in vitro* Dose rates in rads/hr.		O.E.R.		Gain factor Mx/ Mn.
		Ra.229	Cf.252	Ra. 229 Mx.	Cf. 252 Mn.	
Fairchild *et al.* (1970)	Survival of HeLa S₃ cells	32*	16	1·5*	1·3	1·15*
Bushong *et al.* (1970)	Assay of chromosome aberrations in Chinese hamster ovary cells	25	35	2·5	1·75	1·4
Hall and Fairchild (1970)	Impairment of growth of *Vicia faba* root tips	47	16	2·0	1·6	1·25

* The values have been taken from Hall *et al.* (1966) as comparable experiments with radium have not been reported by Fairchild *et al.*

as the ratio of the slopes of the survival curves and with respect to radium was 2·9.

Further studies (Fairchild *et al.*, 1970) showed that at dose-rates above 16 rads per hour cell division was completely inhibited and the biological response was independent of dose-rate. When *Vicia faba* shoots were irradiated at low dose-rates, Hall and Fairchild (1970), found only a small variation in R.B.E. with neutron dose from Californium-252 compared with radium gamma radiation. With radium the biological effectiveness greatly depends on the dose-rate and so the value of R.B.E. for Californium-252 will depend largely on the dose-rate of the radium alone.

SOMATIC RADIOBIOLOGY

PIG SKIN EXPERIMENTS

Atkins *et al.* (1970) have recently reported the results of R.B.E. experiments on pig skin reactions using special surface applicators loaded with Californium-252 or with radium. The applicator (area = 6 × 6 cm, treating distance = 0·5 cm) was sewn on the backs of pigs and was worn for about 7 days. Dose-rates were about 12 rads per hour from the Californium-252 and 35 rads per hour from the radium and the dose distributions were comparable. The early reactions were scored and an R.B.E. of about 5 was determined (Fig. 27). This work implied that even at low dose-rates of about 12 rads per hour there is almost complete inhibition of mitotic activity in the skin. Further experiments using higher dose-rates of radium (so that the appropriate dose levels will be given in the same overall time) are planned, and the R.B.E. is expected to be about 4 under these conditions.

GASTRO-INTESTINAL TRACT

The response of the epithelial cells in the mouse jejunum has been assayed following irradiation with radium and Californium-252 (Withers *et al.*, 1971). Whole body radiation was given by a cylinder arrangement of sources delivering 43·5 rads per hour (26·5 rads neutrons) from Californium-252 and 165 rads per hour from the radium.

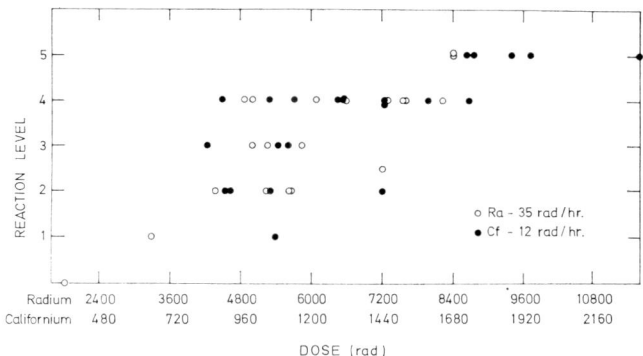

FIG. 9.27. Levels of skin reactions in pigs following treatment with surface applicator of Californium 252 or radium (Atkins *et al.*, 1970).

The numbers of regenerating crypts per circumference of intestine were observed microscopically at about 4 days following various doses of irradiation, and cell survival curves obtained (Fig. 28). Some correction has to be made for the effects of differences in dose-rates, particularly important in the response of intestinal crypt cells, and the radium dose-rates used in the experiments are higher than commonly used clinically. A R.B.E. of 5 is estimated and this may be relevant clinically.

CLINICAL STUDIES WITH CALIFORNIUM-252

Clinical research using after-loading cells of Californium-252 is now in progress at the M.D. Anderson Hospital and Tumour Institute in Houston. Metastatic lesions have been treated by interstitial implants

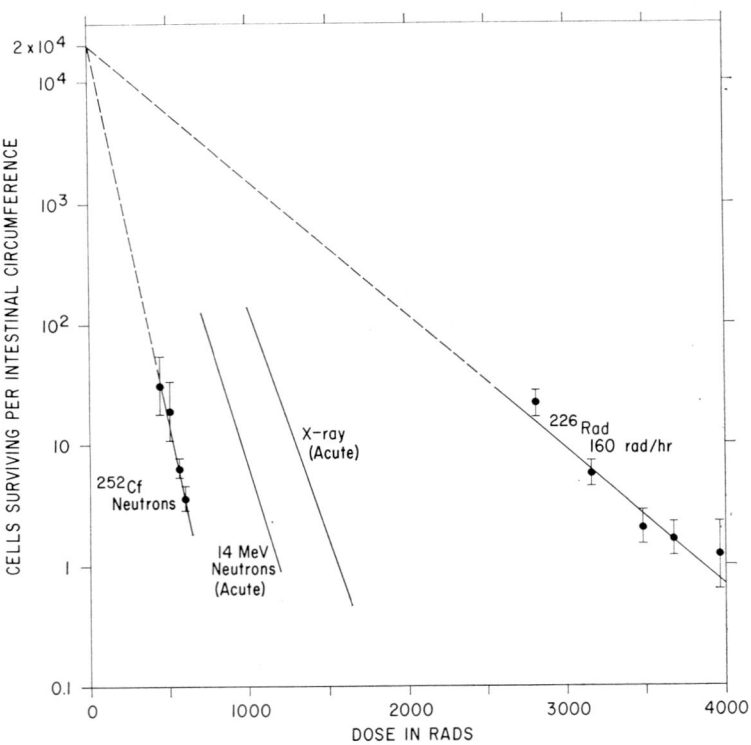

FIG. 9.28. Survival curves of intestinal crypt cells following exposure to Californium
252 14 MeV neutrons and radium (Withers *et al.*, 1969).

and good early tumour regression has been reported with no untoward
response in normal tissues (Californium-252 Progress, August 1970).
Careful clinical assessment is continuing and further studies irradiating
recurrent breast nodules and metastatic cervical lymph nodes are to be
undertaken at the Hospital of the University of Pennsylvania.

THE CURIUM-242/BERYLLIUM SOURCE

In the United Kingdom another possible source of fast neutrons for
plesiotherapy is being developed. The Radio-Chemical Centre at
Amersham is now producing a mixture of Curium-242 and beryllium;
alpha particles impinge on the beryllium, producing fast neutrons. The
neutron energy is higher than from Californium-252 and the gamma ray
contamination is only about 5% of the total emission. The half-life of
these sources is 163 days. These sources may have biological advantages
compared with Californium-252, but as yet fundamental radiobiological
studies have not been undertaken.

THERAPEUTIC IMPLICATIONS OF FAST NEUTRON RADIATION

Much evidence indicates that many malignant tumours contain foci of hypoxic cells which, because of their radioresistance, can be the origin of recurrence after X-ray therapy. The presence in a tumour of only 1% of anoxic cells considerably reduces its radiocurability by X or γ rays; for a 90% chance of cure, twice the dose of radiation would be required for such a tumour compared to a well-oxygenated tumour of the same size. Fast neutrons, having a low O.E.R., deliver a much greater effective dose to the hypoxic tumour cells than do X-rays, for the same effect on well-oxygenated normal tissues around the tumour which limits the dose of radiation which may safely be given.

Munro (1967) has produced a theoretical analysis of the influence of O.E.R. on the relationship of cure rates to dose, considering the response of a simple model tumour to single doses of irradiation. When the O.E.R. is 2·5 the presence of a tiny fraction of 10^{-6} anoxic cells begins to affect the curability of the tumour with radiation. When the O.E.R is 1·5, only fractions of anoxic cells greater than 10^{-3} have a significant effect on the cure rate. In these hypothetical tumours extremely small proportions of anoxic cells are considered to control the curability following single doses of radiation.

When fractionated radiotherapy is used, re-oxygenation occurs in many tumours and undoubtedly is of great importance in determining the success of conventional regimes of X-ray treatment, but we have too little knowledge as yet to suggest an optimum scheme of fractionation. With fast neutrons re-oxygenation is of less importance, and providing large enough doses are given with each fraction, considerable improvement in cure rates should be expected. Even if the expected improvement in cure rates is not realized, fast neutrons may still be of benefit for social and economic reasons, since shorter courses of treatment with neutrons, giving fewer larger fractions, might produce as good results as prolonged fractionated treatments with X-rays.

Experimental evidence suggests that fast neutron therapy may produce a therapeutic gain of about 20–30%. It is important to consider which type of tumour should be selected for trials. Careful thought must be given not only to the biological nature and natural history of the tumour (Kaplan, 1971), but also to its stage of advancement (Duncan, 1971), and adequate numbers of patients must be available to be able to demonstrate the significance of any differences that may be found (Withers, 1971).

Stewart et al. (1969) have analysed the recurrence rate and incidence of necrosis following megavoltage X-ray therapy of laryngeal carcinoma.

Although these results are not derived from a randomly controlled trial, selection into the various dose groups was not predetermined in any way during the period when optimum dosage was being sought. The response of T_1 and T_3 lesions is shown (Fig. 29) and it can be seen that an increase in the dose to the small (T_1) lesions will not produce any improvement in cure rate. However, with T_3 lesions, if anoxia is the only factor determining the response, for the same level of necrosis (8%) an increase of the effective dose of 20% should result in a 20% increase in cures. It is, therefore essential, that the response of locally advanced tumours be examined in the early trials for not only would the inclusion of early lesions seem undesirable on ethical grounds

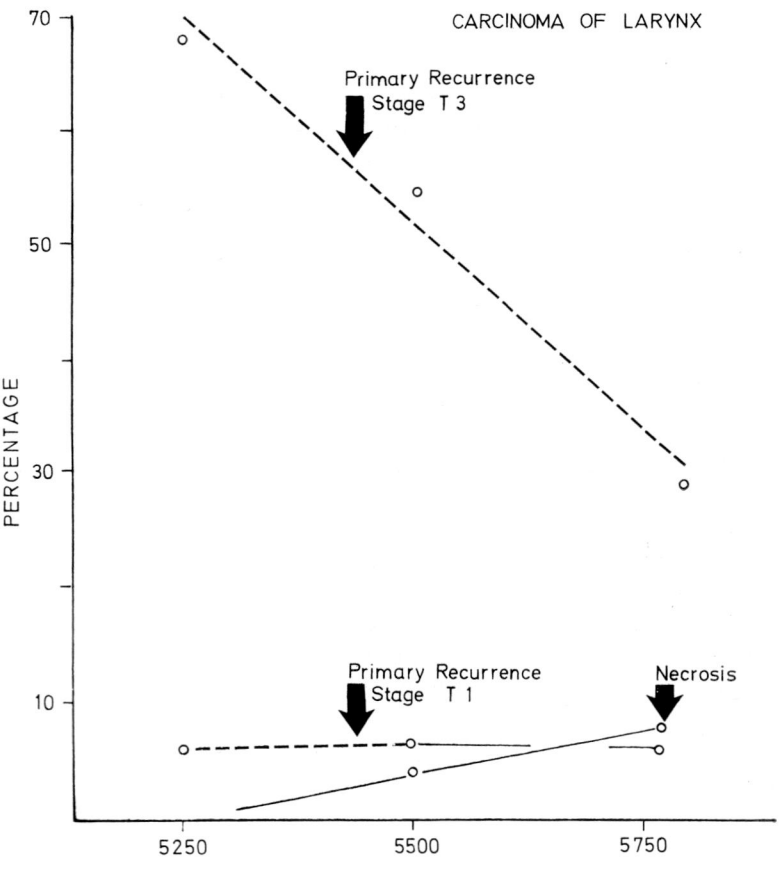

Fig. 9.29. Rates of recurrence of T1 and T3 carcinomata of the larynx treated with various doses in 3 weeks. The rates of necrosis of the larynx are also shown (Stewart *et al.*, 1969).

(where cure rates are already good with X-ray therapy) but it is also unlikely that one could demonstrate any significant improvement in local control of such tumours.

Fast neutrons are of course being evaluated clinically because of their increased effectiveness in treating anoxic tumours, but they may be found to be advantageous in other ways. The variation in response of different mammalian cells in relation to intrinsic sensitivity and recovery from sublethal radiation injury is much smaller with fast neutrons than with X-rays. It is possible that tumours, such as soft tissue sarcomas, which usually respond poorly to X-rays, may be more successfully controlled by fast neutrons.

EXCLUSIVE USE OF FAST NEUTRONS IN CLINICAL TRIALS

It would appear that the greatest advantage of fast neutron therapy should be obtained by their exclusive use throughout the whole course of treatment, but giving a smaller number of larger fractions than normally used with low L.E.T. radiations. A course of fast neutron therapy should be compared with the best one can achieve with X or γ ray therapy. The schemes of fractionation of the radiations to be compared may be quite different in these clinical trials but the treatment technique and particularly the distribution of dose should be as similar as possible. The final analysis should compare the 'therapeutic ratios' of the two treatments in relation to local control rates for the tumour and the incidence of late radiation effects on normal tissue. It is likely that most centres involved in assessing fast neutron therapy will conduct definitive clinical trials with fast neutrons alone compared to X-ray therapy.

Although the main interest in fast neutron therapy is in the possibility of improving cure rates, palliative radiotherapy is also important. It is possible that in centres which now use large single exposures of X-rays as a palliative treatment, fast neutrons may be much more effective because of their greater efficiency in killing anoxic cells. Regression of tumours may be greater and the length of remission could be increased.

There is at present renewed interest in the role of pre-operative radiotherapy in the light of recent radiobiological studies (Powers and Palmer, 1968). The use of *low-dose* irradiation should be considered in certain clinical situations, and in these, fast neutrons should be much more effective than low-dose X-radiation since many of these tumours are likely to contain a high proportion of anoxic cells.

FAST NEUTRONS FOLLOWING A COURSE OF X-RAY THERAPY

Consideration must also be given to the possibility of using fast neutrons at the end of a fractionated course of X-ray therapy. Since the proportion of anoxic cells in a tumour before the last treatment determines the probability of cure, the use of high L.E.T. radiation such as fast neutrons at this time would be much superior to X-rays. Combined therapy should be kept in mind particularly when experimental data are available to help determine the size and timing of the last dose of radiation.

Another prospect for fast neutron therapy is that improved results in treating carcinoma of the uterine cervix may follow the sequential use of fractionated megavoltage X-ray therapy and, intracavitary neutron irradiation. Since the effects of neutron irradiation from Californium-252 are largely independent of dose-rate, the development of a 'Cathetron' type of system for the isotope commends itself from the radiobiological viewpoint in addition to the advantages in radiation protection. It is possible that many radiotherapy departments may be able to obtain such equipment without having the facilities for neutron beam therapy and the optimum combined therapeutic regime may have to be determined.

THE SIMULTANEOUS USE OF X-RAYS AND FAST NEUTRONS

Finally, consideration must be given to the hypothesis of Lawson (1969) that the use of high and low L.E.T. radiations given simultaneously may have a low O.E.R. very close to that of the high L.E.T. radiation alone. His theory postulates that as a result of processes of 'interaction' between the different radiations, the biological response may be greater than a simple additive effect of the radiations considered separately. Experiments are being conducted now to determine the validity of this theory and, if confirmed, the practical importance would be great. Radiotherapy equipment producing mixed beams of neutrons and X-rays could be manufactured which might have considerable physical and economic advantages compared to the neutron generators being developed at the present time.

CONCLUSION

Radiobiological research has provided an understanding of the adverse reactions produced during the original clinical trial of fast neutron therapy and has suggested a reappraisal which may show considerable therapeutic advantages.

The development of sources of fast neutrons for radiotherapy opens up new possibilities of research in physics, in biology and in clinical medicine. Further research into the fundamental action of neutrons and comparison with X-rays and with other low L.E.T. radiations may lead to a better understanding of the basic principles involved in radiation therapy generally. Even if fast neutrons eventually are shown to be of only limited value in cancer therapy, the study of their effects may well result in the more rational use of X-rays and of radium. But there are reasonable grounds for expecting that fast neutron radiation will offer improved cure rates in many of the common cancers and also better palliation for patients with more advanced tumours.

ACKNOWLEDGEMENTS

I would thank Dr. E. C. Easson, the radiotherapy staff and other colleagues of the Christie Hospital and Holt Radium Institute, for their constructive debate on the clinical use of fast neutrons. I am particularly indebted to Dr. David Greene and Mr. Don Major for their advice and information on the physical aspects of fast neutron beams. Dr. Alma Howard, Dr. Ebert and Dr. Nias have always been prepared to discuss the radiobiological problems and have been of great help to me.

I would record my appreciation of Mr. R. Schofield of the Department of Medical Illustration for his advice on the presentation of the illustrations and to his staff for their work of preparation for publication.

I am also grateful to Miss J. Entwistle who undertook the task of typing the manuscript.

REFERENCES

ABELSON, P. H., & KRUGER, P. G. (1949). Cyclotron-induced radiation cataracts. *Science*, **110**, 655.

ADAMS, G. E. (1967). The General Application of Pulse Radiolysis to Current Problems in Radiobiology. *Current Topics in Radiation Research*, Vol. III, p. 36. Ebert and Howard (Eds.). Amsterdam: North-Holland Publ. Co.

ALMOND, P. (1970). Communication at meeting on Fundamental Aspects of Fast Neutrons in Radiotherapy, Rijswijk.

ALPER, T. (1962). The dependence of chemical protective action on oxygen, as studied with bacteria. *Br. J. Radiol.*, **35**, 361.

ALPER, T. (1963). Comparison between the oxygen enhancement ratios of neutrons and X-rays, as observed with *Escherichia coli* B. *Br. J. Radiol.*, **36**, 97.

ALPER, T., & MOORE, J. L. (1967). The interdependence of oxygen enhancement ratios for 250 kV X-rays and fast neutrons. *Br. J. Radiol.*, **40**, 843.

ASHWOOD-SMITH, M. J., ROBINSON, D. M., BARNES, J. H., & BRIDGES, B. A. (1967). Radiosensitization of bacterial and mammalian cells by substituted glyoxas. *Nature, Lond.*, **216**, 137.

ATKINS, H. L., FAIRCHILD, R. G., ROBERTSON, J. S., & LEHMAN, W. P. (1970). Comparison of irradiation by 252-californium and radium on the skin of swine. *Radiology*, **96**, 161.

AUXIER, J. A., SNYDER, W. S., & JONES, T. D. (1968). *Radiation Dosimetry*, Vol. I. Attix and Roesch (Eds.), New York: Academic Press.

BABIB, A. O., & WEBSTER, J. H. (1969). Changes in tumour oxygen tension during radiation therapy. *Acta radiol.*, **8**, 247.

BARENDSEN, G. W. (1968). Responses of Cultured Cells, Tumours and Normal Tissues to Radiations of Different Linear Energy Transfer. *Current Topics in Radiation Research*, Vol. IV. Ebert and Howard (Eds.). London: North-Holland Publ. Co.

BARENDSEN, G. W., & BROERSE, J. J. (1966). Dependence of the oxygen effect on the energy of fast neutrons. *Nature, Lond.*, **212**, 722.

BARENDSEN, G. W., & BROERSE, J. J. (1969). Experimental radiotherapy of a rat rhabdomyosarcoma with 15 MeV neutrons and 300 kV X-rays. I. Effects of single exposures. *Eur. J. Cancer*, **5**, 373.

BARENDSEN, G. W., & BROERSE, J. J. (1970). Experimental radiotherapy of a rat rhabdomyosarcoma with 15 MeV neutrons and 300 kV X-rays. II. Effects of fractionated treatments, applied five times a week for several weeks. *Eur. J. Cancer*, **6**, 89.

BARENDSEN, G. W., KOST, C. J., VAN KERSEN, G. R., BEWLEY, D. K., FIELD, S. B., & PARNELL, C. J. (1966). The effect of oxygen on impairment of the proliferation capacity of tumour cells in culture by ionising radiations of different L.E.T. *Int. J. Radiat. Biol.*, **10**, 317.

BATEMAN, J. L., BIARATI, B. J., & BOND, V. P. (1971). Dose dependence on fast neutron R.B.E. for lens opacification in mice. *Radiology*, in press.

BERRY, R. J. (1969). Growing points in mammalian radiobiology and their implications in radiotherapy. *Radiol. Clins N. Am.*, **7**, No. 2, 281.

BERRY, R. J., BEWLEY, D. K., & PARNELL, C. J. (1965). Reproductive capacity of mammalian tumour cells irradiated *in vivo* with cyclotron-produced fast neutrons. *Br. J. Radiol.*, **38**, 613.

BERRY, R. J., & ELLIS, R. E. (1966). A fast neutron source for radiotherapy. *Nature, Lond.*, **211**, 267.

BEWLEY, D. K. (1963). Physical aspects of the fast neutron beam. Pre-therapeutic experiments with the fast neutron beam from the M.R.C. cyclotron. *Br. J. Radiol.*, **36**, 81.

BEWLEY, D. K. (1970). Fast Neutron Sources for Radiotherapy. *Current Topics of Radiation Research*, Vol. VII. Ebert and Howard (Eds.). Amsterdam: North-Holland Publ. Co.

BEWLEY, D. K., & HORNSEY, S. (1964). Radiobiological Experiments with Fast Neutrons with Reference to the Possible Value of Neutron Therapy. *Proceedings of Symposium on Biological Effects of Fast Neutron and Proton Irradiations*. Upton, Vol. II, p. 173. Vienna: I.A.E.A.

BEWLEY, D. K., FOWLER, J. F., MORGAN, R. L., SILVESTER, J. A., TURNER, B. A., & THOMLINSON, R. H. (1963). Experiments on the skin of pigs with fast neutrons and 8 MV X-rays, including some effects of dose fractionation. *Br. J. Radiol.*, **36**, 107.

BEWLEY, D. K., & PARNELL, C. J. (1969). The fast neutron beam from the M.R.C. cyclotron. *Br. J. Radiol.*, **42**, 281.

BEWLEY, D. K., FIELD, S. B., MORGAN, R. L., PAGE, B. C., & PARNELL, C. J. (1967). The response of pig skin to fractionated treatments with fast neutrons and X-rays. *Br. J. Radiol.*, **40**, 765.

BOND, V. P. (1964). Comparison of the Mortality Response of Different Mammalian Species to X-rays and Fast Neutrons. *Proceedings of Symposium on Biological Effects of Fast Neutron and Proton Irradiations*, Vol. II, p. 365. Vienna: I.A.E.A.

BOULOGNE, A. R., & EVANS, A. G. (1969). Californium-252 neutron sources for medical applications. *Int. J. appl. Radiat. Isotopes*, **20**, 453.

BOUNDEN, J. E., LOMER, P. D., & WOOD, J. D. L. H. (1965). A neutron tube with constant output for activation analysis and reactor applications. *Nucl. Instrum. Meth.*, **33**, 283.

BRENNAN, J. (1969). Fast neutrons for radiation therapy. *Radiol. Clins N. Am.*, **7**, No. 2, 365.

BROERSE, J. J. (1966a). *Effects of Energy Dissipation by Monoenergetic Neutrons in Mammalian Cells and Tissues*. Radiobiological Institute of the Organisation of Health Research T.W.O., Rijswijk.

BROERSE, J. J. (1966b). Dosimetry for fast neutron irradiations of cultured cells and intact animals. Comparison of activation and ionisation methods. *Int. J. Radiat. Biol.*, **10**, 429.

BROERSE, J. J. (1969). Dose mortality studies for mice irradiated with X-rays, gamma rays and 15 MeV neutrons. *Int. J. Radiat. Biol.*, **15**, 115.

BROERSE, J. J., & BARENDSEN, G. W. (1967). Measurements of the biological effects and physical parameters of neutrons from the $^9Be(^3He, n)$ ^{11}C reaction. *Int. J. Radiat. Biol.*, **13**, No. 2, 189.

BROERSE, J. J., BARENDSEN, G. W., & VAN KERSEN, G. R. (1967). Survival of cultured human cells after irradiation with fast neutrons of different energies in hypoxic and oxygenated conditions. *Int. J. Radiat. Biol.*, **13**, 559.

BROERSE, J. J., BARENDSEN, G. W., & VAN PUTTEN, L. M. (1971). R.B.E. values for 15 MeV neutrons for effects on normal tissues. *Eur. J. Cancer*, **7**, 171.

BROERSE, J. J., & VAN BEKKUM. (1969). Communication quoted in 'Dose mortality studies for mice irradiated with X-rays, gamma rays and fast neutrons'. *Int. J. Radiat. Biol.*, **15**, 115.

BROERSE, J. J., DUNCAN, W., ENGELS, A. C., GILBERT, C. W., GREENE, D., HENDRY, J. H., HOWARD, A., LELIEVELD, P., MASSEY, J. B., & VAN PUTTEN, L. M. (1971). The survival of colony forming units in mouse bone marrow after *in vivo* irradiation with D.T. neutrons, X-rays and gamma radiation. *Int. J. Radiat. Biol.*, **19**, 101.

BROWN, D. V. L. (1960). *The Delayed Effects of Whole Body Radiation*, p. 51. Watson (Ed.). Baltimore: Johns Hopkins Press.

BROWNELL, G. L., SOLOWAY, A. H., & SWEET, W. H. (1967). Neutron Capture Therapy. *Modern Trends in Radiotherapy*. Deeley, T. J. and Wood, C. A. P. (Eds.). London: Butterworths.

BUSHONG, S. C., PRASAD, N., BRINEY, S. A., & OLIVER, G. D., Jr. (1970). Radiocytogenic determination of the oxygen enhancement ratio of californium 252. *Radiology*, **96**, 167.

CATER, D. B., & SILVER, I. A. (1960). Quantitative measurements of oxygen tension in normal tissues and in tumours of patients before and after radiotherapy. *Acta radiol.*, **53**, 233.

CATTERALL, M. (1971). Clinical experience with fast neutrons from the Hammersmith cyclotron. *Eur. J. Cancer*, **7**, 227.

CATTERALL, M., ROGERS, C., THOMLINSON, R. H., & FIELD S. B. (1971). An investigation into the clinical effects of fast neutrons. *Br. J. Radiol.* **44**, 603.

CHURCHILL-DAVIDSON, I., SANGER, C., & THOMLINSON, R. H. (1957). Oxygenation in radiotherapy. II. Clinical application. *Br. J. Radiol.*, **30**, 403.

COGAN, D. G., MARTIN, S. F., & KIMURA, S. J. (1949). Atomic bomb cataracts. *Science*, **110**, 654.

DARDEN, E. B., Jr., COSGROVE, G. E., UPTON, A. C., CHRISTENBERRY, K. W., CONKLIN, J. W., DAVIS, M. K., with GOSSLEE, D. G., & KASTENBAUM, B. A. (1967). Late somatic effects in female mice irradiated with single doses of 14 MeV fast neutrons. *Int. J. Radiat. Biol.*, **12**, No. 435.

DAVIES, M. L., DARDEN, E. G., & COSGROVE, G. E. (1965). Early haematological effects of whole body 14 MeV neutron irradiation in mice. *Acta radiol.*, **3**, 87.

DENEKAMP, J., FOWLER, J. F., KRAGT, K., PARNALL, C. J., & FIELD, S. B. (1966). Recovery and repopulation in mouse skin after irradiation with cyclotron neutrons as compared with 250 kV X-rays or 15 MeV electrons. *Radiat. Res.*, **29**, 71.

DOWNTON, D. W., & WOOD, J. D. H. L. (1968). A 10^{11} Neutron per Second Tube for Activation Analysis. *Proceedings of International Conference on Modern Trends in Activation Analysis, Gaithersburg*, p. 1059. National Bureau of Standards, Publication 312, Washington.

DUNCAN, W. (1971). Possibilities for the application of fast neutrons in Manchester. *Eur. J. Cancer*, in press.

DUNCAN, W., GREENE, D., & MAJOR, D. (1971). Radiotherapeutical requirements with respect to depth dose and collimation of fast neutron beams. *Eur. J. Cancer*, in press.

DUNCAN, W., GREENE, D., HOWARD, A., & MASSEY, J. B. (1969). The R.B.E. of 14 MeV neutrons. Observations on colony-forming units in mouse bone marrow. *Int. J. Radiat. Biol.*, **15**, 397.

DUNCAN, W., GREENE, D., & MEREDITH, J. W. (1971). Considerations on the use of 14 MeV neutrons in radiotherapy. *Br. J. Radiol.*, in press.

EDMUNDSON, P. W. (1968). Severe fibrosis of the skin and subdermal tissue of goats after single exposures to fast neutrons. *Int. J. Radiat. Biol.*, **14**, 263.

EDMUNDSON, P. W., BATCHELOR, A. L., & LLOYD, J. P. F. (1967). Eye findings in goats during the three years after acute whole body neutron and gamma irradiation. *Int. J. Radiat. Biol.*, **13**, 147.

ELKIND, M. M., & SUTTON, H. (1960). Radiation response of mammalian cells grown in culture. Repair of X-ray damage in surviving Chinese hamster cells. *Radiat. Res.*, **13**, 556, 593.

ELLIS, F. (1967). Fractionation in Radiotherapy. *Modern Trends in Radiotherapy*. Deeley, T. J. and Wood, C. A. P. (Eds.). London: Butterworths.

EVANS, N. T. S., & NAYLOR, P. F. D. (1963). The effect of oxygen breathing and radiotherapy upon the tissue oxygen tension of some human tumours. *Br. J. Radiol.*, **36**, 418.

EVANS, R. G., PINKERTON, A., DJORDJEVIC, J. M., & LAUGHLIN, J. S. (1971). Changes in biological effectiveness of a fast neutron beam with depth in tissue-equivalent material. *Radiat. Res.*, **45**, 235.

FAIRCHILD, R. G., DREW, R. M., & ATKINS, H. L. (1969). The relative biological effect of ^{252}Cf radiation on HeLa cells in culture. *Radiology*, **93**, 1187.

FAIRCHILD, R. G., DREW, R. M., & ATKINS, H. L. (1970)a. Dose rate effects for various dose rates of ^{252}Cf radiation on HeLa cells in culture. *Radiology*, **96**, 171.

FAIRCHILD, R. G., DREW, R. M., & ATKINS, H. L. (1970b). The oxygen enhancement ratio for protracted irradiation with ^{252}Cf. U.S.A.E.C. Report B.N.L.-14456, Brookhaven National Laboratory, Upton, New York.

FIELD, S. B. (1969a). Early and late reactions in skin of rats following irradiation with X-rays and fast neutrons. *Radiology*, **92**, 381.

FIELD, S. B. (1969b). The relative biological effectiveness of fast neutrons for mammalian tissues. *Radiology*, **93**, 915.

FIELD, S. B., & PARNELL, C. J. (1965). The use of threshold detectors to determine changes in a fast neutron energy spectrum with depth in a phantom. *Br. J. Radiol.*, **38**, 618.

FIELD, S. B., JONES, T., & THOMLINSON, R. H. (1967). The relative effects of fast neutrons and X-rays on tumour and normal tissue in the rat. Single doses. *Br. J. Radiol.*, **40**, 834.

FIELD, S. B., JONES, T., & THOMLINSON, R. H. (1968). The relative effects of fast neutrons and X-rays on tumour and normal tissue in the rat. Part II. Fractionation, recovery and reoxygenation. *Br. J. Radiol.*, **41**, 597.

FOWLER, J. F. (1966). Radiation Biology As Applied to Radiotherapy. *Current Topics in Radiation Research*. Ebert and Howard (Eds.). London: North-Holland Publishing Company.

FOWLER, J. F. (1967a). Fast Neutron Therapy—Physical and Biological Considerations. *Modern Trends in Radiotherapy*. Deeley, T. J. and Wood, C. A. P. (Eds.). London: Butterworths.

FOWLER, J. F. (1967b). Kinetics of injury and repair to mammalian tissue by high L.E.T. radiation. *Radiat. Res.*, Suppl. 7, 276.

FOWLER, J. F., MORGAN, R. L., & WOOD, C. A. P. (1963). The biological and physical advantages and problems in fast neutron therapy. A symposium on pre-therapeutic experiments with the fast neutron beam from the Medical Research Council cyclotron. *Br. J. Radiol.*, **36**, 77.

FOWLER, J. F., MORGAN, R. L., SILVESTER, J. A., BEWLEY, D. K., & TURNER, B. A. (1963). Experiments with fractionated X-ray treatment of the skin of pigs. Fractionation up to twenty-eight days. *Br. J. Radiol.*, **36**, 188.

FOWLER, P. H., & PERKINS, D. H. (1961). The possibility of therapeutic applications of beams of negative pi-mesons. *Nature, Lond.*, **189**, 524.

FLEISCHER, A. A. (1968). The Production of Fast Neutrons by Small Cyclotrons. T.C.C. Report 2003, The Cyclotron Corporation, Berkeley, California.

GAMBINO, J. J., FAULKENBERRY, B. H., & SUNDE, P. B. (1968). Survival studies on rodents exposed to reactor fast neutron radiation. *Radiat. Res.*, **35**, 668.

GILES, N. H., BEATTY, A. V., & RILEY, H. P. (1952). The effect of oxygen on the production by fast neutrons of chromosomal aberrations in tradescantia microspores. *Genetics*, **37**, 641.

GOLDACRE, R. J., & SYLVAN, B. (1959). A rapid method of studying tumour blood supply using systemic dyes. *Nature, Lond.*, **184**, 63.

GRAY, L. H., CONGER, A. D., EBERT, M., HORNSEY, S., & SCOTT, O. C. A. (1953). The concentration of oxygen dissolved in tissues at the time of irradiation as a factor in radiotherapy. *Br. J. Radiol.*, **26**, 638.

GREENE, D. (1964). A fast neutron source for radiotherapy. *Nature, Lond.*, **202**, 204.

GREENE, D., & THOMAS, R. L. (1968). An experimental unit for fast neutron radiotherapy. *Br. J. Radiol.*, **41**, 455.

GREENE, D., & THOMAS, R. L. (1969). The attenuation of 14 MeV neutrons in steel and polythene. *Physics Med. Biol.*, **14**, 45.

GREENE, E., & MAJOR, D. (1971). Collimation of 14 MeV neutron beams. *Eur. J. Cancer*, **7**, 121.

HALL, E. J. (1969). Radiobiological measurements with 14 MeV neutrons. *Br. J. Radiol.*, **42**, 805.

HALL, E. J., BEDFORD, J. S., & OLIVER, R. (1966). Extreme hypoxia: its effect on the survival of mammalian cells irradiated at high and low dose rates. *Br. J. Radiol.*, **39**, 302.

HALL, E. J., & FAIRCHILD, R. G. (1970). Radiological measurements with californium 252. *Br. J. Radiol.*, **43**, 263.

HAM, W. T., Jr. (1960). *Fast Neutron Physics*, Chapter IV. London: Interscience Publishers.

HILLIER, M., LOMER, P. D., STARK, D. S., & WOOD, J. D. L. H. (1967). Performance of Targets in Scaled-off Neutron Tubes. *Proceedings of Symposium on Accelerator Targets Designed for Production of Neutrons*, EUR. 3895 d.f.e., Liège, p. 125.

HILLIER, M., LOMER, P. D., STARK, D. S., & WOOD, J. D. L. H. (1971). A 14 MeV neutron source for radiotherapy. *Br. J. Radiol.*, in press.

HIROSE, F. (1968). Early Effects of 14·1 MeV Neutron Irradiation on Intestinal Mucosa. *Gastro-intestinal Radiation Injury*, p. 331. Sullivan, A. (Ed.). Excerpta Medica Foundation.

HORNSEY, S., (1970). Differences in survival of jejunal crypt cells after radiation delivered at different dose rates. *Br. J. Radiol.*, **43**, 802.

HORNSEY, S., & SILINI, G. (1962). Recovery of tumour cells cultured *in vivo* after X-rays and neutron irradiation. *Radiat. Res.*, **16**, 712.

HORNSEY, S., & SILINI, G. (1963). Studies on cell survival of irradiated Ehrlich ascites tumour. II. Dose effect curves for X-ray and neutron irradiations. *Int. J. Radiat. Biol.*, **4**, 135.

HORNSEY, S., VATISTAS, S., BEWLEY, D. K., & PARNELL, C. J. (1965). The effect of fractionation on four-day survival of mice after whole body neutron irradiation. *Br. J. Radiol.*, **38**, 878.

HORNSEY, S., & VATISTAS, S. (1968). Gut Leakage and Intestinal Death as a Measure of Radiation Damage: R.B.E. Values for Neutrons and the Effects of Fractionation. *Gastro-intestinal Radiation Injury. Report of a Symposium held at Richmond, U.S.A.*, p. 396. Sullivan (Ed.). Excerpta Medica Foundation.

KAPLAN, H. S. (1971). Criteria for the selection of types of tumours for radiotherapy with unconventional radiations. *Eur. J. Cancer*, in press.

KELSEY, C. A., BOONE, M. L. M., HEVEZ, J. M., WILEY, A. L., & SPALEK, G. C. (1971). Gas target source for neutron radiation therapy. *Radiol.*, **98**, 686.

KEMBER, W. F. (1969). Radiobiological investigations with fast neutrons using the cartilage clove system. *Br. J. Radiol.*, **42**, 595.

KRAUS, A. C., & BOND, J. O. (1951). Neutron cataracts. *Am. J. Ophthal.*, **34**, 25.

LAWRENCE, J. H., AEBERSOLD, P. C., & LAWRENCE, E. O. (1936). Comparative effects of X-rays and neutrons on normal and tumour tissue. *Proc. natn. Acad. Sci. U.S.A.*, **22**, 543.

LAWSON, R. C. (1969a). Californium 252 as an external source of neutrons for radiotherapy. *Br. J. Radiol.*, **42**, 714.

LAWSON, R. C. (1969b). Interaction of Radiations of Different L.E.T. *Proceedings of Symposium on the Use of Cyclotrons in Medicine.* London: Medical Research Council.

LAWSON, R. C., & WATT, D. E. (1967). The L.E.T. distribution of the recoil proton dose from D.D. and D.T. neutrons. *Physics Med. Biol.*, **12**, 217.

LAWSON, R. C., & WATT, D. E. (1968). The L.E.T. distribution of the recoil proton dose from polyenergetic neutron sources. *Physics Med. Biol.*, **13**, 619.

LINDOP, PATRICIA J. (1970). Tissue Effects of Radiation in Relation to Radiotherapy. *Current Topics in Radiation Research*, Vol. VII. Ebert and Howard (Eds.). London: North-Holland Publ. Co.

LOMER, P. D., & GREENE, D. (1963). A fast neutron source for radiotherapy. *Nature, Lond.*, **198**, 200.

LUNDBERG, D. A. (1971). The design of a practical fast neutron radiotherapy equipment for routine clinical use. *Br. J. Radiol.*, in press.

McNALLY, N. J., & BEWLEY, D. K. (1969). A biological dose meter using mammalian cells in tissue culture and its use in obtaining neutron depth dose curves. *Br. J. Radiol.*, **42**, 289.

MALLAMS, J. T., FINNEY, J. W., & BALLA, G. A. (1965). Regional oxygenation and radiation therapy. *Am. J. Roentg.*, **93**, 160.

MARION, J. B., & FOWLER, J. L. (1960). Fast Neutron Physics, Part I. New York: Interscience Publishers.

MARSHALL, T. (1970). Private communication.

MASUDA, K. (1968). Effects of 14 MeV neutrons on the reproductive capacity of HeLa S3 cells. *J. Radiat. Res., Japan* 9-3-4, 116.

MORGAN, R. L. (1967). Fast Neutron Therapy—Clinical Applications. *Modern Trends in Radiotherapy.* Deeley, T. J. and Wood, C. A. P. (Eds.). London: Butterworths.

Moroson, H., & Furhan, M. (1968). Can N-ethyl-laleimide preferentially radio-sensitize hypoxic tumour cells *in vivo*? *Int. J. Radiat. Biol.*, **13**, 585.

Munro, T. R. (1967). The influence of the oxygen–nitrogen sensitivity ratio on theoretical dose: dose rate relations. *Br. J. Radiol.*, **40**, 619.

Nias, A. W. H., Greene, D., Margaret Fox, & Thomas, R. L. (1967). Effect of monoenergetic neutrons on HeLa cells and P.388F cells *in vitro*. *Int. J. Radiat. Biol.*, **13**, No. 5, 449.

Nias, A. H. W., & Greene, D. (1971). Changes in the Biological Parameters for Mammalian Cells as a Function of Position in a 14 MeV Neutron Field. *Proceedings of Third International Congress of Radiation Biology, Evian*, in press.

Owen, L. N. (1960). A rapid method for studying tumour blood supply using Nissamine Green. *Nature, Lond.*, **187**, 795.

Oliver, G. D., Jr., & Wright, C. N. (1969). Dosimetry of an implantable ^{252}Cf source. *Radiology*, **92**, 143.

Paris, M. F., Downton, D. W., & Glanford, C. W. (1968). An experimental fast neutron radiotherapy system. *J. R. nav. scient. Serv.*, **23**, No. 4, 232.

Pickering, J. E., Williams, D. B., Melville, G. G., Jr., McDowell, A. A., Heffingwell, T. P., & Zillner, R. W. (1960). *Biological Effects of Nuclear Radiation on the Monkey (Macaca mulatta). A two-year evaluation.* W.T.1542. School of Aviation Medicine, U.S.A.F. Brooks Air Force Base, Texas.

Poppe, E. (1957). Experimental investigations on cataract formation following whole body roentgen irradiation. *Acta radiol.*, **47**, 138.

Powers, W. E., & Palmer, L. A. (1968). Biological basis of pre-operative radiotherapy. *Am. J. Roentg.*, **102**, 176.

Powers, W. E., & Tolmach, L. J. (1963). A multi-component X-ray survival curve for mouse lymphosarcoma cells irradiated *in vivo*. *Nature, Lond.*, **197**, 710.

Randolph, M. L. (1957). Energy disposition in tissue and similar materials from 14.1 MeV neutrons. *Radiat. Res.*, **7**, 47.

Reifenschweiler, O. (1968). A High Output Sealed-off Neutron Tube with High Reliability and Long Life. *Proceedings of International Congress on Modern Trends in Activation Analysis, Gaithersburg*, p. 1066. National Bureau of Standards Publication 312. Washington.

Sawada, S. (1963). Comparative studies on the lethal effects of X-rays, ^{60}Co gamma rays and 14·1 MeV fast neutrons on mice. *Nippon Acta radiol.*, **23**, 1085.

Sawada, S., & Yoshinaga, H. (1963). The relative biological effectiveness of X-rays, ^{60}Co gamma rays and 14·1 MeV fast neutrons for acute death in mice. *Nippon Acta radiol.*, **23**, 1080.

Schlea, C. S., & Stoddard, D. H. (1965). Californium isotopes proposed for intracavitary and interstitial radiation therapy with neutrons. *Nature, Lond.*, **1**, 1059.

Sheline, G. E., Field, S. B., Brennan, J. T., Phillips, T. L., & Raventos, A. (1971). Human tissue changes following neutron therapy. *Am. J. Roentg.*, **111**, 31.

Snyder, W. D., & Neufield, J. (1955). Calculated depth dose curves in tissue for broad beams of fast neutrons. *Br. J. Radiol.*, **28**, 331.

Stewart, J. G., Jackson, A. W., & Chew, M. K. (1969). Private communication.

Stone, R. S., Lawrence, J. H., & Aebersold, P. C. (1940). A preliminary report on the use of fast neutrons in the treatment of malignant disease. *Radiology*, **35**, 3227.

Stone, R. S., & Larkin, J. C. (1942). The treatment of cancer with fast neutrons. *Radiology*, **39**, 608.

Stone, R. S. (1948). Neutron Therapy and Specific Ionisation. Janeway Memorial Lecture. *Am. J. Roentg.*, **59**, 771.

Suit, H. D., & Maeda, M. (1966). Oxygen effect factor and tumour volume in the C3H mouse mammary carcinoma. *Am. J. Roentg.*, **96,** 177.

Tobias, C. A., & Todd, P. W. (1965). Heavy charged particles in cancer therapy. *National Cancer Institute Monograph No. 24,* 1.

Upton, A. C., Christenberry, K. W., Melville, G. S., Firth, J., & Hirst, G. S. (1956). The relative cataractogenic effectiveness of neutrons. *Radiology,* **67,** 686.

Van Putten, L. M. (1968). Oxygenation and Cell Kinetics After Irradiation in a Transplantable Osteosarcoma. *Effects of Radiation on Cellular Proliferation and Differentiation,* p. 493. Vienna: I.A.E.A.

Van Putten, L. M. (1968). Tumour re-oxygenation during fractionated radiotherapy; studies with a transplantable mouse osteosarcoma. *Eur. J. Cancer,* **4,** 173.

Van Putten, L. M., Lelieveld, P., & Broerse, J. J. (1971). The response of a poorly re-oxygenating mouse osteosarcoma to X-rays and fast neutrons. *Eur. J. Cancer,* **7,** 153.

Vastistas, S., & Hornsey, S. (1966). Radiation induced protein loss into the gastrointestinal tract. *Br. J. Radiology,* **39,** 547.

Vogel, H. H., & Jordan, D. L. (1968). A Comparison of the Damage to the Small Intestine by Fission Neutrons on Gamma Rays from Cobalt. *Gastro-intestinal Radiation Injury,* p. 327. Sullivan. (Ed.). Excerpta Medica Foundation.

Wilson, K., & Field, S. B. (1970). Private communication in *Fast Neutron Beams for Therapy* by D. K. Bewley. Current Topics in Radiation Research, Vol. II.

Withers, H. R., Oliver, G. D., & Glenn, D. W. (1971). Response of mouse jejunal crypt cells to low dose-rate irradiation by Californium-252 neutrons and radium gamma rays. *Radiation Research,* in press.

Withers, H. R., Brennan, J. T., & Elkind, M. M. (1970). The response of stem cells of intestinal mucosa to irradiation with 14 MeV neutrons. *Br. J. Radiol.,* **43,** 796.

Withers, H. R., Almond, P. R., & Brown, B. W. (1971). Considerations for clinical trials with fast neutrons. *Eur. J. Cancer,* **7,** 231.

Wright, C. N., Boulogne, A. R., Reinig, W. C., & Evans, A. G. (1967). Implantable californium 252 neutron sources for radiotherapy. *Radiology,* **89,** 337.

Wright, E. A., Bewley, D. K., & Parnall, C. J. (1966). The effects of cyclotron neutrons on the intact mouse thymus under normal and hypoxic conditions. *Br. J. Radiol.,* **39,** 551.

Yamamoto, O. (1967). On the variation of LD-50 in time after 14·1 MeV fast neutrons and 180 kV p X-rays for young and adult mice. *Nippon Acta radiol.,* **26,** 1361.

10 Radiotherapy in Hyperbaric Oxygen

SASHA MORRIS

The potential importance of the oxygen effect in clinical radiotherapy has already been made clear in Chapter 8. One of the most immediate and direct applications has been the use of hyperbaric oxygen to attempt to enhance the effects of radiotherapy. Pure oxygen breathed at atmospheric pressure had been shown to enhance the effect of radiation therapy on skin tumours (Hultborn and Forssberg, 1954). If oxygen could be given at increased atmospheric pressures, then it seemed reasonable that even more anoxic cells would be reached and made increasingly radiosensitive by the permeation of the oxygen under pressure. Churchill-Davidson, Sanger and Tomlinson (1955) were the first to attempt the treatment of human tumours by radiotherapy under hyperbaric oxygen conditions. Histological examination of the tumours, half of each tumour being treated while the patient breathed 3 atmospheres of oxygen, the other half being treated with the patient breathing air at normal atmospheric pressure, showed a greater amount of radiation damage in the oxygenated section. From further cell survival studies, (Powers and Tolmach, 1963) it has been found that the proportion of surviving tumour cells dropped from 1 in 100 to 1 in 1,000 if irradiated under conditions of hyperbaric oxygen.

TECHNIQUES

VICKERS CHAMBER

It is now 16 years since hyperbaric oxygen was first used for patients being treated by radiotherapy, and the Vickers modification of the original hyperbaric oxygen chamber (Emery et al., 1960) has become a feature of many radiotherapy departments throughout the world. Basically, it consists of two six feet long concentric and transparent cylinders of plastic with metal caps at each end, attached to a chassis mounted on spring castors. The inner plastic cylinder holds the gas under the required pressure, which is generally 3 atmospheres absolute (A.T.A.). The outer cylinder, separated from the inner one by an air space, acts as a fail-safe mechanism, holding the pressure temporarily if the inner cylinder should fracture, but not permanently oxygen-tight

so that there would be, under these circumstances, a gradual leak of gas
and fall in pressure. It is also important in that it protects the inner
cylinder from accidental damage by impact with other objects when the
chamber is moved for treatment purposes. One end of the chamber is
permanently sealed by the metal cap. It is to this end that the oxygen
supply and the exhaust duct are connected. The newest model (Fig. 1),
installed recently in Glasgow, has no connection with an electrical
supply, but uses the hovercraft principle, which not only allows the
chamber to be moved with ease but is also geared to adjust the height
of the chamber, bringing the treatment area on the patient to the correct

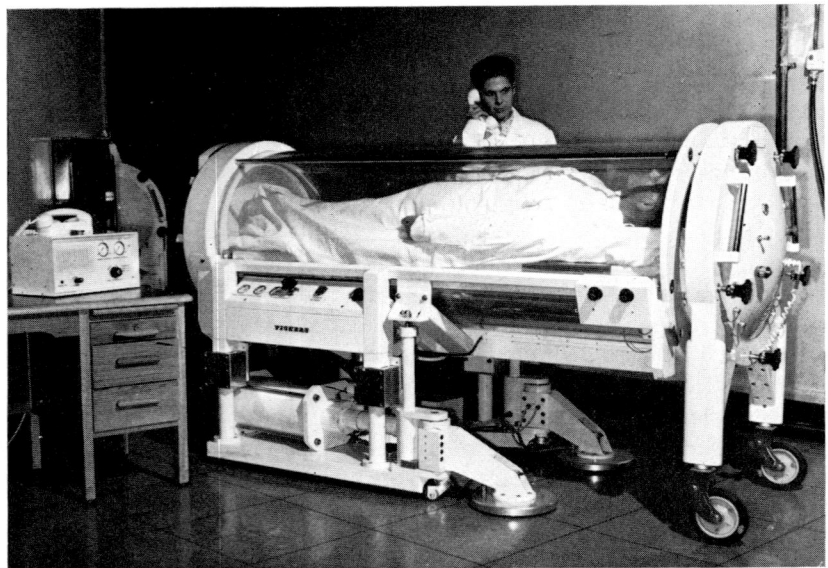

Fig. 10.1. The Vickers Hyperbaric Oxygen Chamber, with 'hoverpads' and pneumatic height adjustment.

distance from the head of the X-ray or Cobalt γ-ray unit. The other
end of the chamber is secured by five screw handwheels which, when
released, permit the door to be opened and the stretcher-bed to be
pulled out on to a trolley.

Two-way communication with the patient, who is slid, feet first, into
the chamber and can be seen to his or her full length, is by microphones
set on the inner side of the door and by a telephone receiver attached
to the control panel on the side of the chamber, the electrical supply
being from a 10 volt battery fitted on to the chassis. There is also a
remote control console with communication for use when the patient
is being treated, and is, therefore, inaccessible to the staff in charge.

Physiological monitoring can be carried out through connections on the door of the chamber. Oxygen flows in at a maximum rate of 400 litres per minute, to be piped out through the exhaust duct only via the motorized spring-loaded valve. This valve can alter the pressure within the chamber by a control from the operator's console which can increase or decrease the spring-loading. Safety devices prevent the pressure from rising higher than 30 lb/sq. inch. As oxygen is constantly flushing through the chamber, carbon dioxide, nitrogen and water vapour are rapidly removed from the patient's vicinity, and the temperature does not vary more than 4°C.

To minimize the danger of fire and actual injury, patients are required to change into proban-treated cotton gowns and to remove all jewellery, dentures, hairpins, and so on before entering the chamber. Sheets on the stretcher are also proban-treated.

OXYGENATION

An essential preliminary to treatment is the time spent by the patient—generally about 20 minutes—in the oxygen chamber. It is not enough to pressurize the patient to 3ATA—a procedure which takes 4–5 minutes in the majority of cases. The patient, at 3ATA, must then be in the chamber for a minimum period of time so that all tumour tissue is thoroughly oxygenated. It is important to take into consideration the fact that tumour tissues appear to take considerably longer than normal tissues to saturate with oxygen (Evans and Naylor, 1963). The Medical Research Council Working Party on Hyperbaric Oxygen have concluded that a minimum of 15 minutes should ensue between full pressurization and the onset of treatment, as suggested by Watson (1968) and Cater and Silver (1960).

BEAM DIRECTION

Setting up the patient for radiotherapy is not a problem. There is no difficulty in defining the area to be treated through the transparent walls of the chamber. The patient lies in the appropriate position, turning over if required to do so. The normal light-positioning mechanism, available in megavoltage units, can be used in combination with the elevating mechanism of the chamber to attain the correct focus-to-skin-distance. For accurate beam direction in the treatment of tumours of the head and neck, where the patient's head is held in a cast, a method has been devised using an extra lens mounted in front of the treatment head of a linear accelerator (Sutherland and Griffiths, 1966, and Sutherland 1968). Curvature of the cylinder wall is too slight to alter the isodose curves used in planning the treatment, but the thickness of the double wall must be taken into account and the dose of radiation to be given increased accordingly to allow for this. The actual treatment time must vary according to the dose of radiation prescribed, but is usually between 1 and 4 minutes for each field irradiated. Naturally, during this time, the patient must lie quite still within the chamber and must be alone in the treatment room. Many centres use closed-circuit television to watch the patient during the course of treatment as well as using the two-way communication system. As soon as the treatment is completed, the chamber is returned to the preparation room and the patient is decompressed over 4–5 minutes.

OTHER METHODS

It is worth mentioning at this stage that other methods have been used for administering hyperbaric oxygen to patients receiving radiotherapy. A chamber developed by Oxygenaire consists of a metal cylinder with a transparent plastic head cap. This has been used in Aberdeen for the treatment of head and neck cancer, in the way already described. In Japan, the 'Ralstron' method of treatment for patients suffering from gynaecological cancer has been developed. This combined the administration of pure oxygen by mask within a chamber pressurized to 3ATA with air, and the insertion of Cobalt-60 by remote control via tubes into applicators which have been inserted into the vagina before treatment. As elsewhere, there needs to be a 'soaking' period of 10 minutes before the irradiation, and the whole procedure takes about 40 minutes (Wakabayashi et al., 1969).

HAZARDS

The primary hazard of using pure oxygen in treatment is a technical one—that of fire. This was demonstrated to the world in a most tragic way when American astronauts lost their lives within one minute of their oxygen chamber catching fire due to an aberrant spark. In the set-up for hyperbaric radiotherapy, electrical points must be kept to a minimum and oxygen leads into and out of the chamber must be leak-proof. Ideally, the exhaust duct should conduct the oxygen to the outside air. As already mentioned, fire-proofing of sheets and hospital gowns for use in the chamber is a highly recommended safety precaution.

In the actual treatment programme, the major complication can be the non-cooperation of the patient. Unless the latter has complete confidence in the doctor and staff in charge, radiotherapy under conditions of hyperbaric oxygen becomes impossible. For doctors and technicians, procedures are simple and straightforward; for the patient, it is a step into the unknown which he or she is most fearful to take. As in all forms of treatment, it is essential to explain what is going to happen and, if possible, to let the patient 'try out' the chamber by lying in it under normal and raised oxygen pressure. By doing this, the patient appreciates that he is not cut off either visually or aurally from those around him. He can see, hear and converse with the doctor and attendants in charge. It is also important that he can accommodate his ears to the changing atmospheric pressure. Often this is no problem for one who has travelled by air or comes from a hilly area of country, and is able to adjust his ears to the increasing pressure. For others, a constant reminder to yawn, swallow, cough or use the Valsalva technique (which should be demonstrated before the patient enters the chamber) will be sufficient to cut down any discomfort which the patient might experience as the oxygen pressure rises. Nasal decongestants are also used to clear the eustachian tubes. It may take as long as 15 minutes to reach the required pressure of 30 lb/sq. inch on the first occasion. But it is almost always possible to speed up the rate of compression to about 4 minutes within one or two treatments as the patient learns to accommodate automatically. Rarely, myringotomy may be required and grommets can be inserted to ensure complete relief during subsequent treatment. Decompression is no problem as the entire treatment is completed within 30–45 minutes and the use of pure oxygen eliminates any danger of the 'bends' developing as could happen with decompression of ordinary air containing nitrogen.

Oxygen does sometimes appear to have a toxic effect leading to convulsions, although the mechanism for this has not been satisfactorily explained. It may be due to oxidation of critical enzyme systems in the body metabolism, or to increased carbon dioxide tension at cellular level, since all available haemoglobin may be taken up by the increased concentration of oxygen (Dickens 1946). It is certainly impossible to foresee which patients will convulse during treatment, or at what point they will do so. In a series of 150 cases in Glasgow, there have been 8 patients each of whom had a single attack of convulsions, 4 during decompression and 4 during treatment. All recovered completely within a few minutes of removal from the oxygen chamber, this being effected within 40 seconds by emergency decompression, and all completed their course of treatment without any evidence of complications.

The other possible hazard to radiotherapy under hyperbaric oxygen conditions is the increased liability of certain tissues to damage if included in the area being treated. These tissues—cartilage, the lens and cornea of the eye, the outer layers of the skin, and scar tissue—have little or no vascularization and normally exist at low oxygen tensions. A state of increased oxygenation increases their response to ionizing radiations, and there might be a relatively higher likelihood of damage or necrosis. In trials so far, this potential hazard has not been of major significance, only a few sporadic cases being reported.

RESULTS

Several sites of tumour have been treated. It should first be mentioned that there have been reports from several centres of uncontrolled series of patients, often with miscellaneous diagnoses (Churchill-Davidson, 1967; Phillips *et al.*, 1966). It has been claimed that encouraging results have been achieved, and some workers, especially Churchill-Davidson, have felt so convinced of the value of hyperbaric oxygen that ethical difficulties have prevented them from undertaking any controlled trial.

MEDICAL RESEARCH COUNCIL TRIALS

However, many workers in Britain believed that controlled clinical trials were necessary to assess the value of hyperbaric oxygen and the Medical Research Council in 1965 appointed a Working Party for this purpose. It was decided that patients entered in the trials should satisfy the following criteria:

1. The age of the patient must be less than 75.
2. The patient must be medically fit to undergo treatment in the oxygen chamber and able to lie flat.
3. The diagnosis of carcinoma must be corroborated by histology before treatment.
4. No metastases other than those in regional lymph nodes must be demonstrable.
5. No previous radiotherapy or surgery other than a diagnostic procedure must have been performed.
6. Radical external radiotherapy using megavoltage units must be considered the most suitable form of treatment for the tumour in question.
7. Individual anatomical or clinical criteria of selection must operate for each tumour site.

When this assessment has been made and the dose and volume of tissue to be treated has been prescribed, the patient is randomly selected for treatment in either air or oxygen according to the content of sealed envelopes supplied by the M.R.C. Thus, there will be only one difference between the two randomly selected groups of patients—the atmosphere in which treatment is given—treatment of the patients will otherwise be identical, from all points of view.

HEAD AND NECK CANCER

Among the trials nearing completion, one showing the most promising results has been that conducted by Henk, Kunkler and colleagues in Cardiff (1970), on tumours of the head and neck. A prospective trial of hyperbaric oxygen in the management of these tumours was begun in 1964, and an interim report was given in October 1969. Two hundred and thirteen patients suffering from carcinoma of the head and neck had been treated up to this time, 112 in air, 101 in oxygen. As close a correspondence as possible was made in these two series regarding age, sex, primary site, using the TNM classification, lymph node involvement, histopathology, haemoglobin level, and tumour treatment dose. It so happened that well-differentiated squamous carcinoma occurred in greater numbers in the oxygen series. As a group, this did less well, as also did males, and patients with lymph node involvement—this last would be expected. All patients in both series were treated to a tumour dose of 3,500 to 4,500 rads on a 4 MeV linear accelerator in ten fractions over 3 weeks. Eighteen patients in the oxygen series received less than 50% of their treatment in this medium, due to convulsion, claustrophobia, or non-cooperation, and were excluded from the final analysis. It must be noted that there is this definite if slight 'morbidity' in oxygen therapy which does not occur with orthodox radiotherapy.

Benefit was clearly demonstrated in a statistically significant increased survival rate of those patients suffering from nasal and oral carcinoma who were treated in hyperbaric oxygen (Fig. 2).

Recurrence-free rates were also calculated. A patient was deemed free of recurrence if there was no clinical evidence of the primary tumour within the irradiated volume on follow-up examination or at death. There was no doubt that patients in the oxygen series, especially in the oral, nasal and laryngo-pharyngeal groups were significantly less liable to recurrence (Fig. 3). Survival rates do not show the same bias in favour of oxygen-treated patients as do the recurrence-free rates. This can perhaps be partly accounted for by the limited follow-up period of the trial. In addition, those patients treated in air, having a greater tendency to local recurrence, required more salvage surgery and this, one is glad to note, effectively improved their survival. The need for surgery applied with particular force to those patients treated for carcinoma of the larynx—7 out of 24 air-treated patients compared with 1 out of 20 oxygen-treated patients required laryngectomy. Thus, the latter were spared the distress of radical mutilating surgery.

The possible control of lymph node metastases has also been considered in an attempt to improve therapy and subsequent survival. Kunkler and colleagues (1970) had made a retrospective study of 151 patients who required treatment for lymph node metastases as well as

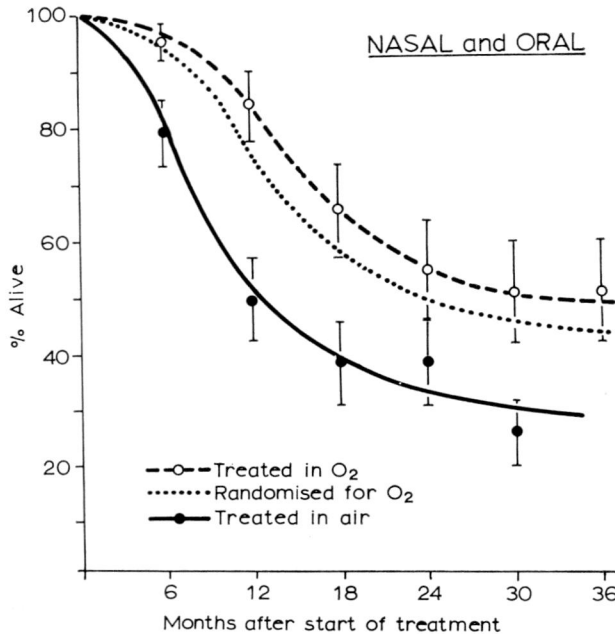

NASAL and ORAL

% Alive

--o-- Treated in O_2
.... Randomised for O_2
--●-- Treated in air

6   12   18   24   30   36

Months after start of treatment

FIG. 10.2. Survival curves for nasal and oral carcinoma reported by Henk and colleagues (1970).

for the primary site in the mouth or oropharynx between 1957 and 1964. Only one third of these cases were treated by surgery, often regarded as the only possible hope of cure for carcinoma at this site. Yet radical radiotherapy, given to 42 cases in the series where lymph node metastases were treated to tissue tolerance levels, gave very similar results to surgery in spite of the fact that the patients selected for radiotherapy were inevitably an older section of the population with more advanced disease. The results were as follows:

Surgery: 5 year survival—27%, failure—48%.
Radical Radiotherapy: 5 year survival—29%, failure 50%.

Only 3 out of 57 cases receiving palliative radiotherapy survived 5 years, showing that the latter can only have a temporary growth restraint effect unless the dose is raised to tissue tolerance levels.

With the employment of hyperbaric oxygen as an adjunct to radical X-ray treatment, still better lymph node control may be achieved. This has been demonstrated with small numbers, so small that the difference is not yet statistically significant. Seven out of 14 patients treated in oxygen were alive and free of recurrence after 1 year, compared with only 2 out of 10 patients similarly treated in air. These cases all had primary sites in the oral cavity or oropharynx. Thus, Kunkler and his colleagues

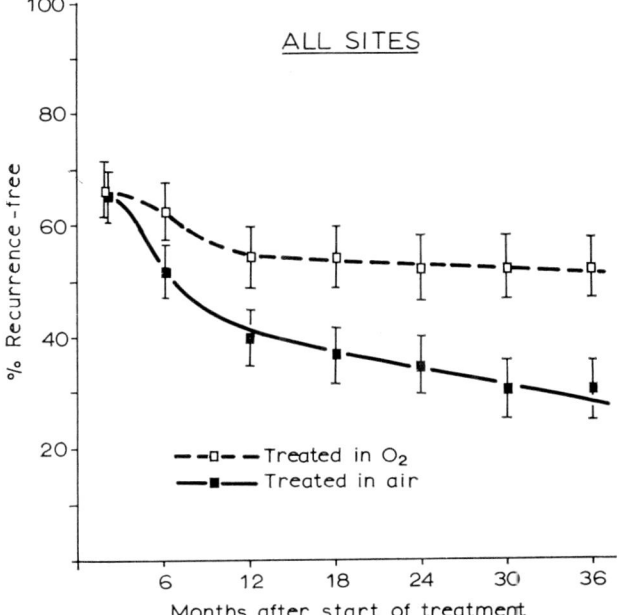

FIG. 10.3. Recurrence-free rates for all patients with head and neck carcinoma reported by Henk and colleagues (1970).

have been able to include more patients for radical treatment to involved nodes who, before this trial, might only have been given palliative doses. In fact, the proportion rose from 42% during the 1957–64 period to 79% between 1964 and 1967 with a slightly higher survival rate after 18 months' follow-up. This has been achieved with a reduction in the number of patients subjected to radical node surgery from 1 in 5 in the earlier period to 1 in 48 in the 1964–67 period. This work clearly suggests an improvement in the results of treatment of lymph node metastases, as well as in local tumour control, by the use of radical radiotherapy combined with hyperbaric oxygen. Similar encouraging results have been noted by other workers (Churchill-Davidson, 1967).

There was no evidence in this trial that hyperbaric oxygen encouraged the spread of metastases, in spite of this suggestion by other workers (Johnson, 1968).

CANCER OF THE UTERINE CERVIX

The second main site to be considered is the uterine cervix. Another controlled clinical trial is being conducted at the present time by Watson and colleagues (1971) in Glasgow, where an oxygen chamber has been in use since 1964. This trial, under similar conditions to Cardiff, was begun in 1966 to assess the value of hyperbaric oxygen in the treatment of advanced carcinoma of the uterine cervix where tumour has already reached the pelvic wall. It has been shown that the oxygen effect is minimal when low intensity radiation is given over a prolonged period of time, but is maximal when high intensity X-rays are used over short periods. These findings have been applied to the treatment of cervical carcinoma, Stages III and IV, confined to the pelvis, in the Glasgow trial. Patients receiving radical therapy from a 4 MeV linear accelerator are treated in air or in 3ATA oxygen according to random selection, and are given localized radium treatment to the cervix at the end of their course of treatment. The criteria for entry to the trial are the same as in Cardiff, and random selection for air or oxygen is only made after a complete assessment of the patient's condition and prescription of treatment. All cases are treated according to a standard technique, one which has been used since the installation of megavoltage equipment in Glasgow in 1962. It consists of a 4 week course of therapy on the linear accelerator during which the pelvis is subjected to a tumour dose of 4,250 rads by means of four fields, two being treated daily over 5 days per week so that each field is given a total of ten treatments. When this has been completed, a single radium insertion is carried out in theatre to increase the tumour dose in and around the cervix, to 7,500 rads at Point A.

An interim assessment of this trial was made in April 1971. One hundred and twenty five patients have been treated, 62 in oxygen and 63 in air. Ninety six of these were Stage III and 29 Stage IV confined to pelvis. Histologically, a total of 110 were found to be squamous cell carcinoma and these were separately analysed. Increased survival for both

TABLE I

HYPERBARIC OXYGEN TRIAL IN GLASGOW. RESULTS AT APRIL 1971

Carcinoma of cervix (Squamous)	Treatment group	Total	Deaths	% Survival
Stage III	Air	48	22	54
	Oxygen	37	13	65
Stage IV (pelvis only)	Air	8	7	12·5
	Oxygen	17	11	23·5

Stage III and IV cases treated in oxygen is clearly shown when compared with the equivalent air series, but the numbers remain too few as yet for conventional statistical significance.

Reports on uncontrolled series of patients have come from St. Thomas's Hospital, London (Bates, 1969) and from Canada (Johnson, 1968). Bates treated 21 patients by a four-field 'brick' treatment to give 3,500 rads maximum tissue dose in six fractions over 3 weeks. All these cases were Stage III, and at the time of report, 14 were alive at periods varying from 3 to 60 months. It was later reported (Bewley, 1970) that all these patients had survived at least 22 months, and it was suggested that this result was significantly better than that of early patients treated in air but with intra-cavitary treatment also. Johnson had also used external ^{60}Cobalt radiation only, treating 25 cases of Stage III and IV carcinoma of cervix, giving 6,000 rads in 6 weeks, and with local failure of 55% at 6 months; it was also suggested that there was an increased number of deaths from distant metastases.

TRIALS IN AUSTRALIA

Valuable studies have also been conducted by Van den Brenk and his colleagues (1968) in Melbourne, where a hyperbaric oxygen chamber has been in use since 1961. Their technique of treatment has been pressurization of patients, using barbiturate anaesthesia, to 4ATA oxygen, to be maintained there for 10–30 minutes before irradiation with 4 MeV X-rays. The course of treatment, consisting of 2–6 fractions, was given over a period of 7–28 days. Only patients with inoperable or recurrent disease were accepted. 10% of these had distant metastases and many had other concurrent organic disease. Van den Brenk's aim, was to show an improvement in the quality of survival, however short-term this might be. In fact, he states that 87% of cases treated for carcinoma of the upper respiratory and digestive passages by this regime were alive at 6 months compared with 50% alive after treatment by conventional daily techniques of irradiation in air. The incidence of sequelae following irradiation dropped from 50% when 3 × 1,000r was used in air or in oxygen to 30% when daily fractionation in air or 3 × 800r in oxygen was used. It fell to 18% when 6 × 500r in oxygen was the treatment given.

Work has also been carried out in Melbourne (Van den Brenk et al., 1968) to estimate the radiosensitivity of the spinal cord under conditions of hyperbaric oxygen—vitally important when attempting to eradicate malignant disease in the head or neck regions without causing radiation myelopathy. It is suggested that there is a higher incidence of this complication after treatment in hyperbaric oxygen than in air, but the data are insufficient to be finally conclusive.

CANCER OF LUNG AND BLADDER

Important clinical trials under the Medical Research Council have also been carried out in Portsmouth using telecobalt treatment on two main sites—the lung or bronchus, and the urinary bladder. Interim reports have been published (McEwan, 1966; Cade and McEwan, 1967; McEwan, 1968). Tumours in both sites have been treated radically, five treatments weekly, to a tumour dose of 6,000 rads over 8 weeks. These trials have been very well done with substantial numbers of patients, and it is all the more disappointing that there are no significant differences in results so far for either site of tumour.

FRACTIONATION

One subsidiary factor of importance is the question of fractionation. The first treatment by Churchill-Davidson was done with a few large fractions of treatment, rather than the conventional daily treatment over several weeks, simply because the first hyperbaric treatments were necessarily elaborate, difficult, and time-consuming. The use of the Vickers Chamber and the realization that a general anaesthetic was unnecessary made daily treatment possible. When the M.R.C. trials were begun, it was thought that the only difference between the two randomly selected groups should be the hyperbaric oxygen, and that there should be identical fractionation of treatment on both sides. However, after it began to be apparent, especially from the Portsmouth results, that improvement in results from hyperbaric oxygen under these circumstances might only be small, perhaps even negligible, it was suggested that the full benefit of hyperbaric treatment might only be achieved with small numbers of large fractions. It has even been suggested that any apparent benefits shown in Cardiff by Kunkler and colleagues might have been demonstrated, *not* because the hyperbaric oxygen results were better, but because the results of treatment of the conventional air series were worse because of the fractionation used (10 fractions over 3 weeks). The question will obviously be difficult to resolve, since the effects of fractionation itself are not yet fully understood, particularly quantitatively. However, further variations of the trials are being suggested.

CONCLUSIONS

Fifteen years have gone by since the publication of the first report on the use of hyperbaric oxygen in radiotherapy and its value continues to remain a subject for debate. One important lesson for us all is the urgent necessity to undertake properly controlled trials from the beginning to assess the value of any further possible advances in treatment. However, it is at least clear that there is no evidence that hyperbaric oxygen has done harm to any patient; and the rationale for its use has a firm basis in experimental fact. Statistically valid evidence on the value of hyperbaric oxygen is just beginning to appear, and it is to be hoped that this evidence will grow more substantial from the trials at present in progress.

ACKNOWLEDGEMENTS

Very sincere thanks for providing much material for this review are due to Professor P. B. Kunkler who was, unfortunately, prevented by illness from undertaking the authorship of this chapter himself, and to Dr E. R. Watson, Dr M. A. C. Cowell and other colleagues in Glasgow for all their help and encouragement.

REFERENCES

BATES, T. D. (1969). The treatment of stage III carcinoma of cervix by external radiotherapy and high pressure oxygen. *Br. J. Radiol.*, **42**, 266.

BEWLEY, D. K. (1970). The treatment of stage III carcinoma of cervix by external radiotherapy and high pressure oxygen. *Br. J. Radiol.*, **43**, 498.

CADE, I. S., & McEwan, J. B. (1967). Megavoltage radiotherapy in hyperbaric oxygen. *Cancer*, **20**, 817

CATER, D. B., & SILVER, I. A. (1960). Quantitative measurements of oxygen tension in normal tissues and in tumours of patients before and after radiotherapy. *Acta radiol.*, **53**, 233.

CHURCHILL-DAVIDSON, I., SANGER, C., & THOMLINSON, R. H. (1955). High pressure oxygen and radiotherapy. *Lancet*, i, 1091.

CHURCHILL-DAVIDSON, I., SANGER, C., & THOMLINSON, R. H. (1957). Oxygenation in radiotherapy. II. Clinical application. *Br. J. Radiol.*, **30**, 406.

CHURCHILL-DAVIDSON, I. (1967). *Modern Trends in Radiotherapy*, pp. 73–91. Wood, C. A. P., and Deeley, T. J. (Eds.). London: Butterworths.

DICKENS, F. (1946). Toxic effects of oxygen on brain metabolisms and on tissue enzymes. *Biochem. J.* **40**, 145.

EMERY, E. W., LUCAS, B. G. B., & WILLIAMS, E. G. (1960). Technique of irradiation to conscious patients under increased oxygen pressure. *Lancet*, i, 248.

EVANS, N. T. S., & Maylor, P. F. D. (1963). The effect of oxygen breathing and radiotherapy upon the tissue oxygen tension of some human tumours. *Br. J. Radiol.*, **36**, 418.

HALL, E. J., BEDFORD, J. S., & OLIVER, R. (1966). Extreme hypoxia; its effect on the survival of mammalian cells irradiated at high and low dose rates. *Br. J. Radiol.*, **39**, 302.

HENK, J. M., KUNKLER, P. B., SHAH, N. K., SMITH, C. W., SUTHERLAND, W. H., & WASSIF, S. B. (1970). Hyperbaric oxygen in radiotherapy of head and neck carcinoma. *Clin. Radiol.*, **21**, 223.

HULTBORN, K. A., & FORSSBERG, A. (1954). Irradiation of skin tumours during pure oxygen inhalation. *Acta radiol.*, **42**, 475.

JOHNSON, R. J. R. (1968). Gynaecological Cancer Treated with Cobalt under Hyperbaric Conditions. *Frontiers of Radiation Therapy and Oncology*, Vol. 1, pp. 149–55. Basel and New York: Karger.

KUNKLER, P. B., HENK, J. M., SHAH, N. K., SMITH, C. W. (1970). Radiotherapy and Hyperbaric Oxygen in Malignant Tumours of the Oral Cavity and Oropharynx with Lymph Node Metastases. Gann Monograph No. 9. Tokyo: Maruzen.

McEWAN, J. B. (1966). Clinical trial of radiotherapy and high pressure oxygen. *Ann. R. Coll. Surg.*, **39**, 168.

McEWAN, J. B. (1968). Hyperbaric oxygen and radiotherapy. *Archivo Patol.*, **40**, 49.

PHILLIPS, D. L., MORRIS, S., & ORR, J. S. (1966). Report on the first year's use of hyperbaric oxygen in supervoltage radiotherapy at the Western Infirmary, Glasgow. *Clin. Radiol.*, **17**, 173.

POWERS, W. E., & TOLMACH, L. J. (1963). A multicomponent X-ray survival curve for mouse lymphosarcoma cells irradiated *in vivo. Nature, Lond.*, **197**, 710.

SUTHERLAND, W. H., & GRIFFITHS, D. (1966). Beam direction in hyperbaric oxygen therapy. *Br. J. Radiol.*, **39**, 696.

SUTHERLAND, W. H. (1968). A new method of beam directions with particular applications in hyperbaric oxygen therapy. *Br. J. Radiol.*, **41**, 633.

VAN DEN BRENK, H. A. S., MADIGAN, J. P., & KERR, R. C. (1968). Experience in Melbourne with the Use of Hyperbaric Oxygen Combined with Megavoltage Radiation in 614 Cases of Advanced Malignant Disease. *Frontiers of Radiation Therapy and Oncology*, pp. 162–74. Basel and New York: Karger.

VAN DEN BRENK, H. A. S., RICHTER, W., & HURLEY, R. H. (1968). Radiosensitivity of the human oxygenated spinal cord based on analysis of 357 cases receiving 4 MeV X-rays in hyperbaric oxygen. *Br. J. Radiol.*, **41**, 205.

WAKABAYASHI, M., OHSAWA, T., & SUGAWARA, T. (1969). Intracavitary Radiation Therapy under the Hybaroxic Condition. XIIth International Congress of Radiology, Tokyo.

WATSON, E. R., HALNAN, K. E., & MORRIS, S. (1971). A Controlled Clinical Trial of Hyperbaric Oxygen in the Radiotherapy of Advanced Carcinoma of the Cervix Uteri. *Modern Trends in Radiotherapy*, Vol. II. Deeley, T. J. (Ed.). London: Butterworths.

WOOTTON, P. (1968). An Approach to the Determination of Individual Patient Soaking Times in Hyperbaric Oxygen Radiation Therapy. *Frontiers of Radiation Therapy and Oncology*, Vol. 1, pp. 90–7. Basel and New York: Karger.

11 Endolymphatic Radiotherapy

GERALD E. FLATMAN

A vital factor in the emergence of present day scientific medicine from the witchcraft of the Dark Ages was the ability to study human anatomy, a subject so long inhibited by the Church which frowned upon dissection of any but the executed criminal. Modern knowledge of the anatomy of the lymphatic system dates from Aselli's work in 1627 although Trapnell (1965) attributes the earliest observations to Herophilus in 335 B.C.

That it is necessary to treat the lymphatic field as well as the primary site of a carcinoma has been recognized by oncologists for many years. Paterson (1952) in his Mackenzie Davidson Memorial Lecture showed that the cure rate is higher if the volume of tissue treated by radiotherapy is limited to that involved by the disease. Basing his principles upon the anatomy as well as the natural history of cancer, Green (1959) designed a method of 'tracking' the disease along the course of lymphatics in the abdomen using orthovoltage X-ray therapy and later gamma radiation from ^{60}Co. Cannulation of lymphatic channels now makes it possible to irradiate lymphatic tissue from within and to obtain dosage concentration far in excess of that reported by Green.

In 1952 Kinmonth described a practical method of lymphatic injection upon which its clinical application in 1954 formed the basis of present day lymphography. A further logical development of this procedure was the use of peripheral lymphatic channels as routes through which radioactive material might reach and destroy malignant cells within the lymphatic system. Jantet (1958) first described the use of radioactive colloidal gold (^{198}Au) for lymphatic perfusion when he treated 4 patients suffering from advanced lymph node disease due to secondary carcinoma, lymphosarcoma and follicular lymphoma. He reported further experience of this in 1962 and in 1964 applied it to the treatment of malignant melanoma.

The value of diagnostic lymphography in the treatment of malignant disease has been pointed out by Macdonald (1969) and Mahaffy (1965, 1969) amongst others but it earlier became clear that there would be an advantage in being able to visualize the lymphatic tissue which was being subjected to radiation and Seitzman (1963), Chiappa (1964), Edwards et al. (1968) and Gibson et al. (1968) reported the use of

[131]I Ultrafluid Lipiodol. Later [32]P Ultrafluid Lipiodol was introduced and Lord *et al.* (1968) have compared the relative merits of these two substances. Ariel (1964) used ceramic microspheres of diameter $1-4\,\mu$ coated with yttrium-90, and Edwards (1969) ion exchange resin particles also coated with yttrium-90.

TECHNIQUE OF ENDOLYMPHATIC RADIOTHERAPY

The technique whereby the chosen radioactive material is infused is essentially that described by Kinmonth (1954, 1955) for diagnostic lymphography but with the addition of anti-radiation precautions.

If [131]I Lipiodol is to be used the patient is given 5 minims of Lugols iodine three times a day for 2 days before and 3 days after the infusion in order to block the thyroid gland and prevent the uptake of [131]I.

Skin preparation is the same as for any surgical procedure and the patient is usually given standard premedication; although some may prefer a general anaesthetic, the procedure is commonly carried out under local anaesthesia. Whilst no discomfort will be experienced, the procedure may be tedious for the patient may be required to lie still for well over an hour. However, some patients sleep, others may relieve the tedium by reading a book (Fig. 1).

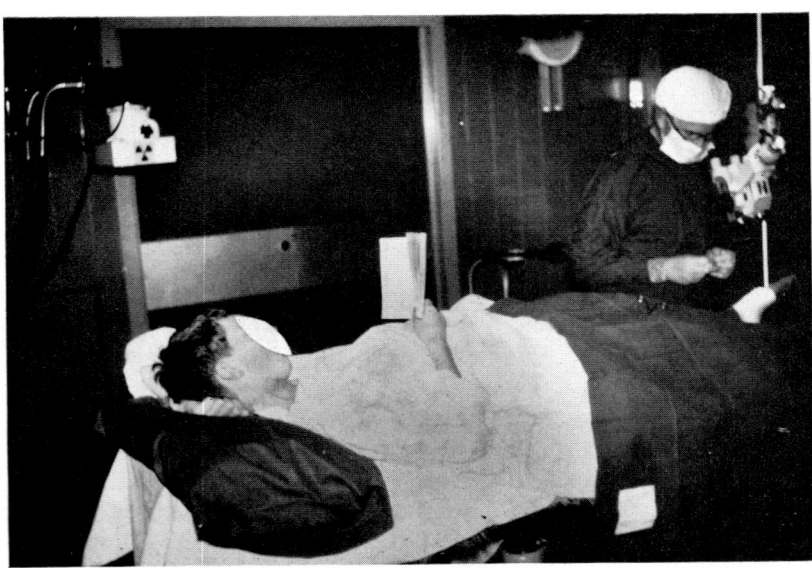

FIG. 11.1. Patient relaxed and reading a book whilst undergoing endolymphatic radiotherapy.

The lymphatics are visualized in the usual way by injecting 0·5 ml Patent Blue, part intradermally and part subcutaneously, and distributed between the four toe or finger webs. Roo (1964) recommends that the webs should be subsequently massaged but this is usually unnecessary and in a few minutes lymphatic channels containing the dye are seen through the skin, converging at the ankle or wrist to form

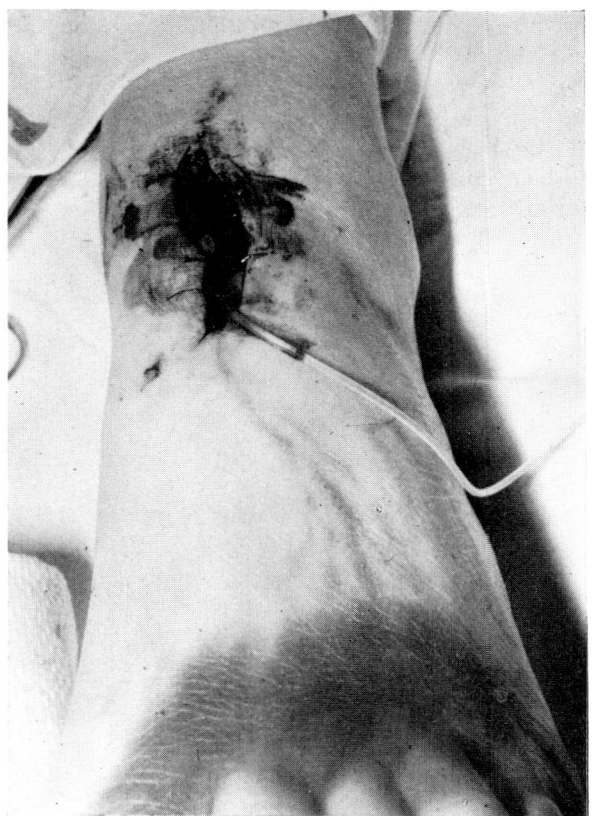

FIG. 11.2. Patent Blue injected between the toe webs outlines the lymph trunks over the dorsum of the foot and a longitudinal S-shaped incision enables enlargement to facilitate exposure of a lymphatic and cannulation.

two or more main cords (Fig. 2). These are exposed under local anaesthesia. The choice of incision is an individual matter, but Gibson *et al.* (1968) recommend a shallow S-shaped incision running longitudinally. This has the advantage over a straight transverse or longitudinal incision in that it gives broader access and can be readily extended upwards or downwards if the first lymphatic is found unsuitable or is unavoidably damaged. Mahaffy (1965) in carrying out the procedure for diagnostic purposes advised that the lymphatic should not be dissected out entirely because it collapses and is then difficult to cannulate. The experience of others contradicts this view since mobilization enables a clamp to be applied to the proximal end of the exposed portion of lymphatic following which centripetal massage distends the lumen. It can then be supported on a flat surface to facilitate cannulation. Adequate exposure to facilitate manipulation is essential as a precaution against the risk of spillage of the radioactive material with the possible consequence of tissue necrosis. White (1964) used a soft polythene cannula introduced through a hole made in the wall of the lymphatic by a 26 gauge dental needle and rendered rigid by means of a 30 second cold blast of oxygen which dries the tissue. This is particularly applicable to infusions of cytotoxic drugs since the polythene

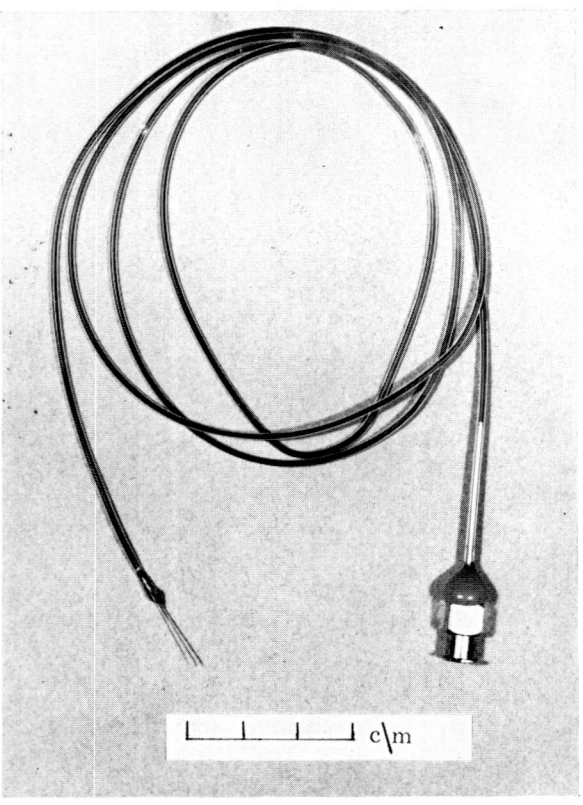

Fig. 11.3. Disposable lymphangiography set.

tube may be left *in situ* for periods of up to 2 weeks thus allowing repeated infusions. An operating microscope can be of great value. *The Lymphography Set.* This consists of a No. 30 S.W.G. needle 30 mm long swaged on to 900 mm of translucent vinyl tubing with a bore of 0·63 mm (Rutt *et al.*, 1964) (Fig. 3). This tubing in turn is swaged on to a No. 14 needle which has had its point ground off and this is fixed to a Luer syringe for radiological lymphography. A strong polypropylene syringe is equally satisfactory (Edwards, 1968; Gibson *et al.*, 1968) and has the advantage of being disposable (Fig. 4).

Rutt *et al.* (1964) primed the lymphography set with radioactive Lipiodol, which has the disadvantage that radioactive material may be liberated into the tissues if cannulation has not been satisfactory. Gibson *et al.* (1968) originally injected 0·2 ml of non-radioactive Ultra-fluid Lipiodol so that an X-ray picture of the lower part of the limb could be taken to confirm the success of cannulation. This had the obvious disadvantage that the material which first came into contact with any malignant cells had no therapeutic value and might have

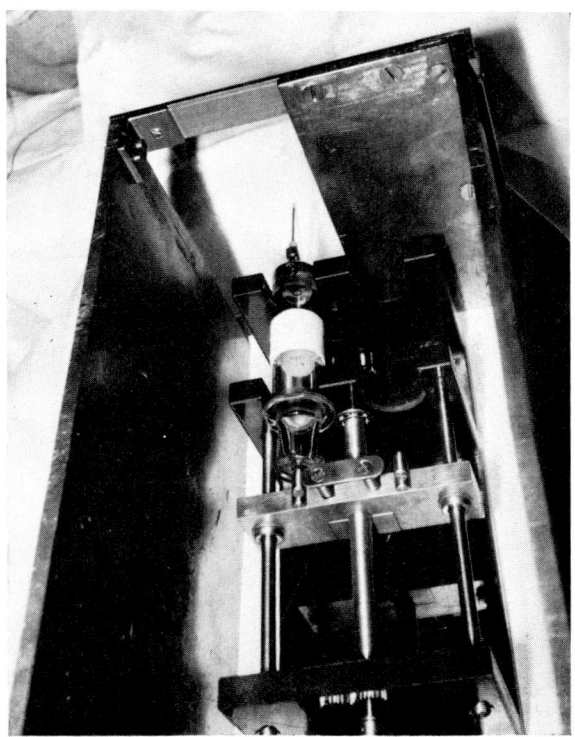

FIG. 11.4. Syringe mounted in an electrically driven pump surrounded by protective lead shield.

328   GERALD E. FLATMAN

displaced such cells into situations which the subsequent [131]I Lipiodol did not reach. Subsequent experience has shown that saline is adequate as a priming solution. If the lymphatic has been successfully cannulated there is no leakage, and the saline can be visualized running along the lymphatic by any of the bubbles which are invariably present. The saline-containing syringe is then replaced with another containing the infusion. This latter has previously been prepared and loaded by a member of the physics staff and stored in readiness within easy reach but behind a lead safety shield. When required it is transported to the operating table by long handled tongs.

The syringe is placed in, and the infusion given, by means of an electrically driven injector (Fig. 4) surrounded by a casing of 1 cm lead. The rate of injection varies. Gibson *et al.* (1968) use a standard rate of 0·2 ml per minute, and Edwards *et al.* (1968) inject, slowly initially, 0·1 ml per minute in order to avoid extravasation around the nodes, but the last 0·5 ml is injected rapidly in order to achieve extravasation from the afferent lymphatics and thereby produce a perilymphatic dose.

Radiography. As soon as the radio-opaque radioactive material is

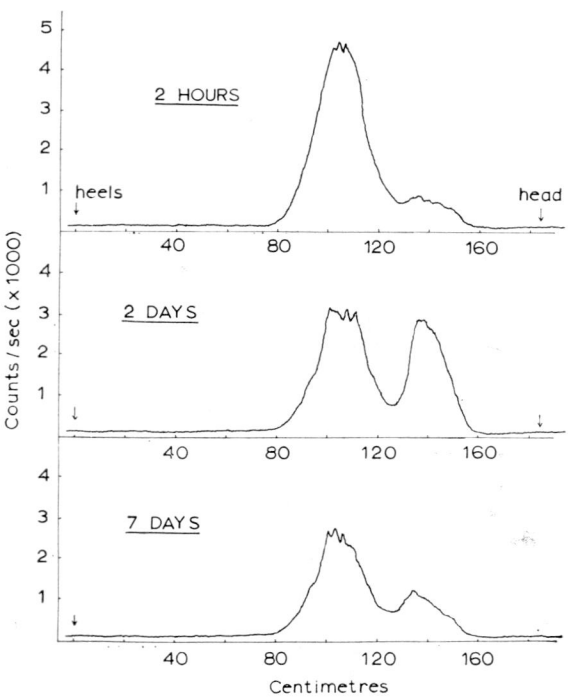

FIG. 11.5. Profile scans showing peak uptake in lungs 2 days after endolymphatic perfusion of the foot with ^{131}I-Lipiodol.

flowing satisfactorily into the lymphatic, a radiograph of the appropriate portion of the limb is taken to confirm satisfactory cannulation.

Monitoring. Edwards *et al.* (1968) monitor the course of the infusion using two collimated Geiger counters, one of which is fixed over the regional node area being treated, and the other being mobile and tracing the course of the isotope along the limb. This second counter is also used to scan the lung fields.

In the event of early high readings due to unsatisfactory cannulation, inadvertent venous injection, or possible lymphovenous connections in involved nodes, the infusion can be stopped. In the experience of the author, however, immediate scanning of the lungs is of little value since the lung dose did not reach its peak until 2 days after injection (Fig. 5).

Gibson *et al.* (1968) defer scanning until immediately after the wound has been closed. Scanning includes a count over the site of the injection, along the lymphatics of the limb, the major lymph node sites, the lungs and the thyroid gland. Scanning is repeated in 24 and 48 hours and a full set of diagnostic films are taken at 24 hours (Fig. 6). Blood and urine samples are counted daily until the patient is discharged and leucocyte and platelet counts are made at intervals for 6 months.

Radiation protection. Precautions are taken in accordance with those adopted at all times when radioactive materials are in use.

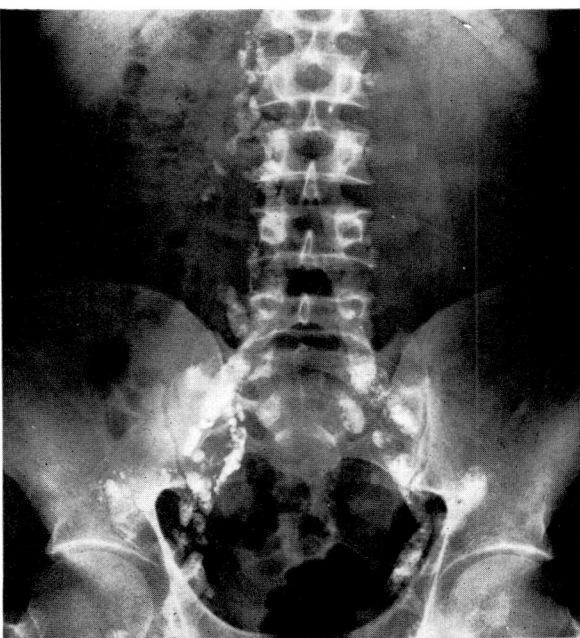

FIG. 11.6. 24-hour film of patient suffering from Hodgkin's disease.

All staff are badge monitored. The syringe, preferably disposable, is loaded with the radioactive liquid remotely and behind lead screens by the physics staff. It is brought to the operating table only at the time required for the infusion to commence, being handled with long handled tongs and carried in a lead container. During the infusion the syringe and the injection pump are surrounded by a thick lead screen (Fig. 3). All materials such as towels, swabs and gloves are monitored for contamination in the usual way and all contaminated items stored in appropriate containers until their radioactivity has fallen low enough to permit disposal. Whilst it is not necessary for the patient to be nursed in a single ward he or she may remain radioactively 'hot' for up to 7 days, and consequently must be nursed in approved premises with facilities for monitoring clothing and excreta and for disposal of radioactive waste.

RADIOACTIVE MATERIALS USED FOR ENDOLYMPHATIC RADIOTHERAPY

Jantet (1958) first used a colloidal solution of radioactive gold of particle size 6 mμ injecting between 50 and 80 mCi into the foot lymphatics. He subsequently changed to a solution of particle size 30 mμ which caused less overflow into the liver and confined the activity to the course of the injected lymphatic trunk and to the regional lymph nodes (Figs. 7 and 8). Seitzmann et al. (1963), on the other hand, having initially used radioactive colloidal gold, discarded it because they considered its diffusion out of the lymphatics into the soft tissues to be too rapid.

The advantages of visualizing the lymphatic system as well as the applications of radiotherapy were soon appreciated. Lipiodol was the ideal opaque medium and the criteria laid down by Seitzmann et al. (1963) for the ideal isotope and its carrier in combination were:

1. Homogeneity in ultra-fluid lipiodol (ethiodol).
2. Confinement to the lymphatic system.
3. Uniform distribution within the lymph nodes.
4. Primary beta emission.
5. Innocuous degradation products.

[131]I-Lipiodol fulfils the requirements since it remains within the lymphatic system and there is no significant uptake by liver, spleen, kidneys or thyroid. More recently ^{32}P-Lipiodol, with its more penetrating beta radiation, has been used by Edwards et al. (1968). Ariel (1964) reported the use of ceramic microspheres 1–4 μ in diameter coated with yttrium-90, and Edwards (1969) ion exchange resin particles with adherent

yttrium-90. Nevertheless oil media have the advantage that they are retained in the lymph nodes for a much longer time than are water media. Animal experiments have shown this not to be harmful and consequently the use of oil media proves to be a safe method of obtaining fuller information about lymph channels and nodes over a period of time.

RELATIVE EFFICIENCY OF ^{131}I AND ^{32}P

Lord and Kinmonth (1968) compared the effect of ^{131}I and ^{32}P labelled lipids on rabbit lymph nodes containing VX_2 tumours. In a controlled series the ^{32}P treated group survived significantly longer than the ^{131}I group. The effects on the iliac lymph nodes showed the ^{32}P to be marginally superior to ^{131}I though not statistically significant. Survival time was considered to be a more sensitive index of superiority than histological comparisons.

The radiation characteristics of the two isotopes are shown in the following table:

Emission	^{32}P Beta only	^{131}I Beta particles and gamma rays
Beta energy (meV)		
Maximum	1·7	0·61
Mean	0·68	0·187
Beta range (mm)		
Maximum	8	2
Mean	1·8	0·4
Half-life (days)	14·3	8·0
K beta factor		
(rad/μCi/gm)	730	110

Experimenting with the same tumour Edwards et al. (1966) had shown, by microscopy and by survival times, that ^{131}I Lipiodol was effective in treating nodes involved with microscopic metastases. The concentration of the Lipiodol was maximum in the lymph nodes and next highest in the lungs. However, by judicious control of the volume infused, spillover to the lungs could be kept to a minimum. Both in the experimental animal and in the human, rapid elimination from the lungs takes place (Gibson et al. 1968).

DISEASES SUITABLE FOR TREATMENT BY ENDOLYMPHATIC RADIOTHERAPY

Liebner (1965) pointed out that for endolymphatic radiotherapy (therapeutic lymphography) to be of significant help the primary growth must metastasize in such a manner that intralymphatic injections can follow the possible spread of neoplastic cells. The response will depend upon the histology and consequently the radiosensitivity, as well as on the energy of the radiation and the density of the tumour.

TESTICULAR TUMOURS

Liebner's requirements are fulfilled by testicular tumours, and using ^{131}I-Lipiodol Seitzmann et al. (1963) reported on endolymphatic radiotherapy through the feet as an adjunct to surgical treatment, since diagnostic lymphography has demonstrated the difficulty of removing all retroperitoneal tissues. He did not at the same time, however, acknowledge the accomplishments of external irradiation in these conditions. Naulleau (1966) and Chiappa et al. (1966) used similar material and techniques for post-operative irradiation of the ilo-inguinal and paraortic lymph nodes following epididymo-orchidectomy for seminoma and teratoma. Chiappa makes the point that where the nodes appear to be inadequately filled, supplementary external radiotherapy should be given by means of a supervoltage technique to a tumour dose of 2,000 to 3,000 rads in 2 to 4 weeks. Seitzmann had shown that where lymph node material was obtained for subsequent histological study the effect varied from none to complete destruction of tissue.

MALIGNANT LYMPHOMA

Jantet (1957) first treated abdominal lymphosarcoma and follicular lymphoma by endolymphatic radiotherapy using radioactive colloidal gold. Other workers including Unslenght (1965, 1968), Romieu et al. (1966), Bennadonna et al. (1968), Chiappa et al. (1966) and Coeur et al. (1969) have treated both these conditions and also Hodgkin's Disease. Chiappa et al. (1964) gave unilateral foot endolymphatic radiotherapy to a series of patients suffering from lymphosarcoma and receiving systemic cytotoxic chemotherapy. They compared the response of involved paraortic lymph nodes on the side receiving irradiation with the side under the influence of the cytotoxic drug alone. A more rapid and more lasting effect was produced by the combined therapy and in no case did the association of these two forms of treatment prejudice other forms of treatment.

Bennadonna *et al.* (1968) reviewed a series of 285 patients suffering from malignant lymphomata of whom 143 had Hodgkin's disease. 10 cc ^{131}I-Lipiodol (0·2–2·5 mCi/ml) was injected into each foot and in some cases this was repeated later. They found that the destruction of lymphomatous material was often incomplete because the ^{131}I was not adequately distributed throughout the lymph nodes. At the same time recurrences were seen most often in adequately filled nodes. In these cases external radiotherapy was indicated.

Seventeen patients suffering from chronic lymphatic leukaemia and having ilo-inguinal and retroperitoneal adenopathy were treated with [131]I Lipiodol by Chiappa (1966). He reported a good response in all cases but recommended that the endolymphatic radiotherapy should be combined with alkylating agents when attempting to control 'aggressive varieties' of the disease. It is not recommended for the asymptomatic form of the disease.

FEMALE GENITAL NEOPLASMS

Vecchietti (1967) reported the treatment of 200 patients suffering from carcinomas of the corpus and cervix uteri, vagina and vulva using ^{131}I-Lipiodol and ^{32}P-Lipiodol. He pointed out that the greater penetrating power of the ^{32}P beta radiation leads to rapid and massive histological damage in involved lymph nodes. Only 5% of the total dose of ^{32}P is excreted in the first 5 days compared with 40% in the case of [131]I. Vecchietti concludes that the method is especially valuable when combined with surgery.

BLADDER NEOPLASMS

Chiappa *et al.* (1966) used ^{131}I-Lipiodol in an attempt to control lymph node involvement from carcinoma of the bladder, but reported it to be of doubtful value.

MALIGNANT MELANOMA

In Britain much of the investigative work into the value of endolymphatic radiotherapy has been applied to the field of malignant melanoma, led by Kinmonth and his co-workers, and a number of centres are co-operating with an M.R.C. working party with a view to ultimate assessment of the long term results.

The treatment of malignant melanoma in which there are no palpable regional lymph nodes, is still controversial. Fortner *et al* (1964) carried out routine prophylactic block dissection of regional nodes after excision and grafting of the primary tumour. They found that 38% of regional nodes were in fact infiltrated with tumour although this was not detectable clinically. Routine prophylactic dissection of regional lymph nodes is frequently complicated by delayed healing and sometimes by sepsis. Scarring frequently leads to oedema and this may discourage some surgeons from carrying out the procedure.

Endolymphatic radiotherapy offers an alternative in that, whereas microscopic metastases in nodes may be destroyed, subsequent block dissection for residual disease is still possible, and where there are no metastases present there are no adverse effects upon the patient. There is also the great advantage that the lymphatics between the primary site and the regional nodes also receive irradiation.

Jantet (1964) reported the treatment of 13 patients suffering from malignant melanoma with radioactive gold. The basic technique has been described above and the volume of colloidal gold solution used varied from 0·25 ml to 2·8 ml. The injection was given over an approximate period of 5 minutes, but in some of the later cases the latter half of the volume was given as rapidly as possible in order to produce more extravasation through the walls of the lymph trunks.

Lymph nodes excised from two patients enabled direct calculations to be made and showed a dose range from 26,500 to 35,000 rads in nodes of the groin from a full dose of 59·4 mCi. Ten of these 13 patients, all with Stage I disease, were alive 5–9 years after treatment.

Edwards et al. (1968) and Gibson et al. (1968) reported the use of ^{131}I-Lipiodol for the treatment of malignant melanoma, both as a prophylactic treatment in Stage I, and as an adjuvant to surgery in Stage II. Both groups of workers have used the same techniques. They aim to give a dose of 40–45 mCi in 4 ml for the lower limb, and 35 mCi in 2 ml for the upper limb. Occasionally these dosages have been given to both limbs and on one occasion Edwards et al. infused all four limbs in a patient who had had a melanoma on the back. This is the sum total of treatment carried out 3 weeks after excision and grafting of a Stage I tumour. Where nodes subsequently become involved, or when treating a Stage II tumour, block dissection of the regional lymph nodes is carried out 4 weeks after infusion.

Edwards et al. (1968) reviewed a series of 50 patients, 31 with Stage I disease and 19 with Stage II disease, treated from one and a half to four years previously, and attempted a comparison of results with another group of patients treated entirely by surgery by another surgical team in the same hospital. The 'surgery alone' group consisted of 52 patients of whom 24 survived 3 years (46%), and of the 50 'surgery and [131]I' group, 39 survived one and a half to four years (78%). Survival figures for the stages are Stage I, 55% and 93%; and Stage II, 10% and 52·6%. However, Edwards agrees that the groups are dissimilar in several ways and a true assessment of the value of the method cannot be made until the working party of the Medical Research Council reports on its nationwide controlled trial in several years' time.

Gibson *et al.* (1968) in a report on early experiences with 17 patients stated that 5 out of 11 remained clinically free from disease for periods ranging from 9 to 20 months.

Ariel *et al.* (1967) reported that 6 patients remained well and free from evidence of melanoma for periods ranging from 12 to 53 months after endolymphatic infusion of ^{131}I and ^{198}Au. They also reported the use of ceramic microspheres of diameter 1–4μ coated with yttrium-90 in 7 patients with malignant melanoma.

DOSAGE DISTRIBUTION

Radioactive colloidal gold (^{198}Au) has a relatively short half life of 2·7 days. Whilst it emits beta and gamma rays, 95% of its activity is due to the beta radiation and the contribution from gamma radiation can be ignored. The maximum beta particle range is about 5 mm. Jantet (1962) carried out total body scanning following direct intralymphatic injection of colloidal gold in one foot, carrying out surface counts and drawing up contour lines (Figs. 7 and 8).

Hine and Brownell (1956) and Brownell (1961) have shown in animal experiments that after injecting amounts of 63 μCi to 250 μCi, quantities of from 4·2 μCi to 85 μCi were present in the popliteal nodes giving doses of 5,600 to 67,000 rads. The iliac nodes contained from 2·2 μCi to 32 μCi giving a proportionally lower dosage. It was noted by them that to increase the proportion of the administered dose in the nodes it was necessary to keep the total volume small and to inject it slowly.

Jantet (1962) excised nodes from the inguinal region after giving a small test dose of 1·41 mCi radioactive colloidal gold into the foot, and was able to measure the dose in two nodes as 6,000 and 7,200 rads respectively. In another patient given a full dose of 59·4 mCi he calculated doses of 35,000 rads and 26,500 rads in nodes in the right and left groins respectively. With experience the dose level aimed at has been gradually raised to 70,000 rads, requiring a dose of 70 mCi ^{198}Au.

Radioactive Iodine-131 has a half life of 8 days and emits gamma rays as well as beta particles of maximum range of 2 mm. Gibson *et al.* (1968) assessed node volumes from stereoscopic radiographs and shift films, from which they calculated an activity ranging from 500 to 1,000 microcuries per gram, giving a mean dose of 50,000 to 100,000 rads. The half life in the nodes as measured with the scanner was found to be 7·5 days. This compares with the 6 days calculated by Seitzmann *et al.* (1963), who used the following formula to calculate dosage to individual nodes removed:

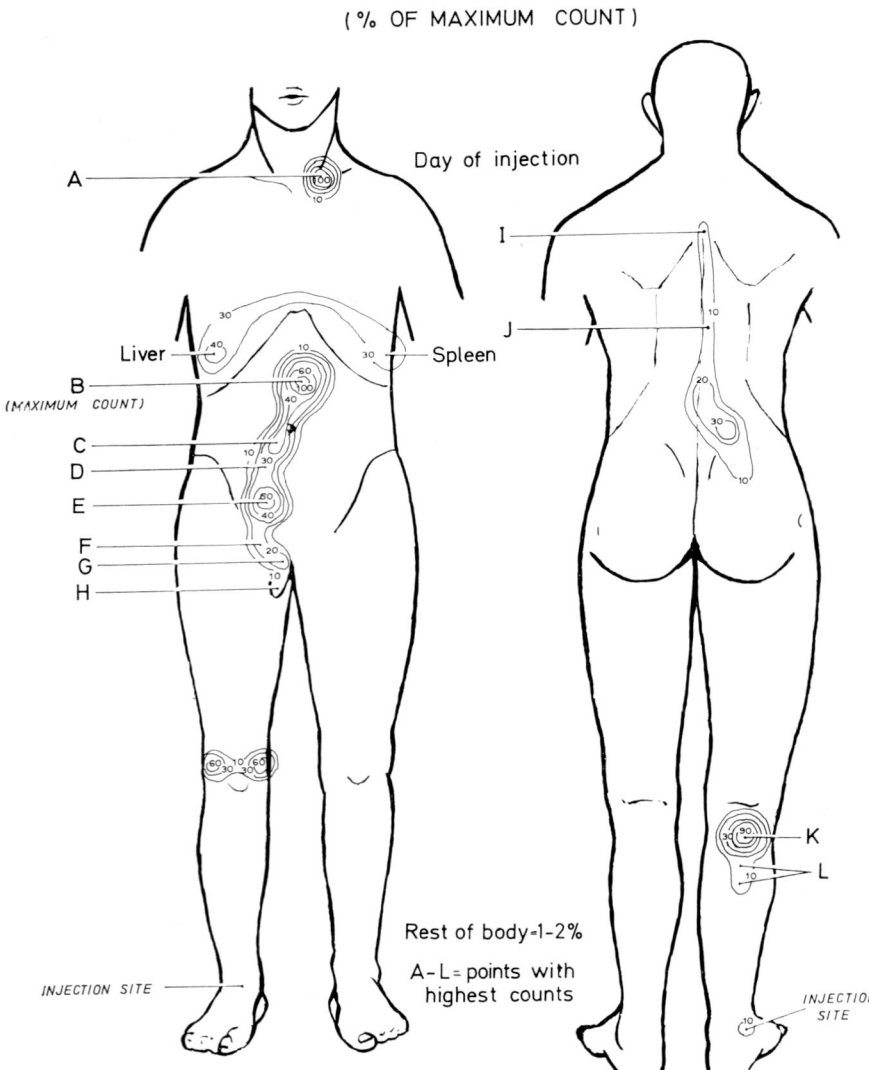

FIG. 11.7. Contour lines drawn after total body scanning following direct intralymphatic injections of colloidal [198]Au in the foot. The count at point A
is 60% of the maximum count. (By courtesy of Mr. G. H. Jantet and the
Editor, *British Journal of Radiology*.)

SURFACE COUNTS

(Counts/second corrected for background)

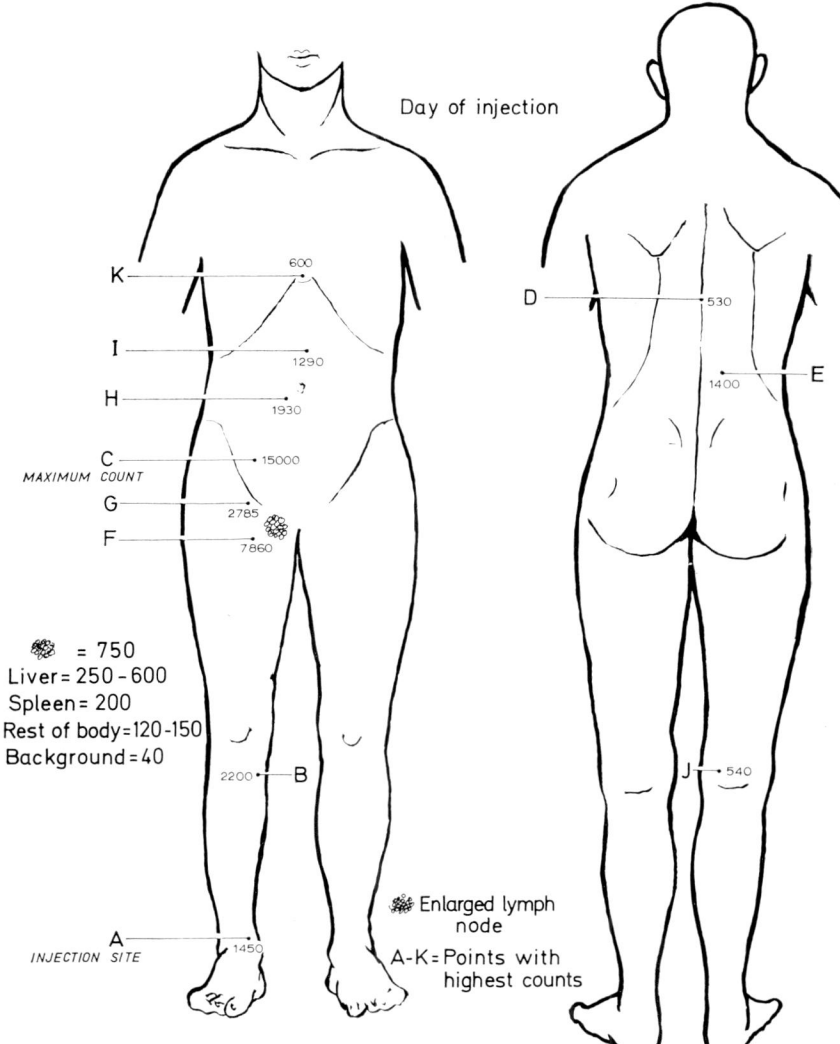

Day of injection

K — 600
I — 1290
H — 1930 ?
C — 15000
MAXIMUM COUNT
G — 2785
F — 7860

= 750
Liver = 250 - 600
Spleen = 200
Rest of body = 120-150
Background = 40

B — 2200

A — 1450
INJECTION SITE

D — 530
E — 1400
J — 540

Enlarged lymph node
A-K = Points with highest counts

FIG. 11.8. Surface counts obtained after total-body scanning following direct intralymphatic injection of colloidal [198]Au in the right foot. (By courtesy of Mr. G. H. Jantet and the Editor, *British Journal of Radiology*.)

Dose (in beta rads to total decay *in vivo*) = 73·8 × concentration in μCi/Gram × 0·187 (E_β for ^{131}I) × T_{eff}. (effective half life).

The formula makes no allowance for possible inhomogeneity of the distribution of the isotope within the node. Since the isotopes currently in use emit radiations of very limited penetrating power, the dose distribution within a node will cover only a few cells or clones in thickness. Thus a small tumour deposit may be effectively irradiated whilst the inadequate penetration of a larger deposit may render the method completely ineffective.

The levels of both Lipiodol and ^{131}I in blood and urine are measured daily following the infusion until the patient is discharged from hospital. This is usually at the end of a week, when the total body radioactivity has fallen below 30 millicuries, and in accordance with the standards laid down by the Code of Practice patients may travel by private transport. Gibson *et al.* (1968) carried out measurements for a longer period of time and recorded their findings graphically. Fig. 9 represents both the percentage of the total injected radioactivity excreted daily in the urine (scale on the left), and the percentage of the total injected radioactivity circulating in the blood (scale on the right). The same curve represents both because within the accuracy of measurements, the urine concentration follows that of the blood, but at a higher level. The upper curve shows the percentage of the total injected Lipiodol. This curve is obtained from the lower one by making allowance for the radioactive decay of the ^{131}I. Peak activity in the blood and urine is at

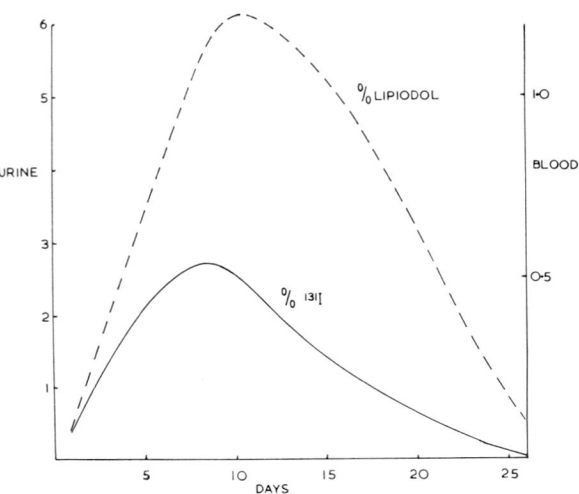

FIG. 11.9. Post-operative levels of Lipiodol and ^{131}I in blood and urine.

8 days, but Seitzmann *et al.* (1963) found this to be variable between 2 and 6 days, and at the same time estimated the effective half life of the ^{131}I to be 6 days.

COMPLICATIONS

Jackson (1966) listed the sequelae of diagnostic lymphography in women with pelvic malignancies:

1. Elevation of pulse rate or temperature after 24–72 hours.
2. Shivering attacks.
3. Aches and pains.
4. Nausea and vomiting.
5. Delayed healing or infection of wound in foot.
6. Oedema of the ankle or even of the whole limb.
7. Deep venous thrombosis.
8. Cough.
9. Blood in sputum.

These occurred in patients who had received perfusions of up to 16 ml of Lipiodol delivered at the rate of 1 ml in 10 minutes, and the total time taken for bilateral lymphography was 3–4 hours. Jackson refers to 4 deaths recorded in the literature by 4 separate groups of workers and attributed to oil embolism. He concludes that lymphography must be considered to be potentially a dangerous procedure, but goes on to suggest that if proper precautions are taken no serious complications should develop.

An additional complication seen by the author on two occasions is that of an allergic reaction to the Patent Blue dye, giving rise to oedema of the foot in one case and of the whole leg in another. The perfusion was not commenced.

Complications of endolymphatic radiotherapy are potentially the same as those due to the diagnostic procedure (although the volumes used are much smaller than those quoted by Jackson), but in addition there are those inherent in the use of radioactive materials.

RADIATION HAZARDS

The risk of radiation damage to tissues other than the lymph nodes under treatment may occur either from spillage of the ^{131}I-Lipiodol into the blood stream, via the thoracic duct or by abnormal lympho-venous communications (Edwards and Kinmonth, 1969), or by leakage into the tissues through a ruptured or open lymphatic. The damage is thus most likely to affect the blood forming cells, the lungs, the thyroid gland or the subcutaneous tissues.

EFFECT ON HAEMOPOIETIC SYSTEM

Yoffey and Courtice (1956) studied the effect on the bone marrow of animals, of the irradiation of lymphatic tissues including the effect of internally deposited radio-isotopes. Although they failed to find primary stimulation of haematopoiesis there were compensatory increases in certain of the cellular constituents of the peripheral blood invariably preceded by a reduction for varying periods. Warren *et al.* (1950) had earlier observed a preliminary depression, followed by hyperplasia of lymphoid and myeloid tissues, in mice treated with a minimal dose of radioactive phosphorus.

Edwards *et al.* (1967) in the course of their clinical studies of endolymphatic radiotherapy, noted that a selective lymphopenia was likely to occur in patients, particularly after single lower limb infusions. They pointed out the large volume of lymphatic tissue irradiated in what might be regarded as a 'hind quarter volume' plus para-aortic nodes. The lymphopenia lasted for periods up to 5 months in some patients and the possible value of endolymphatic infusion of radioactive substances as a method of immuno-suppression in relation to tissue transplantation was postulated.

Jantet (1962) quoted the case of a patient who developed a temporary aplastic anaemia lasting 3 weeks and from which she recovered, following the injection of 51 mCi ^{198}Au solution for malignant melanoma in the calf. She had previously received radiotherapy for nasopharyngeal lymphosarcoma.

Gibson *et al.* (1968) reported only one patient who developed any significant degree of leucopenia. The white blood cell count fell to 2,400 and the platelet count to 80,000 per cu mm 3 weeks after the injection of 45 mCi ^{131}I-Lipiodol into the foot. There was a spontaneous return to normal within a month.

LUNGS

Lahneche *et al.* (1967) calculated that frequently 33% or more of ^{131}I was taken up by the lungs. Gough *et al.* (1964) in a series of 40 patients found that none developed pulmonary symptoms. Gibson *et al.* (1968) reported that lung scans showed a variable uptake with an effective half life of 4 days. In all cases the total activity in the right lung was higher than the left, irrespective of the foot injected and the activity was distributed in a patchy or blotchy manner, the regions of higher activity being 1–2 cm apart (Fig. 10). About 50% of the radioactive Lipiodol appeared in the lungs of one patient giving a beta dose of over 1,000 rads and a total beta and gamma dose of 1,500 rads. This patient had, however, a previous block dissection of the groin and

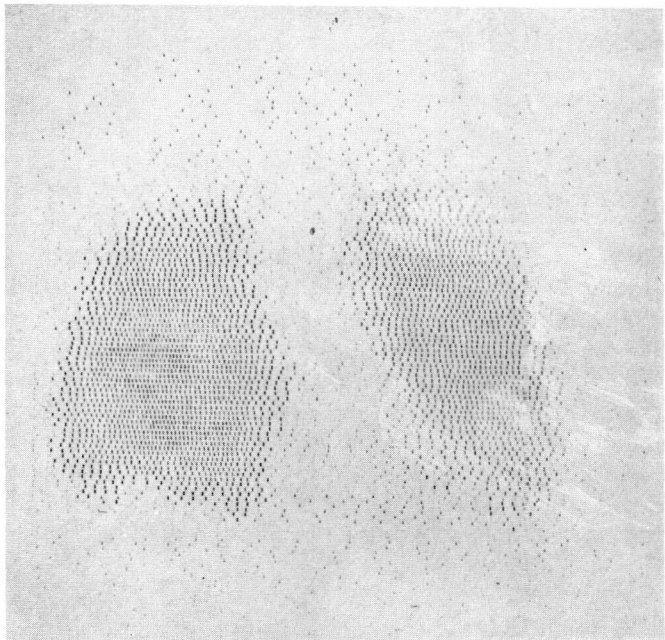

FIG. 11.10. Scanning 3 days post-operatively illustrates the relatively high concentration of the isotope in the lungs; in all cases it has been greater on the right.

may have had abnormal lymphatic connections. Other patients received mean beta doses of between 100 and 900 rads and in all cases the gamma doses to the lungs amounted to about 50% of the beta dose. The radioactivity in the lungs of all patients in which this was closely followed, including the patient with the highest lung dose, did not reach its peak until 1–2 days after the injection as shown by the profile scan (Fig. 4). This suggests that most of the Lipiodol reaching the lungs does so by normal lymphatic channels and not by abnormal lympho-venous connections. The routine scanning of the lungs during infusion carried out by Edwards *et al.* (1968) would therefore not pick up the highest dose in the routine case.

Koehler *et al.* (1968) showed experimentally in dogs that excess radioactive medium can be prevented from spilling over into the lungs by thoracic duct cannulation to remove excess oil. Liebner *et al.* (1965) argued that most workers using Lipiodol give a larger volume for injection than is necessary, resulting in frequent spillage into the venous system with an increase in dosage to lungs and thyroid. Nevertheless no serious symptoms referable to lung damage due either to the oil or to the associated radioactive material have been reported. Seitzmann *et al.*

(1963) had carried out autopsies on some patients, but found no significant radioactivity in the lungs which adds weight to the subsequent experience of other workers that there is no serious hazard to the patient's lungs.

THYROID

Before endolymphatic radiotherapy with ^{131}I-Lipiodol, all patients are given Lugol's iodine 5 mg t.i.d. orally. This limits the uptake of ^{131}I by the thyroid gland and no case of hypothyroidism has been reported as a consequence of the procedure. Gibson *et al.* (1968) reported two patients in whom scans showed some uptake. In one, Virchow's node showed clearly in a radiograph and scan (Fig. 11a and 11b) 4 hours after injection but had disappeared by the next day. Moderate activity appeared in the thyroid 3 weeks later. In another patient Virchow's node was active for 2 days after injection, but 4 days later activity had cleared from the node and had appeared in the thyroid.

SUBCUTANEOUS LEAKAGE

This can occur under any of three circumstances:

1. At the site of injection, resulting from faulty technique.
2. From open ended lymphatics, at the site of a skin graft.
3. From open ended lymphatics within a lymphoedematous limb.

In the event of extravasation of radioactive material around the cannula the infusion must be stopped, the lymphatic tied, and the wound washed out with saline before closing. Where the dye shows the presence of open ended lymphatics (Fig. 12) no attempt should be made to proceed with the infusion from a point distal to that site, though it may still be possible to cannulate a lymphatic proximal to the affected area. It appears that open ended lymphatics persist for a short time under a skin graft and leakage is to be expected if the cannulated site is distal to the graft, and the lymphatics run near to it. Similar open ended lymphatics were seen in a lymphoedematous arm (Fig. 13) and would certainly have resulted in leakage if the infusion had been given.

Jantet (1962) had one case of radionecrosis of skin measuring 2·5 cm diameter which followed leakage of ^{198}Au. This was successfully excised and grafted. Gibson *et al.* (1968) had the same experience in two patients after leakage of ^{131}I. In one, excision and grafting was successful, but the second patient died before surgery became possible.

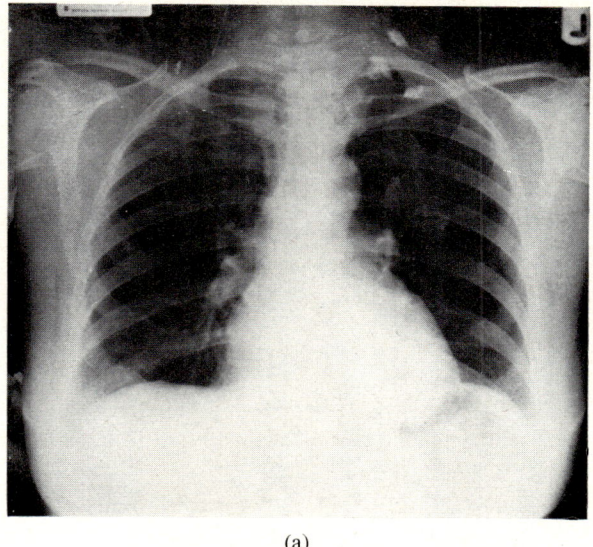

(a)

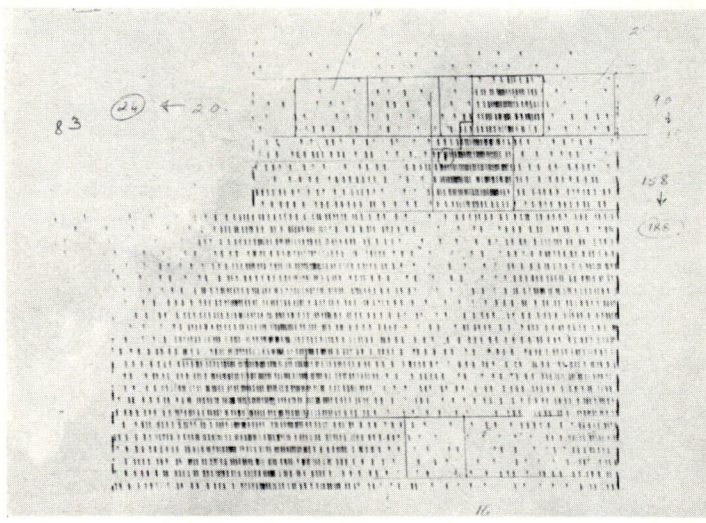

(b)

FIG. 11.11. (a) Radiograph and (b) scintiscan 4 hours after perfusion of foot lymphatic with ^{131}I-Lipiodol. Note the high level of dosage in the left supra-clavicular nodes.

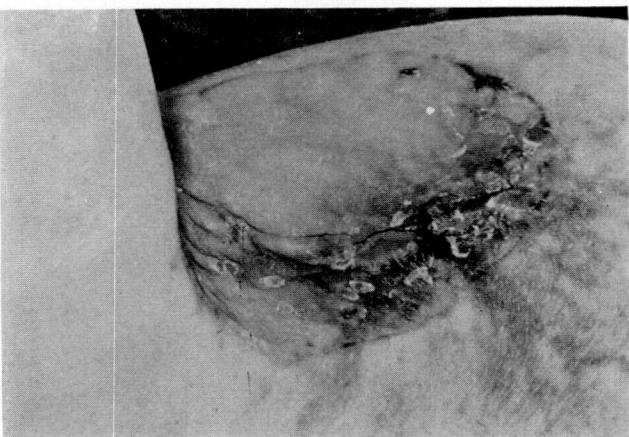

FIG. 11.12. Skin graft applied to back of knee in which Patent Blue dye is diffusing through open-ended lymphatics.

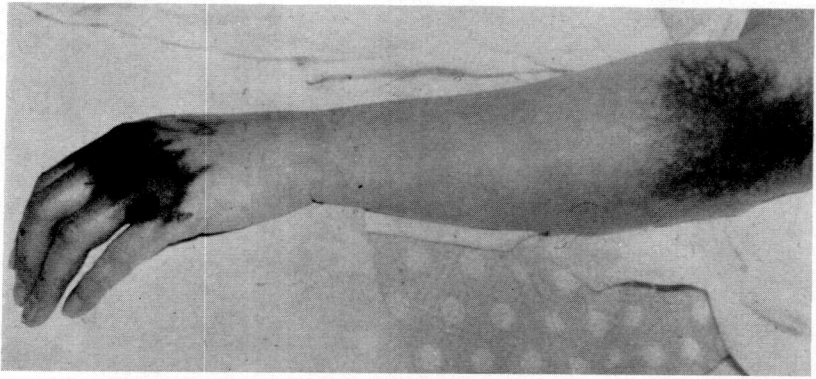

FIG. 11.13. This patient had a recent block dissection of her axilla resulting in a mild degree of lymphoedema of the forearm. Dye has leaked from apparently open-ended lymphatics near the elbow and three smaller areas on the upper arm were noted. The demonstration of open-ended lymphatics is an absolute contraindication to infusion unless a lymphatic can be cannulated proximal to the graft.

LYMPHOEDEMA

A mild degree of oedema of the ankle or forearm is common following perfusion. Its duration and severity can be minimized by applying a crêpe bandage to the ankle or wrist on top of the wound dressing. This should be applied on the operating table, and when the patient returns to the ward the limb should be kept horizontal for 48 hours postoperatively. The majority of patients are free from oedema within two or three months.

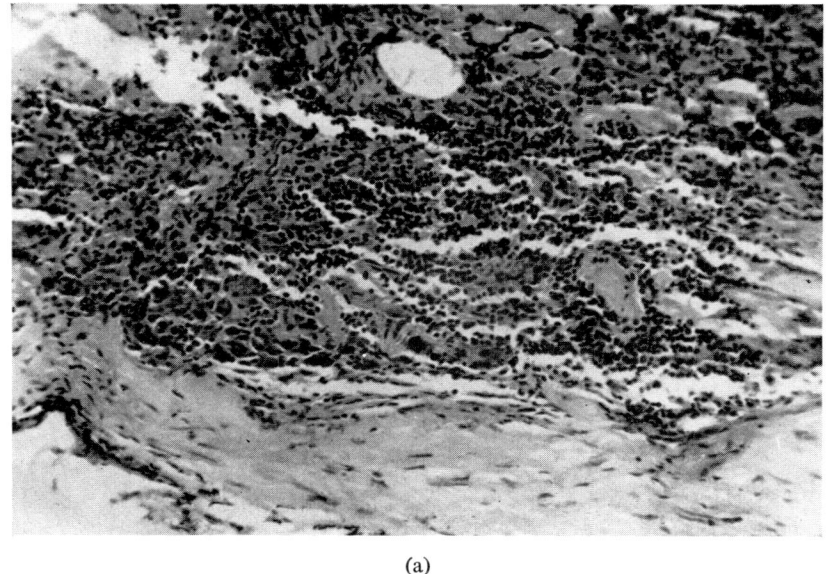

(a)

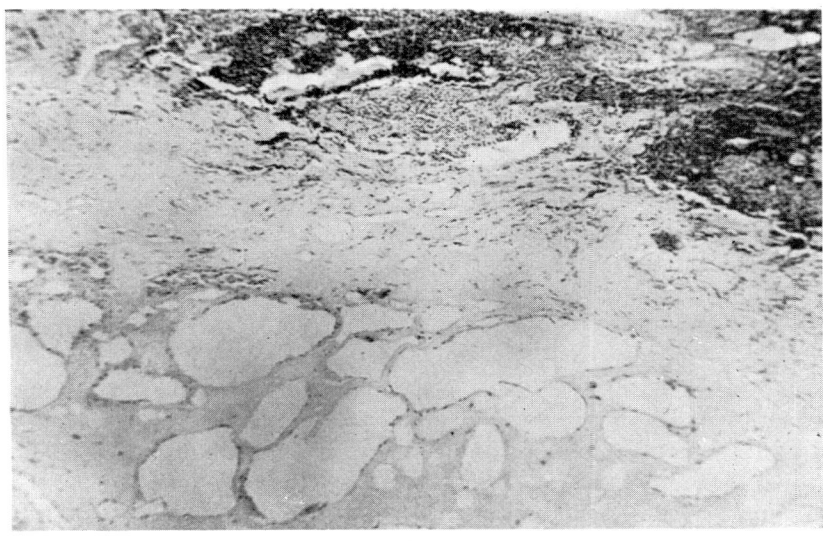

(b)

FIG. 11.14. (a) Section of node prior to perfusion. (b) Section of node removed 1 month after perfusion with ^{131}I-Lipiodol and showing central necrosis with a few possibly viable cells remaining at the periphery.

12*

HISTOLOGICAL CHANGES IN LYMPH NODES
RESULTING FROM RADIOACTIVE PERFUSION

Lord et al. (1969) described experiments in rabbits with VX_2 tumour metastasis in lymph nodes. After infusion with ^{32}P or ^{131}I the rabbits were killed 1–250 days later, and histological examination showed that there was rapid necrosis of all cells within the physical range of the isotope. After cellular debris had been removed there remained a fibrous framework of the node. Progressive fibrosis followed, eventually leading to the formation of a contracted sclerotic massun recognizable as a normal node. No specific effects of radiation were found in other organs.

Seitzmann et al. (1963) studied the response of lymph nodes to ^{131}I-Lipiodol, and reported that the histology varied from no response to complete destruction.

In a patient studied by the author, in whom block dissection of inguinal nodes was carried out one month after ^{131}I-Lipiodol perfusion for Stage II malignant melanoma of leg, the histology of a node showed major destruction of the normal architecture, though there remained some doubt about the viability of a few remaining pigmented cells at the region of the sinus (Figs. 14a and 14b).

Vecchietti (1967) considered ^{32}P to produce a more rapid and thorough histological destruction of lymph nodes than ^{131}I.

CONCLUSIONS

Endolymphatic radiotherapy is based upon two sound principles; first that the cure rate is likely to be higher if the volume irradiated is limited to that involved by the disease, and secondly that the anatomy of the lymphatic system is such that perfusion will reach those tissues along which certain tumour types are known to spread. In less than two decades lymphography has become commonplace and there are obvious advantages in being able to visualize the extent and volume of tissue irradiated.

Doubtless other materials will become available in the future, but to date those exploited are limited in number. Colloidal gold has been shown to be effective radiotherapeutically, though it has the same disadvantage as radioactive microspheres and resin particles (of ^{131}I-Lipiodol and ^{32}P-Lipiodol) of not being radio-opaque. Whilst the relative merits of ^{198}Au, ^{131}I, and ^{32}P depend partly upon the energy and penetrating power of their radiations, other factors such as the ready diffusibility of radioactive colloidal gold, affecting the volume of perilymphatic tissue irradiated, and the capacity for absorption of the solution by lymph nodes, must be taken into account. Experimental comparison of ^{32}P and ^{131}I in irradiation of tumours in rabbits, has shown ^{32}P to be superior in terms of survival and of histological effect. Clinical experience, however, appears to be greater with ^{131}I, from which the beta radiation has a maximum penetration of 2 mm. With this isotope doses of up to 100,000 rads have been reported with apparently no detrimental effect to the patient. Similar dosage from ^{32}P with a maximum beta range of 8 mm might, however, produce severe localized nerve damage if a concentration of the isotope should chance to lie in a node adjacent to a nerve trunk in the abdomen or pelvis.

The types of malignant disease treated by this method are either those peculiar to the lymphatic system such as lymphosarcoma, or those known to spread predominantly via the lymphatics such as testicular tumours and malignant melanoma. Lymphosarcoma is an example in which the method is used for active treatment, possibly combined with external irradiation and cytotoxic drugs. Testicular tumours and malignant melanoma of the skin present circumstances under which both active and prophylactic treatment may be given, and in malignant melanoma the surgeon may be enabled to spare a proportion of patients the operation of block dissection, which has a high morbidity rate.

Already a claim has been made for an improved survival rate in the treatment of malignant melanoma, but care must be taken to ensure that the use of endolymphatic radiotherapy as adjuvant treatment is not less effective than established methods, such as the routine post operative irradiation of abdominal and pelvic nodes for testicular tumours by megavoltage radiotherapy. However, failure of response to the endolymphatic method does not appear to preclude the subsequent use of external irradiation.

Dosage distribution, measured and calculated by various workers, suggests that more than half the injected radioactivity is concentrated in the perfused lymphatic tissues (Fig. 15), but in some cases a third or more may find its way into the lungs via the normal lymphatic channels. Rapid excretion of the isotope takes place and no lung damage has been reported. No permanent damage to the haemopoietic system has been reported, though a selective lymphopenia lasting up to 5 months has been noted in some patients perfused with ^{131}I.

Effectiveness as measured by histological damage is extremely variable and will depend not only upon the radiosensitivity of the tumour material, but also upon its volume, and upon the distribution of the radioactive material within the node itself.

The complications are theoretically those of diagnostic lymphography, together with others consequent upon the use of radioactive materials. In practice the complications appear to be few, but special

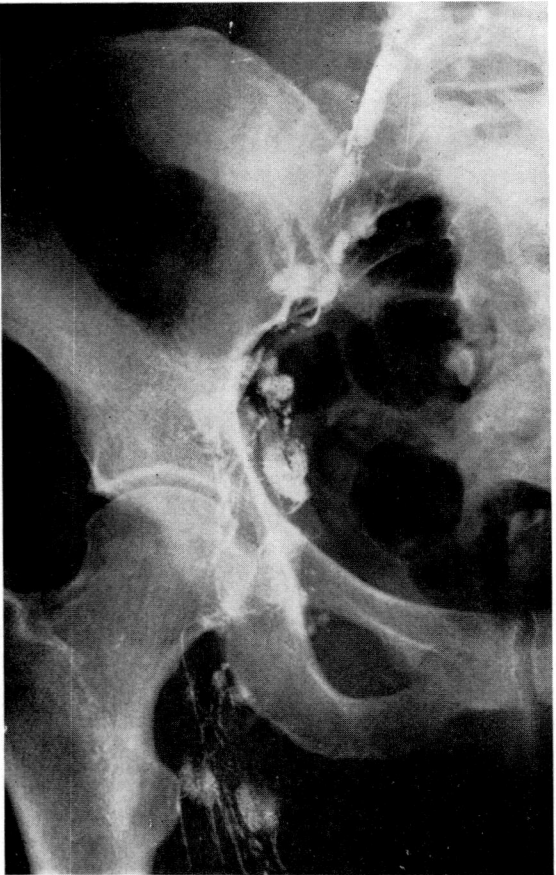

FIG. 11.15. Nodes perfused with ^{131}I-Lipiodol in patient with stage II malignant melanoma of the leg.

mention must be made of the risk of ulceration of the skin if subcutaneous leakage of radioactive isotopes takes place. The initial fear that the application of a high pressure to the perfusate might dislodge and disseminate malignant cells has not been supported by experience.

Monitoring of staff has failed to show any radiation hazard. For the patient it must be admitted that the technique could prove temporarily tedious though, if necessary, this can be overcome by using a general anaesthetic.

The scope of endolymphatic radiotherapy has so far been limited by the accessibility of lymphatics suitable for cannulation, together with the pattern of their distribution relative to the natural spread of the disease under treatment. The greater proportion of work has been done on leg and arm lymphatics, but if the method proves to be superior to other forms of treatment there seems no reason why lymphatics in other parts of the body should not be perfused. A more major surgical approach might be required, but this might well be used to facilitate a major surgical attack supported by active or prophylactic endolymphatic radiotherapy.

It is abundantly clear, however, that the true value and proper place of endolymphatic radiotherapy in the present day management of cancer has yet to be fully assessed.

APPENDIX

^{131}I-Lipiodol and ^{32}P-Lipiodol are obtainable from The Radiochemical Centre, Amersham.

^{131}I-Lipiodol contains 100% ^{131}I, the amount present as labile iodine being $0.1–0.3\%$. It is packed in vials of 45 mCi in 4.5 ml for lower limb infusion and 37.5 mCi in 2.5 ml for brachial infusion.

^{32}P-Lipiodol contains tri-n-octyl phosphate in which the radioactive concentration is not greater than 2 mCi/ml. It is available in bottles containing activities up to 10 mC. 6 mCi of the ^{32}P product is equivalent to 45 mCi of the ^{131}I product.

REFERENCES

ARIEL, I. M., RESNICK, M. I., & GALEY, D. (1964). The intralymphatic administration of radioactive isotopes and cancer chemotherapeutic drugs. *Surgery*, **55**, 353.

ARIEL, I. M., FLYNN, W., & PACK, G. T. (1967). Current possibilities of radioactive ceramic microspheres labelled with yttrium-90. *Minerva med.*, **58**, 4496.

ARIEL, I. M., RESNICK, M. I., & OROPEZA, R. (1967). The intralymphatic administration of radioactive isotopes for treating malignant melanoma. *Surg. Gynec. Obstet.*, **124**, 25.

BLAKE, J. (1968). Difficulty in clinical assessment of lymph nodes after endolymphatic radioiodine. *Postgrad. med. J.*, **44**, 336.

BONADONNA, G., & CHIAPPA, S. (1968). Endolymphatic radiotherapy in malignant lymphomas. A clinical evaluation of 285 patients. *Cancer*, **22**, 885.

CHIAPPA, S., GALLI, G., & PALMIA, C. (1964). Observations on intralymphatic radiotherapy and general chemotherapy. *Clin. Radiol.*, **15**, 202.

CHIAPPA, S., UNSLENGHT, C., & GALLI, G. (1966). Lymphangiography and endolymphatic radiotherapy in testicular tumours. *Br. J. Radiol.*, **39**, 498.

CHIAPPA, S., & UNSLENGHT, C. (1966). Intralymphatic radiotherapy in the treatment of lymph node metastases of carcinoma of the bladder. *Minerva radiol.*, **11**, 686.

CHIAPPA, S., BONADONNA, G., UNSLENGHT, C., MARANO, P., & MOLINARI, R. (1966). The role of endolymphatic radiotherapy in the treatment of chronic lymphatic leukaemia. *Br. J. Cancer*, **20**, 480.

CHIAPPA, S., & VERONESI, U. (1967). Intralymphatic radiotherapy in the treatment of lymph node metastases of the retroperitoneal lymphatic chain. *Minerva med.*, **58**, 4510.

COEUR, P., CHASSARD, J. L., PAPILLON, J., & LAHNECHE, B. (1969). Apropos of regular and radioactive lymphography in chronic lymphocytic leukaemias. *Nouv. Revue Fr. Hémat.*, **9**, 409.

DELLEPIANE, G., & TETTI, A. (1965). Endolymphatic isotope therapy in uterine carcinomas. *Minerva med.*, **56**, 2016.

EDWARDS, J. M., & GIMLETTE, T. M. (1966). Endolymphatic therapy of tumours with particular reference to the VX$_2$ tumour in *Lepus cuniculus*. *Br. J. Surg.*, **53**, 969.

EDWARDS, J. M. (1967). Intralymphatic treatment of lymph node metastases with Lipiodol labelled with ^{131}I with special reference to malignant melanoma. *Minerva med.*, **58**, 4512.

EDWARDS, J. M., LLOYD-DAVIES, R. W., & KINMONTH, J. B. (1967). Selective lymphopenia in man after injection of radioactive I[131]. *Br. med. J.*, **1**, 331.

EDWARDS, J. M., & KINMONTH, J. B. (1968). Endolymphatic radiotherapy for malignant melanoma. *Br. med. J.*, **1**, 18.

EDWARDS, J. M. (1969). Malignant melanoma treatment by endolymphatic radio-isotope infusion. *Ann. R. Coll. Surg.*, **44**, 237.

FISCHER, H. W. (1965). Intralymphatic therapy for lymph node metastases of carcinoma of the cervix. An analysis of the proposition and presentation of pertinent experimental data. *Cancer*, **18**, 1059.

FLATMAN, G. E. (1968). Lymphography and its adaptation for endolymphatic radiotherapy. *Nurs. Times*, **64**, 1400.

GREEN, A. (1959). A technical advance in irradiation technique. *Proc. R. Soc. Med.*, **52**, 344.

GIBSON, T., FLATMAN, G. E., & ORR, J. S. (1968). Endolymphatic infusion of ^{131}I in the treatment of malignant melanoma: early experiences. *Scott. med. J.*, **13**, 226.

GOUGH, M. H., GUINEY, E. J., & KINMONTH, J. B. (1963). Lymphangiography. New techniques and uses. *Br. med. J.*, **i**, 181.

HINE, G. J., & BROWNELL, G. L. (1956). *Radiation Dosimetry*. New York: Academic Press.

JACKSON, R. J. A. (1966). Complications of lymphography. *Br. med. J.*, **i**, 1203.

JANTET, G. H. (1958). 9th Scientific Meeting, Surgical Research Society, London.

JANTET, G. H. (1962). Direct intralymphatic injections of radioactive colloidal gold in the treatment of malignant disease. *Br. J. Radiol.*, **35**, 692.

JANTET, G. H., EDWARDS, J. M., GOUGH, M. H., & KINMONTH, J. B. (1964). Endolymphatic radiotherapy with radioactive gold for malignant melanoma. *Br. med J.*, **i**, 904.

KEY, J. (1968). Perfusion of established melanomata with nitrogen mustard. *Canad. Med. Ass. J.*, **99**, 11.

KINMONTH, J. B. (1952). Lymphangiography in man. Method of outlining lymphatic trunks at operation. *Clin. Sci.*, **11**, 13.

KINMONTH, J. B. (1955). Lymphangiography in clinical surgery and particularly in the treatment of lymphoedema. *Ann. R. Coll. Surg.*, **15**, 300.

KINMONTH, J. B., TAYLOR, G. W., & HARPER, R. K. (1955). Lymphangiography. A technique for its clinical use in the lower limb. *Br. med. J.*, **i**, 940.

KOEHLER, P. R., & POTCHE, E. J. (1968). Experimental studies of intralymphatic administration of radiotherapy with particular emphasis on lymphatic dynamics and lymph node response to lymphography. *Radiology*, **90**, 495.

LAHNECHE, B., & VEROT, R. (1967). Dosimetric problems in intralymphatic radiotherapy. *Minerva med.*, **58**, 4509.

LIEBNER, E. J. (1965). An appraisal of radioactive therapeutic lymphography. *Am. J. Roentg.*, **93**, 110.

LIEBNER, E. J., HAAS, R. E., & LEROY, E. P. (1965). Experimental therapeutic lymphatic studies. *Cancer*, **18**, 827.

LORD, R. S., & KINMONTH, J. B. (1968). Comparison of endolymphatic ^{32}P labelled and ^{131}I labelled lipids in the VX$_2$ involved lymph nodes of the rabbit. *Am. J. Roentg.*, **103**, 856.

LORD, R. S., & KINMONTH, J. B. (1969). Histologic effects of endolymphatic radiotherapy. *Cancer*, **23**, 440.

MACDONALD, J. S. (1969). The value of lymphography to the radiotherapist. *Clin. Radiol.*, **20**, 447.

MAHAFFY, R. G. (1965). Surgical aspects of lymphography. *Jl R. Coll. Surg. Edinb.*, **10**, 125.

MAHAFFY, R. G. (1969). The value of diagnostic lymphography to the surgeon. *Clin. Radiol.*, **20**, 440.

NAULLEAU, J. (1966). The value of radioactive lymphography in the treatment of cancer of the testis. *Bull. Cancer, Paris*, **53**, 433.

PATERSON, R. (1952). Studies in optimum dosage. The Mackenzie Davidson Memorial Lecture. *Br. J. Radiol.*, **25**, 505.

RATTI, A., CHIAPPA, S., & FAVA, G. (1965). Principles and indications of endolymphatic radiotherapy with Lipiodol F labelled with ^{131}I. *Minerva med.*, **56**, 2013.

RATTI, A. (1966). Administration by the lymphatic route of radioactive isotopes for therapeutic purposes. *Minerva med.*, **57**, 4440.

RAVEL, R. (1966). Histopathology of lymph nodes after lymphangiography. *Am. J. clin. Path.*, **46**, 335.

ROO, T. DE (1965). An improved simple technique of lymphangiography. *Am. J. Roentg.*, **98**, 948.

RUTT, D. L., GOUGH, M. H., & KINMONTH, J. B. (1964). Disposable lymphangiography set. *Lancet*, **i**, 475.

RUTTIMANN, A. (Ed.) (1967). *Progress in Lymphology*. Proceedings of the International Symposium on Lymphology, Zurich, Switzerland, 1966. Stuttgart: Georg Thieme Verlag.

SCHEURLEN, H., HERZFELD, U., IMMICH, H., FRASCH, M., & TERES, H. (1969). Endolymphatic radiotherapy in malignant lymphoma. *Strahlentherapie, Sonderb.*, **69**, 174.

SEITZMANN, D. M., WRIGHT, R., HALABY, F. A., & FRIEMAN, J. H. (1963). Radioactive lymphangiography as a therapeutic adjunct. *Am. J. Roentg.*, **89**, 140.

STRICKSTROCK, K. H., WEISSLEDER, H., PFANNENSTIEL, P., & AFKHAN, I. K. (1969). Indication and preliminary results of endolymphatic isotope therapy in malignant diseases of the lymphatic system. *Strahlentherapie, Sonderb.*, **69**, 197.

SURYANARAYAN, C. R. (1966). Intralymphatic radioactive gold-198 perfusion in malignant diseases. *Indian J. Cancer*, **3**, 116.

TRAPNELL, D. H. (1965). Man's understanding of the lymphatics with particular reference to the lung. *Proc. R. Soc. Med.*, **58**, 37.

USLENGHT, C., MUSUMECI, R., & CHIESA, A. (1968). Report of seven years of endolymphatic radiotherapy in the treatment of malignant lymphomas. *Quad. Radiol.*, **33**, 571.

VECCHIETTI, G. (1967). Lymphatic therapy with ^{32}P for female genital neoplasms. *Minerva med.*, **58**, 4511.

WHITE, W. F. (1964). A simple method of lymphatic cannulation for intralymphatic infusion for malignant disease. *Clin. Radiol.*, **15,** 326.

WINKEL, K., BECKER, J., JANNS, E., SCHEURLEU, H., & HERZFELD, U. (1967). Indications, establishment and dosimetry in endolymphatic therapy with [131]I Lipiodol. *Strahlentherapie*, **133,** 481.

YOFFEY, J. M., & COURTICE, F. C. (1956). *Lymphatics, Lymph and Lymphoid Tissues.* 2nd edition. London: Edward Arnold.

.

12 Afterloading Methods in Radiotherapy

C. A. JOSLIN

INTRODUCTION

Despite the advances made in megavoltage therapy, which has led to a decline in the use of radium, the introduction of other types of artificial radioactive isotope has maintained the interest of radiotherapists in this form of treatment. Brachytherapy, or short distance therapy, may be achieved by surface applicators, interstitial implantation, or intracavitary insertion, of a radioactive isotope. The isotopes are usually sealed and the treatment requirements determine the type of isotope used.

One major therapeutic advantage is that of being able to deliver, to a limited volume of tissue, an extremely high integral dose of ionizing radiation whilst maintaining the quality of radiation. These high integral doses, delivered to a restricted treatment volume, are possible because of the rapid fall-off in dose obtainable within a short distance from a treatment source. This also has the effect of limiting the dose of radiation to the surrounding normal tissues. In addition, this 'inverse square law' effect will limit the exposure dose received by medical and other attending staff, but this will not be sufficiently reduced to be disregarded and particular attention has to be given to the treatment technique used.

Existing methods, which usually involve the loading of applicators before treatment is given, can cause a potential radiation hazard to the staff involved. Among the techniques developed to reduce the exposure dose are the methods of 'afterloading' of treatment applicators with a radioactive source.

The applicators are first placed in the treatment region and fixed into position. Each treatment applicator contains a series of tubes into which a radioactive source may be placed. The tubes can then be loaded, either manually or automatically, with a radioactive isotope.

Whatever the technique used, an ideal afterloading system should:

—eliminate radiation exposure to staff
—allow dosimetry to be easily and accurately controlled
—be simple in every respect
—cause the minimal inconvenience to patients.

353

The sources used for afterloading may be of low activity, measured in millicuries, or of higher activity, of the order of Curies.

A disadvantage for afterloading systems utilizing low activity sources (Henschke, 1960; Henschke et al., 1963; Walstam, 1962; Martenson and Vikterlof, 1962) is that treatment times are prolonged, which entails an inconvenience to the patient. It is also difficult to eliminate radiation exposure to nursing staff involved in ward care and patients may have to remain attached to the treatment apparatus for several hours at a time. Attempts to overcome these disadvantages by using high activity sources for afterloading have now been developed (O'Connell et al., 1965, 1967; Joslin et al., 1967; Joslin and Smith, 1970).

THE ELIMINATION OF RADIATION EXPOSURE TO STAFF

As pointed out by Taylor (1958), radiation protection can be very costly and therefore standards of protection will vary in accordance with our risk acceptance. The radioactive emission cannot be switched off, collimation is difficult, and sources have to be continuously accounted for. The early developments, designed to reduce the exposure dose of radiation when using radium, included improved instrumental procedures for source loading and unloading of treatment applicators; reduction in the time taken for the placing and positioning of the treatment applicators, and their removal at the end of treatment. Nursing procedures have also been tailored to reduce the time spent by the patient's bedside to a minimum, and particular emphasis given to instrumental handling of source applicators at the time of removal, and to the use of protective screens at the patient's bedside (Ellis, 1961; Trott and Taylor, 1961; Taylor, 1958; Fallon, 1960; Gallaghar and Saenger, 1957; Suit, Moore, Fletcher and Worsnop, 1963).

Because of the quantity of radium used, the treatment of gynaecological malignancy can result in fairly high doses of radiation to the various members of staff involved, and is responsible for the major proportion of exposure dose received. The way in which this affects the individual staff members will vary with the part they play in patient management. Thus, the greater proportion of radiation received by theatre staff, particularly to their fingers, is from loading ovoids and tubes for gynaecological treatment. Alternatively, where several patients having treatment may be cared for in the same ward at one time, the nursing staff can receive quite high body doses of radiation. Fig. 1 illustrates the exposure dose at various points around the bed of a patient having treatment for gynaecological cancer with radium. The effect of a 5 cm thickness lead shield on the one side of the bed is seen to reduce the exposure dose by approximately 4 to 1.

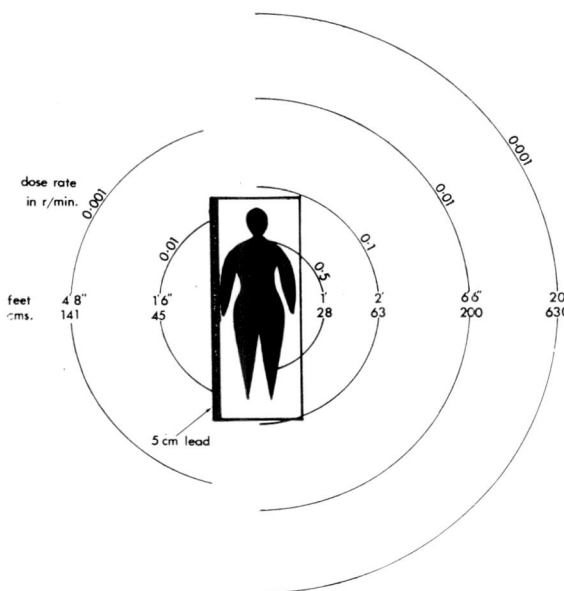

FIG. 12.1. The exposure dose from 75 mg of radium at various distances from a patient's bedside. The effect of shielding with 5 cm of lead and the reduction in exposure dose are shown on the left.

The use of protective lead screens around the bedside has also been extended to loading the treatment applicators from behind lead screens (Ellis, 1961). However, this does not effectively reduce the level of exposure to the medical staff concerned with the actual treatment procedure. Only by loading the treatment applicator after it has been placed in position can the exposure dose be effectively reduced. Although the significance for protecting the user of ionizing radiation was not fully appreciated, 'afterloading' techniques were first described by Strebel (1903) and Abbé (1910) in an effort to improve the practicality of treatment. Abbé was described as using a technique which involved incising a tumour mass and inserting a number of celluloid tubes. These were in different parts of the tumour, but all converging toward the centre. The incision was then closed leaving the ends of the tubes protruding in order to facilitate the insertion of glass radium capsules. The radium was then inserted into each tube in turn and retained for as long as necessary. This principle of afterloading interstitial tubes allows a far greater degree of accuracy, in terms of source position and controlled dosimetry, to be carried out without undue risk to the operator.

Among the early methods of reducing exposure dose to staff are those described by Morphis (1960) in which Teflon tubing is spaced and aligned as for a radium implant. The radium needles are then loaded into these tubes once their position is ascertained as satisfactory, the ends of the tubes being then sealed until the prescribed treatment has been given.

This simple afterloading technique has also been extended to intracavitary and surface mould therapy. Suit *et al.* (1963) described the modifications necessary to allow afterloading of the Fletcher ovoid system for the treatment of cervical cancer. The system used hinged ovoids attached to a central carrier and Teflon tubing is used to carry the radium or other isotope. Loading and unloading of the applicators takes place in the ward, thereby eliminating radiation exposure to the operating theatre staff.

An alternative method of reducing radiation exposure is to use an isotope such as Caesium-137, which simplifies and reduces the problem of radiation protection because of its lower penetrating properties (Horwitz *et al.*, 1964). The beta energy is easily absorbed by encapsulating the source material, leaving a gamma ray energy of 660 KeV available for use. The latter energy is less penetrating than the gamma component (1·0 MeV) for radium, and can therefore be more easily shielded. Table I shows the level of radiation expressed as percentage from various gamma source materials shielded by 2 cm of lead. It can be seen that because of its lower gamma energy, shielding for Caesium-137 will produce a lower exposure dose than from radium or from Cobalt-60.

However, despite the use of less penetrating forms of radiation the main problem of radiation exposure remains. This is due to the fact that low activity sources, which necessitate prolonged treatment times, do not completely remove the problem of radiation exposure during actual treatment. As already mentioned, systems have been devised to help resolve this problem and more elegant arrangements are now

TABLE I

SUITABLE NUCLIDES FOR AFTERLOADING METHODS

Nuclide	^{60}Co	^{222}Ra	^{182}Ta	^{137}Cs	^{192}Ir	^{198}Au
% Transmission through 2 cm Pb.	39	30	28	12	1·9	1·4
Gamma energy Component	1·17 MeV and 1·33 MeV	1·0 MeV	1·2 MeV	0·66 MeV	0·3 to 0·6 MeV	0·41 MeV
Half life	5·3 yrs.	1620 yrs	115 days	30 yrs	74 days	2·7 days

commercially available, being designed to carry automatically the radio-active source pencils from a storage safe to the treatment applicator. Some equipment has been further developed so that the source capsules are returned to the storage safe in the event of any person entering the treatment ward (Cardis and Kjellman, 1967).

An alternative afterloading system operated by a remote control mechanism (the Cathetron), described by O'Connell *et al.* (1965), entails using high activity sources, thereby reducing treatment times to the order of minutes. Patients are confined to a radiation protected treatment room for only a few minutes, thereby completely eliminating radiation exposure to all members of staff and patients. Table II shows

TABLE II

COMPARATIVE RADIATION EXPOSURE USING RADIUM AND THE CATHETRON

	Year	1965	1966	1967	1968	1969
Number of Patients	Radium	141	132	127	96	38
	Cathetron	—	—	31	73	111
	Total	141	132	158	169	149
Finger dose, rem.		72	80	71	44	31
Total body dose in rems.		8·7	10·1	3·2	4·7	2·1

Radiation exposure dose in rems received by 4 members of theatre staff using radium or 'Cathetron' for treating patients. The fall-off in body dose is in the same proportion as patients treated with radium. The finger dose does not fall in the same proportion suggesting that because of the reduced numbers of patients, staff are less worried about finger dose!

the body exposure dose and finger dose received by four members of theatre staff during the treatment of gynaecological cancer and the dose reduction which can be achieved by using the Cathetron for some of the treatments. It is seen clearly that, for about the same total number of patients being treated each year, the exposure dose is reduced in direct proportion to the increase in the number of patients treated on the Cathetron rather than by radium.

DOSIMETRY CONTROL

In order to obtain some element of control over the isodose distri-bution in *intracavitary* or *surface mould* therapy the design of the source applicator is important and this has led to the development of many different systems, each of which is suggested as having some new advantage. Horwitz *et al.* have pointed out that the personal ideals of many a radiotherapist are not fulfilled until he has designed his own applicator for the treatment of cervix cancer.

The introduction of afterloading does not affect the design of such applicators except that some form of access is necessary to allow the carrier system for transporting the radioactive sources to be connected to the applicator.

TREATMENT APPLICATORS

The applicator's design will affect the dose distribution considerably and various types are therefore available. The main object of all of these systems is to increase the dose of radiation laterally towards the pelvic wall, while limiting the antero-posterior doses to protect bladder and rectum.

Design considerations for afterloaded systems are similar to those of before-loaded systems, and only simple modifications are required. One example is the Fletcher system already described; others, O'Connell *et al.* (1967), have modified the Manchester system so as to facilitate afterloading. The latter entails replacement of the normal vaginal pack, which retains the radium in position and protects the anterior rectal wall, with a fixed type of rectal wall retractor (Fig. 2). This retractor is thickened beneath the vaginal ovoids in order to space them away from the posterior vaginal epithelium, thereby reducing the radiation dose to these tissues.

Other systems have been modified to replace radium by Cobalt-60, Iridium-192 or Caesium-137 (Henschke, 1960). The main advantage of these materials comes from their higher specific activity, which allows a reduction in the size of the source element and so facilitates the intro-

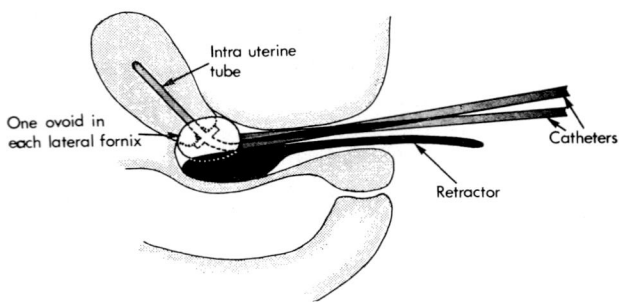

FIG. 12.2. Afterloading is achieved by modifying the Manchester radium system so that the radioactive sources can be passed along catheters to the treatment applicators.

duction of shielding materials. Also, for a given applicator, a smaller size of source element will increase the source to tissue distance and allow much tighter curvatures to be negotiated by the carrier tubes of afterloading systems. Alternatively the source activities can be increased to levels many times that of radium and treatment times reduced accordingly.

The use of different forms of shielding material to control isodose distribution has been described by Neary (1947) and by McLaren and Blomfield (1959). Neary used sources in tandem from the intra-uterine canal down the vagina with shields built into the applicator to protect the bladder and rectum. Another arrangement uses a combination of shielding and low energy gamma emitters, and was described by Tudway (1953) and Tudway et al. (1954) for the treatment of cervix carcinoma with Iridium-192. Similarly Caesium-137 has been used with a shielded applicator (Kottmeir and Walstam, 1962). These methods were designed originally for *before-loaded* applicators which employed low intensity sources, but the principle has now been extended to *afterloaded* applicators by Henschke et al. (1963), who used lead or Tungsten shields to protect the bladder or rectum, and Foley bag catheters as spacers between sources at the vaginal vault.

An alternative to vaginal ovoids is the ring-shaped applicator designed to carry Caesium sources. These are distributed evenly within the applicator (Walstam, 1965). Recent developments by Joelsson and Bäckström (1970) protect adjacent tissues with 18 carat gold discs, attached at intervals around the periphery of the carrier tube between the radiation sources. These discs limit laterally the surface dose on the vaginal applicator at points close to the radiation source. But as the distance increases, this unidirectional effect is lost and all sources effectively irradiate a given volume. Additional gold shielding is also used on the anterior and posterior portions of the ring to protect the rectum and bladder, the whole assembly being made up in araldite. The source loading has been modified to carry 600 mCi of Caesium-137 in the vaginal applicator and 600 mCi in the intra-uterine tube. This increase in activity of the sources used enables treatment times to be reduced to 6 or 8 hours.

An alternative method of controlling the isodose distribution is to continually change the position of the source pencil within a treatment applicator. One such method employs a small high-activity Cobalt-60 source designed to cycle back and forth slowly during treatment (Henschke et al., 1966). Control is achieved by altering the velocity of the source capsule and the overall length of movement.

A similar system, using surface applicators for the treatment of skin tumours (Joslin et al., 1969), is to alter the relative position of a source capsule, contained within a plastic or stainless steel catheter, in a series of steps; the source remaining stationary for a few minutes in each position. Cobalt-60 source trains of several Curies give dose-rates of one hundred or more rads a minute, at treatment distances of 1–3 cm from the sources. This system allows areas of large size and odd shapes to be treated, giving homogeneous dosimetry even where the surface is curved or irregular. One isodose problem to be taken into account with large area moulds is the effect of oblique screenage and tissue absorption, which may reduce the skin surface dose by up to 8%. Attention to source-skin distance is particularly important, since an error of only 1 mm may produce a 5% change in dose. Joslin and colleagues suggest that both preliminary calculations and confirmatory measurements are advisable with this form of treatment; if measurements do disclose any marked irregularity, the treatment schedule can be altered so as to improve dose uniformity to better than that achieved by the Paterson-Parker (1934) system.

A cylindrical applicator may be indicated for intracavitary treatment of regions such as the vaginal vault. By using a single central midline source of 1–2 cm active length within a vaginal obturator of up to 3 cm diameter, and by moving the source in a series of steps, the isodose distribution can be controlled. The system described by Joslin *et al.* does this in three steps, which are manually controlled.

A method of automatically positioning the source capsule in each treatment position has also been described (Twiss and Bradshaw, 1970). In general, such systems require either:

(1) *a large number of source pencils of different active lengths*, which may be individually retained in a stationary position during treatment, and used successively in one or more different treatment tubes on any given treatment applicator.

or, (2) *a small number of very short source capsules* capable of being moved in steps of 1–2 cm each during a course of treatment, thereby acting as an equivalent long source pencil. The time for a source to be retained in any one position needs to be adjustable, thus allowing dosimetric control.

Interstitial therapy, as normally carried out using radium needles, depends upon good spatial positioning of the source elements in order to achieve a satisfactory dose distribution. By using hollow stainless steel tubes, capable of being afterloaded with radium needles, radio-active gold seeds, or radioactive wires, several workers claim an improved implant geometry. The technique of using hollow steel tubes or cannulae allows check radiographs to be taken before treatment begins and therefore enables the spatial distribution to be corrected where necessary, without the operator receiving any radiation or the patient receiving treatment. The implant geometry can, therefore, be carefully controlled in a manner impossible for radium needles.

The nature of the anatomical sites treated by interstitial implants makes it somewhat difficult to apply remote afterloading methods, especially when controlling the relative position of an individual source, as in intracavitary or surface applicators. Among the reasons for this is that interstitial tubes are, by necessity, of small diameter and several centimetres long. Because of the site, it is often difficult to retain these tubes in position without some form of harness and it can be equally difficult to connect supply tubes to them. It would be impracticable for a patient to be connected to a storage safe for more than a few minutes. However, it is a relatively simple matter to use manual afterloading, especially if small diameter wires of radioactive material are used, the lengths of which are chosen to suit the guide tube. The source position can be fixed by some form of 'end' stop at the exit end of the tube and most existing systems rely on this simple principle.

Similar arrangements to those previously discussed can also be applied to the time that individual source elements are left in a treatment tube in order to control isodose distribution.

Some interstitial afterloading methods utilize plastic guide tubes instead of stainless steel. Unless great care is taken, the flexibility of these tubes may be such, especially when they are long, that it is difficult to obey the Paterson-Parker rules. Dutreix et al. (1970) have suggested certain rules for planning this type of implant in order to improve dose distribution. They suggest a reference isodose of not less than 75 % of the basal dose; dose variation within a treatment volume to be within 25 % of the dose in the treatment plane; the distance from a source at which the isodose is twice the reference dose not to exceed 1 cm and the separation between line sources to be not less than 5 mm. A series of graphs are used to select the best arrangement and check radiographs are taken to carry out confirmatory calculations. Although methods of source reconstruction, including computer calculations, are in use to calculate dose distributions, these are usually done in retrospect.

INTRACAVITARY AFTERLOADING FOR GYNAECOLOGICAL CANCER

The simplest application of the afterloading principle is one in which radium, as normally used in a 'before-loaded' applicator, is modified for afterloading. Such a system has been described by Silverstone (1963) in which an afterloaded radium tandem made of stainless steel is used. The tandem, with its introducer handle, resembles an intra-uterine sound and remains permanently loaded. One advantage deriving from such an afterloading technique is that it becomes a simple matter to introduce and remove the source pencils and to fractionate therapy.

Ridings (1963) has described a similar technique using small diameter afterloaded intra-uterine radium sources. He claimed that it was radiobiologically sound to fractionate radium therapy; this gives the advantages of reduced morbidity, reduced exposure dose, precise application and consistency in treatment schedules. The introduction of foam plastic packing in his cases was also said to reduce the incidence of 'pressure' ulceration within the vagina.

The Fletcher system, as modified by Suit, uses Teflon tubing to carry the radium sources. Setting up can be carried out in theatre, and only after check X-rays have been done and the patient returned to the ward is manual loading carried out.

Another system, described by Horwitz *et al.* (1964), utilizes Caesium-137 which reduces problems of radiation protection. Afterloading is carried out manually in the treatment ward, the source units being selected from a range of units which are stored within a lead safe.

A more sophisticated arrangement, which allows afterloading in the ward, has been termed 'Selectatron' (Green, 1970). The system consists of a storage safe which houses up to 36 Caesium-137 or Iridium-192 source elements, which can be individually selected once the treatment requirements for a particular patient are known. The selected sources are then transferred to a protective transport box by pushing the source along a flexible guide tube. The patient is prepared for treatment in theatre and an empty applicator inserted; this in turn is connected to a flexible tube passing down the vagina to the exterior. On return to the ward the transport box is taken to the patient and connected to the flexible tube. The source element is driven from the transport box into the source applicator by an electric motor. The method allows individual afterloading on several patients to be carried out in turn. At the completion of treatment the transport safe is again taken to each patient and the source elements returned to the storage safe.

More recently a remote control system for Caesium-137 has been introduced in an afterloading device called the Curietron (Chassagne *et al.*, 1969). The device allows up to four separately controlled radioactive source elements to be used, which are normally stored within a shielded container. A remote control switch allows the sources to be driven into the treatment applicator. These can be individually withdrawn at any time, giving some degree of treatment flexibility.

Fig. 3 illustrates a remotely controlled system suitable for the treatment of gynaecological malignancy. Such a system must allow for the source capsules to be delivered to the treatment applicators within the patient in a safe and reliable manner. The basic essentials are a storage safe to retain the source elements, and a mechanism to propel the source or sources from the safe to the treatment site, and to return them at the completion of treatment. The design of these systems should be

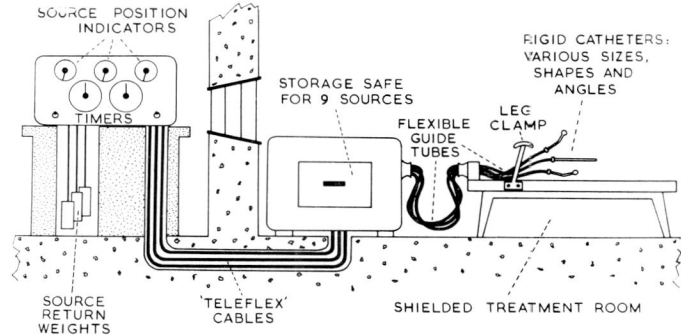

FIG. 12.3. This illustrates a remote after-loading system (e.g. the Cathetron) to facilitate treatment for cervix carcinoma.

such that it satisfies stray radiation leakage requirements. The number of sources stored should also allow for some flexibility in treatment method. One machine (Cervitron-II) provides for the treatment of two patients at any one time. Six flexible cables connect the treatment applicators to a remote-controlled device which contains a control desk and storage safe. A particular advantage is that each line source can be composed individually, by selection at the control panel, before treatment begins. This allows increased flexibility in terms of source loading and dose distribution.

The versatility of these machines is increased if each source is contained by individual control circuits, a function that is available in most of the afterloading machines already in use. This also provides for greater safety in the event of a source sticking and permits each source position to be individually monitored. This last function is important since an alteration in source position of only a few millimetres may make a considerable difference in dose distribution. One important factor, if relying upon a source position indicator, is that it must be extremely accurate. This requires a linkage with the source drive circuit in order to give the true source position at any time. However, among the disadvantages is backlash in the drive circuit which is not necessarily reflected by the monitoring circuit, and this is discussed by Liversage et al. (1967).

SOURCE PENCIL SYSTEMS

In order to allow accurate control of dosimetry the position of the treatment applicators must be maintained throughout the treatment period. It is also important that each individual source element is accurately positioned within the applicator. One method of achieving this is to use some form of spring loading to compress the individual source elements against the extreme ends of the treatment catheters when in the loaded position. In addition, the source pencil itself must be sufficiently flexible so that it will follow the various lines of curvature of the carrier tubes. An example of this is the bend produced in passing from the central axis of the vagina into the uterine canal, where the radius of curvature may be less than 3 cm.

The basic design of a source pencil will depend upon its intended use. However, the maximum length and diameter for any source pencil is determined by the anatomical limitations, whereas the minimal length and diameter for each source pencil is usually determined by the isotope chosen, the strength of source required, and its specific activity. Within these limitations, and using various spacer capsules between source elements, it is possible to choose the type of loading and dose distribution required.

The encapsulating material for an individual source will depend upon the type of screening required. Where absorptive screening is not necessary, a protective sheath will still be needed to prevent contamination from the active source material.

Usually spheres, rods with hemispherical ends, or rods with spherical spacers at either end, containing the isotope are used. These may be placed end to end or separated by spacers, in order to build up the desired length of source pencil. The use of Caesium-137, Cobalt-60 or Iridium-192 as source elements in the treatment of cervix cancer has been discussed in detail (Walstam, 1965).

A method used by Horwitz is one in which disposable plastic applicators are used to simulate the Paris colpostat, suitably modified for afterloading. A selection of source pencils are available. Each source pencil consists of a series of stainless steel cylinders containing ceramic microspheres of Caesium-137. These microspheres provide a high specific activity which reduces the source dimension. Each source unit is permanently sealed and is supported on a flexible cable. The source units are stored within a lead safe which is mobile and can be taken into the ward where loading of the applicators takes place.

One system, Cervitron-II (Cardis and Kjellman, 1968), uses spherical sources of Caesium-137 of diameter 2·5 mm, with neutral spheres of the same dimension as spacers between the active pellets. This arrangement provides source pencils of adjustable linear activity, ranging from 7·5 to 40 mg radium equivalent per centimetre, to be constructed. The variability of linear activity is achieved by preselection of a number of source or neutral pellets whose distribution can be controlled. This allows source pencils of up to 12 cm length with a minimum radius of curvature of approximately 1 cm over 180°. Treatment times can be prescribed for periods ranging up to 100 hours and the whole system is an extremely versatile one.

Another system (the Cathetron) described by O'Connell *et al.* (1967) uses Cobalt-60 source capsules contained within stainless steel cylinders 8·0 mm long and outer diameter 3·2 mm (Fig. 4). In order to make up a source pencil a series of capsules and spacers are loaded into a closed-ended helical spring 12 cm long. In order to maintain the accuracy of position of the individual source elements within the source envelope a short length of compression spring is included; an alternative would be a plastic spacer. Up to three source pencils may be used simultaneously from nine available sources. However, the source pencil lengths are predetermined and can only be altered when the sources are changed and since high activity sources are used this is a specialized procedure.

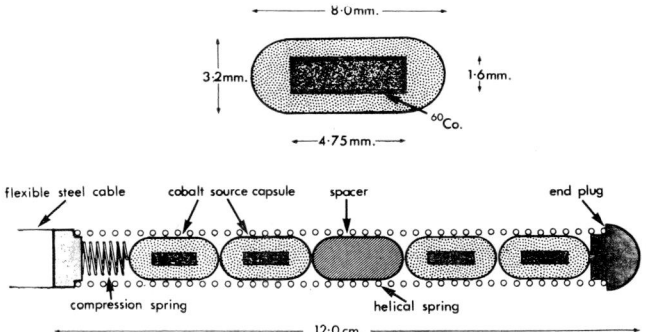

FIG. 12.4. The top diagram shows the type of source capsule used in the Cathetron. Each capsule contains a ^{60}Cobalt solid cylindrical source clad in nickel of 0·26 mm thickness. The lower diagram shows how several source capsules can be used to construct a source pencil. The source pencil illustrated is designed to simulate the Manchester system. Tandem pairs of capsules are used with spacers between each pair of $(x - 1)$ cm length; where x is the total number of source capsules used.

The form of fixation between source pencil and drive cable will vary with the system; a typical one terminates in a threaded screw which can then be connected to the drive cable. The cable has to be flexible in order to allow tight curvatures to be negotiated and unless the degree of flexibility is high, undue wear of the carrier tubes will occur at the various bends. An alternative system (Cervitron-II) depends upon the sources being moved pneumatically by means of compressed air, without the use of drive cables. Six separate control circuits are available and the pneumatic system allows each source pencil to be built up individually according to the required distribution. However, it suffers from the disadvantage of possible failure in the pneumatic system.

RECTAL DOSE MEASUREMENTS

When high activity sources are to be used for treatment it is necessary to be able to pre-determine rectal dose rates, and to do this monitoring source pencils are employed. These are identical in size to the treatment source pencils and produce the same shaped isodose, only at much lower activity. The sources are carried on short flexible lengths of cable attached to fixed lengths of steel rod, which in turn terminate in handles (Fig. 5). It is then a simple matter to measure the rectal dose at various points by means of a suitable measuring probe. The actual source strengths will depend upon the sensitivity of the measuring apparatus. One device incorporates a Cadmium Sulphide crystal within a suitable rigid metal tube and this allows dose-rates to be measured at set points within the rectum.

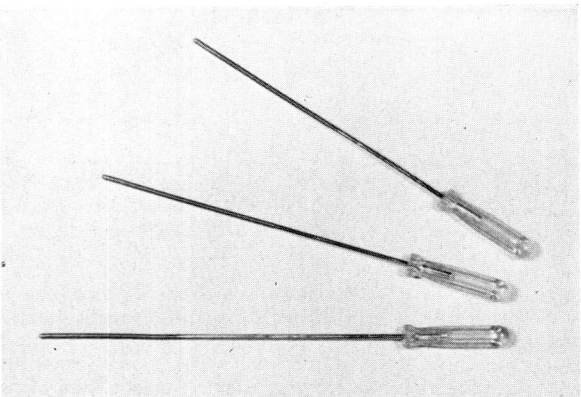

FIG. 12.5. Monitoring source pencils for use with the Cathetron to enable rectal dose measurements to be made before actual treatment.

TRANSIT DOSE

The transfer of source materials from the storage safe to the treatment applicator inevitably results in the patient's tissues being irradiated during transit. The extent of dose received at the surface of the catheter as it passes through normal tissues such as the vulva will depend upon the number of treatment fractions given, the velocity of the source and the source activity. Walstam (1965) derived a formula from which this dose may be calculated:

$$Xt = \frac{A\Gamma}{rv} \cdot \frac{\phi_2}{\phi_1} \mathrm{e} - \frac{\Sigma\mu_1 d_1}{\cos\phi} \cdot d\phi$$

where Xt is the transfer dose at a distance r from the centre of the carrier tube, A is the source activity which moves at velocity y, Γ is the specific γ ray emission, μ_1 is the linear attenuation coefficient of absorber of thickness d_1, and ϕ_1 and ϕ_2 the angles subtended at the beginning and end of the source movement.

Using these data, Liversage *et al.* (1967) calculated, as a result of experimental measurements for the Cathetron, a transfer dose of approximately 130 R at the introitus. This calculation was done for a 5 Ci source moving in and out 15 times with a velocity of 25 cm sec.

Since these calculations were applicable to high activity sources, even when slowly moving, the transit dose can be ignored for the various afterloading systems currently available.

COMBINATION THERAPY

The control of intracavitary dosimetry depends upon being able to place and maintain the treatment sources accurately in position. Most of the afterloading systems described allow this to be done, but unless high activity sources are used treatment times are long and this can produce practical difficulties. Another advantage of using high activity sources is that the short treatment time (measured in minutes) will allow concurrent external and intracavitary therapy.

Combined therapy makes it possible to treat the lymph nodes on the pelvic wall to a much higher dose than is possible with intracavitary treatment alone, so that a high lateral dose becomes much less important, although the bladder and rectal tissues will still require protection.

A suitable wedge in the external treatment beam makes it possible to deliver much higher doses to the pelvic wall lymph nodes than would be the case with simple parallel opposed fields and by arranging the wedge to shield the intracavitary treatment volume the latter can be used independently to deliver very high doses of radiation to the limited volume containing the primary tumour.

Daily fractionation becomes possible, and allows normal tissue recovery to take place between treatments. In one such system intracavitary treatment (Joslin) is given once weekly on four occasions, and external beam therapy four times weekly over the same overall period.

Since the dose-rates obtainable from the two modes of therapy are similar there should be no radiobiological difference between them. A combined isodose plan (Fig. 6) therefore has a more significant radiobiological meaning than that produced by adding conventional radium doses to external beam therapy doses.

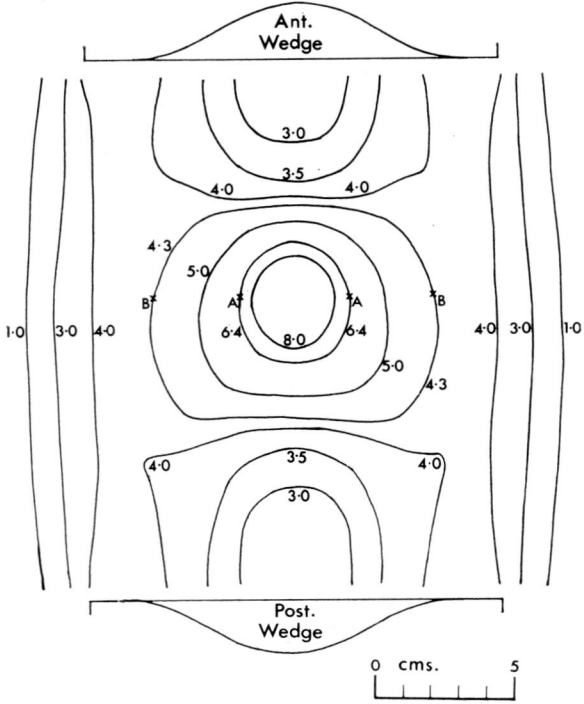

Fig. 12.6. Combined intracavitary and telecobalt isodoses.

CLINICAL CONSIDERATIONS

Where patients are treated with low activity sources for prolonged periods of time it is essential that they can lie comfortably in bed in a supine position. The catheters which connect the patient to the storage apparatus must therefore be long and flexible in order to allow the patient some movement. At the same time they must be sufficiently strong to prevent kinking or compression, which could cause a source pencil to stick, as discussed by Walstam (1965). For high activity sources treatment times are reduced to minutes and as a result it is possible to retain the patient in a lithotomy position on the treatment couch. The catheters can therefore be fixed, relative to the treatment couch, and may be short, semi-flexible, and thick walled.

It is important to maintain the patency of the catheter lumen, since the jamming of a source pencil within a catheter can produce serious exposure hazards to staff where high activity sources are in use. Fig. 7 illustrates a method for the treatment of cervix cancer by means of the

Cathetron. The applicators, in the form of an intra-uterine tube and vaginal ovoids, follow the Manchester system (Tod and Meredith, 1953). Each stainless steel catheter is maintained in position during treatment by means of a simple clamp. The insertion of intra-uterine catheter and vaginal ovoids in an anaesthetized patient is a simple process, which only takes a few minutes. The simplicity of the technique is also partly due to the rectal wall retractor used (O'Connell *et al.*, 1967). The relative positions of the catheters within the pelvis are maintained by their rigidity and allow control of their positions relative

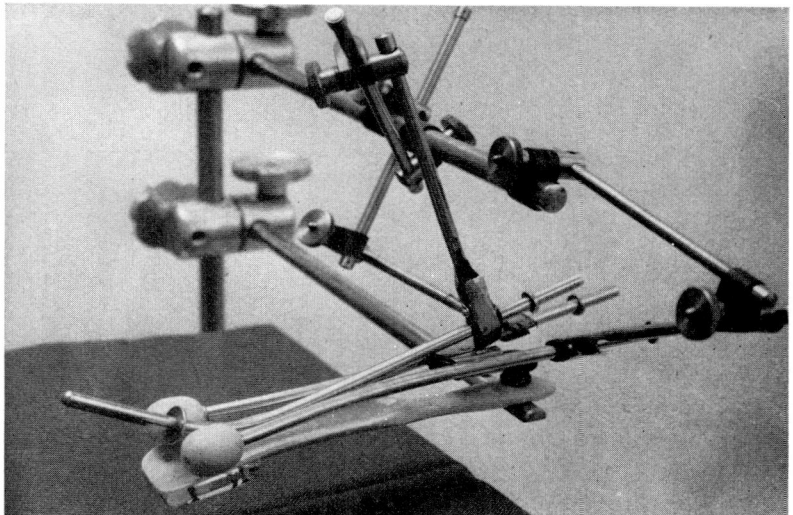

FIG. 12.7. An afterloading arrangement for use with the Cathetron. The uterine tube and ovoid catheters are held in position by spring-loaded clips. The rectal wall retractor also acts as a speculum.

to the pelvic tissues. The availability of different sizes of rectal retractor permits the dose of radiation to the anterior rectal wall to be minimized.

RADIOBIOLOGICAL IMPLICATIONS

One problem which has to be faced when substituting high activity for low activity sources is the radiobiological implication of the change in dose-rate. It is well known that doubling the activity of radium used for treatment will result in a greater radiobiological effect for the same overall dose. This fact remains true up to dose-rates of approximately 20 rads per minute, after which the effect appears to be negligible clinically. It is also important to realize that the inverse square law causes a considerable fall in dose-rate as the treatment distance increases within the pelvis and this may result in a much greater reduction in radio-biological effects than is otherwise apparent.

Table III shows the dose-rates obtainable within the pelvis for both forms of treatment. It can be inferred that the radiobiological effects for radium will differ at various points because of the low dose-rates; whereas the dose-rates from the Cathetron exceed 30 rads a minute and no change in radiobiological effect is likely. The implications have been reviewed (Liversage, 1966; Joslin et al., 1967; Joslin and Smith, 1970), and one suggestion made is that the prescribed doses will have to be reduced below those for conventional radium therapy by a factor of about 0·65 at point A.

TABLE III

PELVIC DOSE-RATES FROM RADIUM AND FROM THE CATHETRON

Source of radiation	Vaginal vault tissues	Manchester points		Pelvic wall
		A	B	
Low activity radium rads/min.	2·5	1·0	0·3	0·15
High activity ⁶⁰Cobalt rads/min (Cathetron)	500	200	55	30

Dose-rates obtainable from radium compared with those from high activity sources (Cathetron) at various points within the pelvis.

Joslin and Smith calculated for their treatment regime that the equivalent single dose at point A was 2,550 rads, which is almost identical with the 2,400 rads calculated for the conventional Manchester radium system. However, this approximate balancing of the single equivalent dose at point A does not imply that it will balance at other points within the pelvis. The radiobiological problems become even more complex when different tissues are to be considered, as discussed by Liversage.

THE POST-OPERATIVE TREATMENT OF VAGINAL VAULT
    TISSUES

Among the methods described for the post-operative treatment of uterine corpus carcinoma are those involving a vaginal obturator in the form of a tube loaded with source pencils in tandem down the vagina. The method is usually a modification of an existing radium technique, such as those described by Dobbie (1953) and by Kottmeir (1959).

In one system of afterloading (Joslin and Smith, 1971) the vaginal applicator, 2–3 cm in diameter, carries a central stainless steel catheter. The catheter is afterloaded by means of a short source pencil of activity 4·3 Ci Cobalt-60 and the applicator is shaped to follow an isodose 0·5 cm from its surface. A typical isodose distribution is shown in Fig. 8. This is uniform for the first 4 cm and decreases towards the end corresponding to the introitus. The source pencil loading is shown, being similar to a loading of 25 + 10 mg of radium in tandem.

VAGINAL APPLICATOR

3 cm. diameter

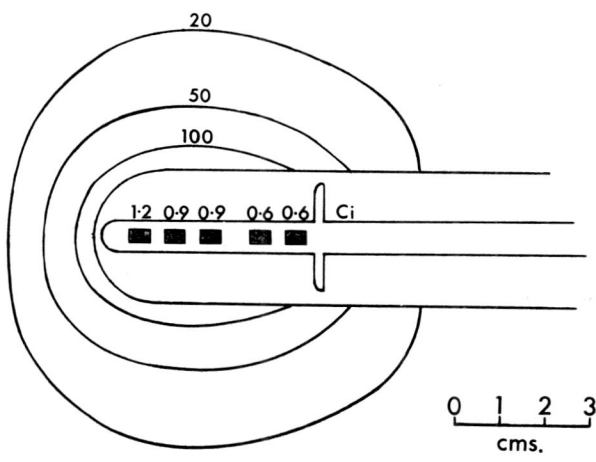

FIG. 12.8. The isodose distribution for a cylindrical applicator suitable for treating vaginal vault tissues.

This type of applicator may be secured in the treatment position by a clamping device attached to the treatment couch. A similar technique, which involves the movement of a source pencil in sequential steps along the applicator in order to treat the whole vagina has also been described (Joslin, Liversage and Ramsey, 1969). A further development, in which the source pencil is automatically moved to each treatment position by a programming system, has been described by Twiss and Bradshaw (1970).

From the patient's viewpoint the principal advantage of high dose-rate techniques is that they cause less personal inconvenience, since she does not have to be confined to bed for treatment lasting only a few minutes. It is also simple to use fractionation regimes, and to combine these with external beam therapy in order to treat the whole pelvis.

OESOPHAGEAL CARCINOMA

The well known technique of using radium bougies suffers from difficulties in accurate positioning of the source pencil, maintaining the source applicator in position for the necessarily long periods of time, and achieving a satisfactory depth dose in the region of the tumour. These disadvantages can to some extent be offset by using high activity sources and an afterloading technique. The technique used by O'Connell (1970) involves initial shrinkage of the oesophageal lesion by external beam therapy. An oesophagoscope is then passed through the resolving tumour and a 'cathetron' source pencil passed down the centre of the oesophagoscope. This will allow a short but reasonable treatment distance between the source and the surface of the oesophagoscope, thereby producing a relatively better depth dose. Treatment times are short and dose-rates of several hundred rads a minute are possible.

LARYNGEAL CARCINOMA

The use of an afterloading type apparatus (Gamma Med) for the treatment of laryngeal cancer by intracavitary therapy was described by Feine and Koburg (1969). The apparatus consists essentially of a storage apparatus designed to carry Iridium-192 sources with an activity of up to 150 Ci or 30 Ci of Cobalt-60. The source pencil dimensions are 1 mm diameter and 1–16 mm long. The source is contained within a stainless steel jacket, 1·8 mm diameter and 10–25 mm long. The dose-rate obtainable from a 150 Ci source of Iridium-192 at 5 mm distance in tissue is 400 rads/sec, and at 2 cm 40 rads/sec.

Feine and Koburg described a technique for the treatment of carcinoma of the laryngeal cord in which endoscopic application of a treatment applicator is made adjacent to the area to be treated. In order to afford protection to adjacent normal tissues a tungsten screen is introduced to shield the major segment of the treatment volume and takes the form illustrated in Fig. 9. Treatment is given to a radical dose level of 7,000 rads at a distance of 4 mm from the central axis of the source in a single fraction which takes less than 5 minutes.

BRAIN TUMOURS

Some brain tumours can be removed leaving a cavity into which it is possible to introduce a spherical applicator. Surgical introduction is obviously necessary and a skull fixing plate is required to maintain

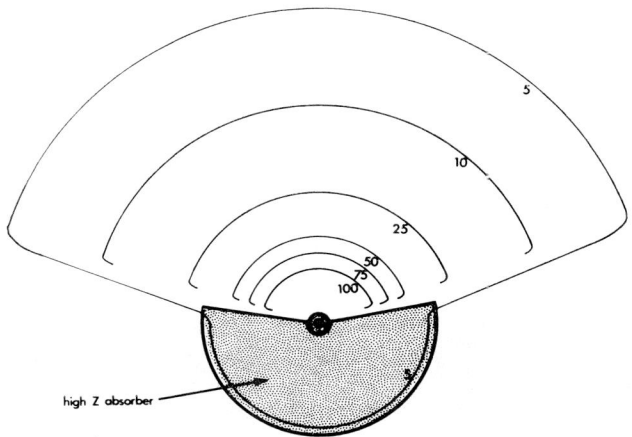

FIG. 12.9. In order to protect adjacent tissues and treat a segmental volume a high 'Z' absorber is used.

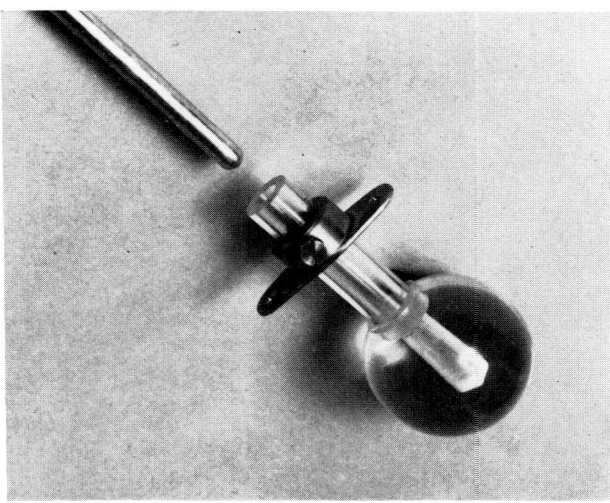

FIG. 12.10. A cylindrical applicator for post-operatively treating brain tumours. The fixing plate can be adjusted to enable the applicator to be placed at any depth. (By courtesy of J. M. Henk, Velindre Hospital, Cardiff.)

the applicator in position. Treatment times may last from days to weeks depending upon the source activity and fractionation regime used. Fig. 10 shows a device used in conjunction with the Cathetron machine. The isodose distribution will obviously depend upon the loading of the source applicator and its shape.

TREATMENT TECHNIQUE FOR BONE CAVITIES

The methods used are again usually modified radium techniques, involving the introduction of an obturator into a cavity. This technique

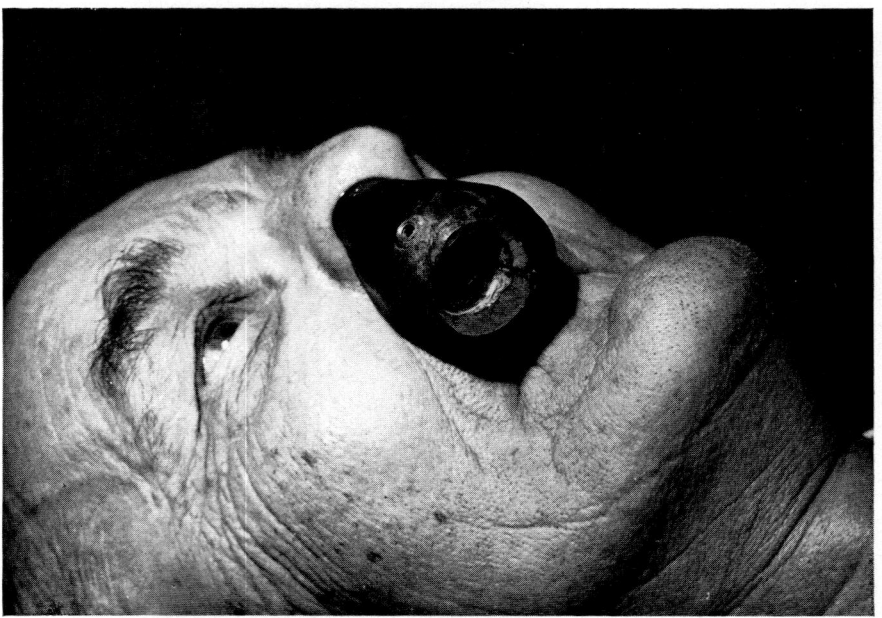

FIG. 12.11(a) The applicator enables a central stainless steel catheter to be held accurately in position.

allows treatment to be planned, in conjunction with external beam therapy, so that the central portions of the tumour volume, in this case the cavity surface, can receive very high doses of radiation. A suitable obturator is shown in Fig. 11(a) and (b) (Kunkler, 1968), for treating in a concurrent manner, with intracavitary and wedged external beam therapy, a carcinoma of the nasal vestibule.

METHODS OF INTERSTITIAL AFTERLOADING

The problem of radiation exposure in the interstitial implantation of radium is similar to that for gynaecological radium. Although the activity of the sources is generally lower, the radiotherapist may receive a high finger dose because of the need to feel the ends of the needles when adjusting their course through the tissues. The needles may also require suturing into position.

In order to achieve better implant geometry, a technique involving mechanical needle stabilizers for radium implants has been described

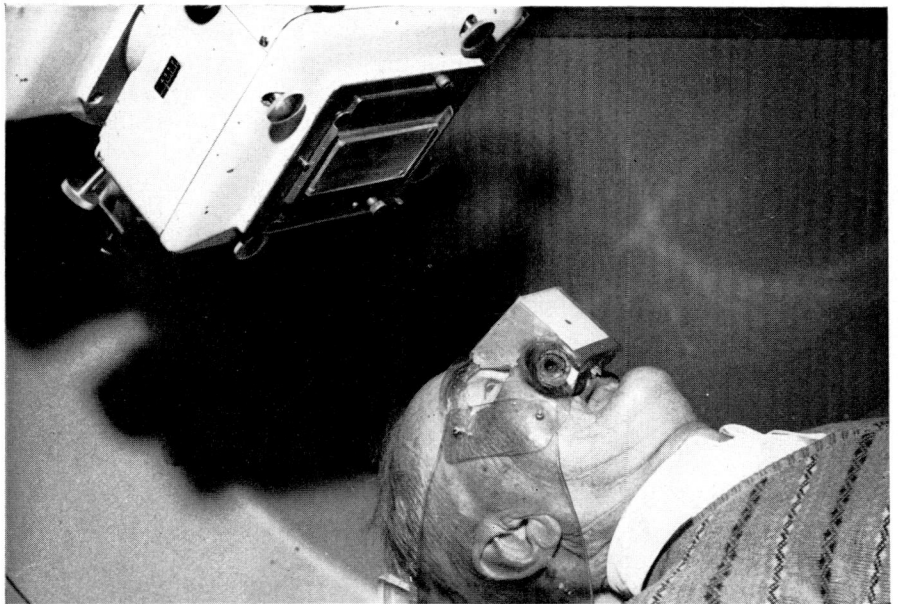

Fig. 12.11(b) Used in conjunction with external beam therapy the applicator allows concurrent treatment with the two modalities.

(Green and Jennings, 1951) which reduces the exposure dose to the operators' fingers. This can be further improved by using hollow stainless steel tubes for the implant and then afterloading these with radium needles. A similar system, using hollow rigid needles afterloaded with various radioactive materials, has also been described by Suit *et al.* (1961).

In order to bring about a reduction in the exposure dose Morphis (1960) described a technique of afterloading in which Teflon tubing, fixed to a steel needle up to 15 cm or more in length, is inserted through the tumour base in the desired configuration. The tubes are pulled through the tissues and positioned accurately with the fingers. The far end of each tube is sealed with a Michel skin clip and radium needles inserted into the open end with special 'holding' forceps. The radium is pushed into the desired position with a stylette, and the open end of the tubing sealed until treatment is complete, the procedure for removal being made in the reverse manner. The clinician is said to receive less than 50 mR using this technique.

Mowatt and Stevens (1956) describe a system whereby stainless steel tubes, of outside diameter 2·4 mm and internal diameter 1·7 mm, are implanted through a perspex stabilizer. The position of these tubes is checked, following which they are activated by means of radon seed inserts. One end of each hollow tube is closed and the other terminates in a screw lock device which retains the insert in position. The radon seeds are each 0·5 mm long and only 0·3 mm in diameter. They are contained within a tube of polyvinyl chloride and normally stored within a lead block. One insert slides into each tube and is manually loaded. The average loading time is said to be only 7 seconds, giving only a small dose to the loader's fingers.

Several similar methods have been described for interstitial implantation either directly or in combination with open surgery (Pierquin, 1964). The surgical removal of a tumour might be followed by the placement of plastic tubes into the tumour base. The wound is then closed with the free ends of the tubes remaining exposed. These are fixed by retaining clips, adjacent to the skin, so that no movement takes place and then loaded post-operatively. The technique described by Ellis (1970) involves loading the tubes 5 days after surgery with Tantalum-182 or Iridium-192 wire inserts, and Ellis *et al.* (1970) have also described an apparatus which enables afterloading to be carried out while the operator remains protected.

Brasfield and Henschke (1958 and 1961) and Henschke (1960), described a system of inserting unloaded nylon tubes in and around a tumour. Various modifications were illustrated including open and closed-end techniques. Loading is carried out with radioactive seeds contained in nylon ribbons using Gold-198, Cobalt-60, Radium-222, Iridium-192, and Tantalum-182, treatment extending to two plane and volume implants. Pierquin and Chassagne (1962) modified an earlier technique to use Iridium-192 wires for afterloading. These are only 0·3 mm diameter and extremely flexible. The length of wire required is determined by inserting a non-radioactive wire first. Iridium wire is then cut to length and sheathed in a thin plastic tube which can then be afterloaded into the interstitial guide tube.

An ingenious method using Iodine-131 was presented by Harper and

Lathrop in 1954 for the treatment of intra-abdominal tumours. Poly-ethylene tubing of only 0·61 mm diameter and bore 0·28 mm is threaded around and through the tumour, following as closely as possible the rules of Paterson and Parker. The length of tubing used, the spacing between turns and the final configuration are carefully controlled. The ends of the tube are brought out from the treatment site and the wound closed. The tubing is then filled with mercury and radiographs taken to ascertain the volume of tissue to be irradiated and dose calculations made. Iodine-131 is used as a source of gamma energy, the beta energy being mostly filtered out by the walls of the tubing. It is injected as silver iodide dissolved in potassium iodide. (Harper calculated that approximately 1 mc. of ^{131}I allowed to decay completely, produces the same tissue dose as 76 mgm hours of radium.) The ends of the tubing are heat sealed and later cut short and allowed to retract beneath the skin.

THE INTERSTITIAL TREATMENT OF BRAIN TUMOURS

Brain tumour tissue remaining after surgical excision has been treated by interstitial afterloading techniques (Mundinger, 1969). An Iridium-192 cylindrical source is passed into successive treatment tubes, the treatment time in each position being determined by the required isodose plan. The treatment is given by remote control, with protective lead screens around the patient's head to allow access, and delivers a dose chosen between 2,500 rads and 3,500 rads at each session, depending upon the histological type of tumour.

An alternative arrangement used for inoperable tumours deeply situated, such as those of the pituitary, is to irradiate after surgical healing has taken place. An accurate approach becomes possible using a stereotactic device (Reichert and Mundinger, 1956, 1959) and an accuracy of ± 0·5 mm is claimed. The method used depends upon the type of tumour and its accessibility.

METHODS OF SURFACE MOULD AFTERLOADING

Although radium has been replaced by superficial X-rays for the treatment of most superficial skin cancers, radium treatment moulds are still preferred for certain tumour sites, where cartilage and tendons are involved, or where the superficial tissues are thin and overlie bone. Other possible indications include post-operative radiation after mastectomy for breast carcinoma, and after excision of superficial soft tissue sarcomas.

Afterloading for surface applicators has not received as much attention as for interstitial and intracavitary techniques, partly because of the
practical difficulties and partly because of the availability of short
distance Cobalt-60 and Caesium-137 therapy units. However, afterloading can offer the advantages of accurately controlled hard
γ-radiation limited to the tumour volume.

One of the difficulties encountered with short distance radium moulds
is that of being able to produce homogeneous dosimetry. For an area

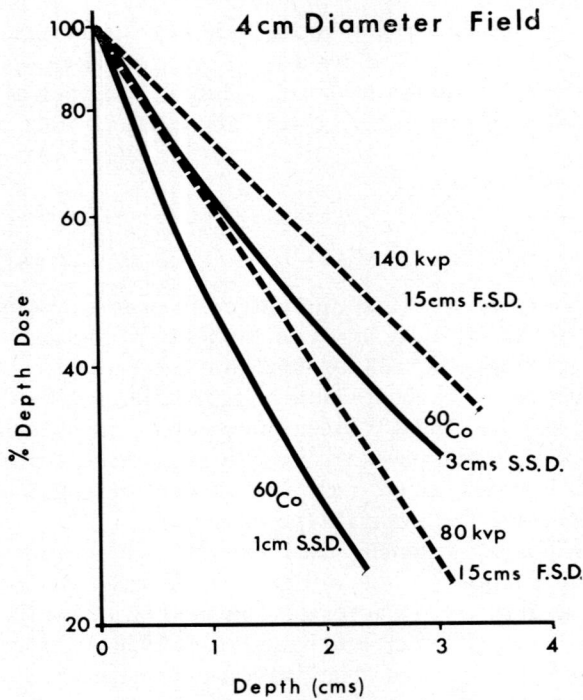

FIG. 12.12. Depth dose data for 80 KVp and 140 KVp (supplement 10, *Brit. J. Rad.*
1961) which is seen to be similar to that for short-distance gamma rays.

of more than 2 sq. cm at a treatment distance of 1–3 cm, it is necessary
to use more than one source of radiation, spatially distributed, in order
to obtain homogeneity of dose. In practice the source dimensions have
to approximate to those of the treatment area as discussed by Paterson
and Parker (1934).

For short treatment distances a rapid fall-off in dose occurs and the
normal tissues beneath the tumour bed will receive a greatly reduced
dose of radiation. The fall-off in dose is shown in Fig. 12 for two

different applicators and for superficial X-rays. It can be seen that the fall-off in dose with distance is similar for the two methods.

The replacement of conventional low activity radium with high activity Cobalt for afterloading surface applicators has been described (Joslin, Liversage and Ramsey, 1969; Joslin and Smith, 1970). Because of the high dose-rates possible with this system, fractionation regimes and treatment times follow those used for conventional superficial X-ray techniques. Therefore, any difference of relative biological efficiency can be allowed for when prescribing treatment, and the dose modified.

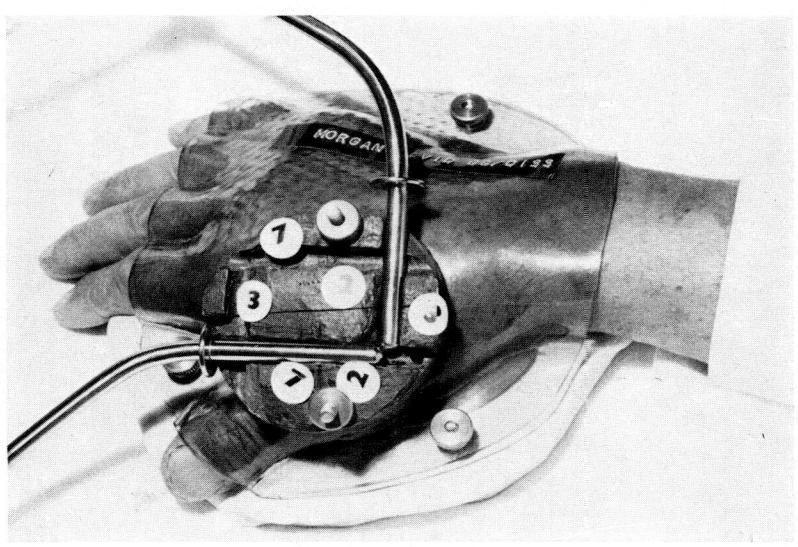

FIG. 12.13(a)

FIG. 12.13(a) and (b). A method of treating a superficial tumour of the dorsum of the hand using the Cathetron at a treatment distance of 1·5 cm. The numbers signify the source pencils used.

A typical treatment set up (Fig. 13) shows an arrangement for treating the dorsum of the hand. A lead tunnel around the treated volume serves to reduce the patient's body dose. For the treatment of lesions such as the pinna it becomes necessary to protect adjacent tissues (Fig. 14) by surrounding the treatment area with lead of suitable thickness. The line sources can be spatially positioned to produce an isodose distribution to fit the Paterson and Parker rules. However, the uniformity of dose set by these rules, which may be 5–10% lower in the central positions

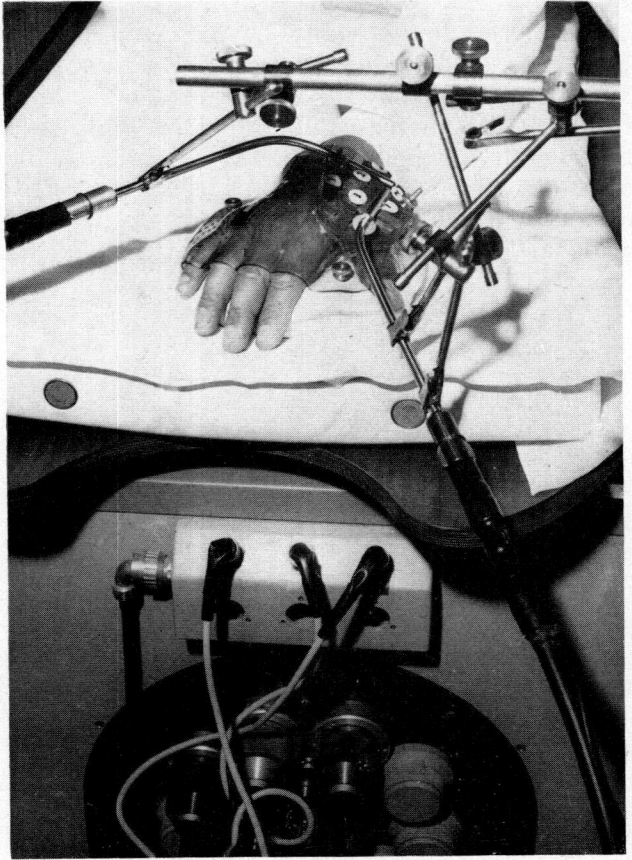

FIG. 12.13(b).

of the mould, can be improved by altering the position of the Cathetron
source pencils and adjusting treatment times. It then becomes possible
to treat surface areas as large as 150 or 200 sq. cm without loss of
uniformity in dose.

FUTURE DEVELOPMENTS

It has been suggested that the only advantage of afterloading is the
consequent reduction or elimination of exposure dose to staff. Despite
the recommendations of the International Atomic Energy Agency (1967),
there are many who feel that the occupational hazards of radiation

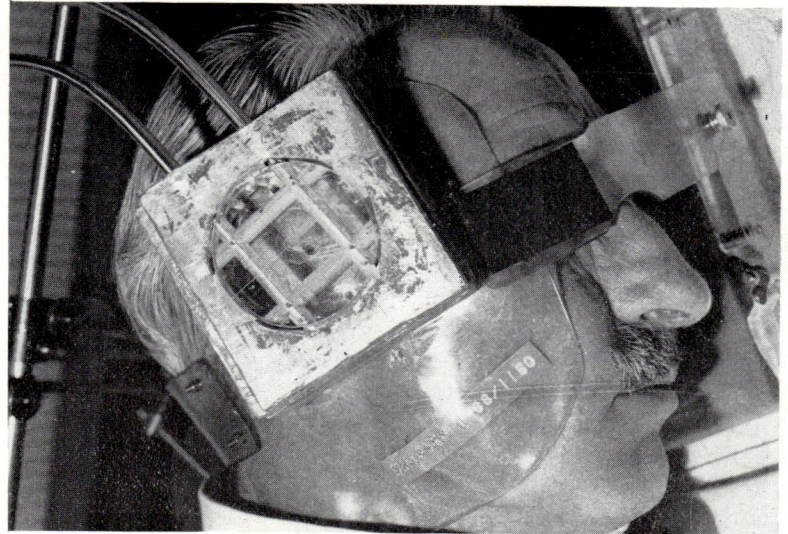

FIG. 12.14(a).

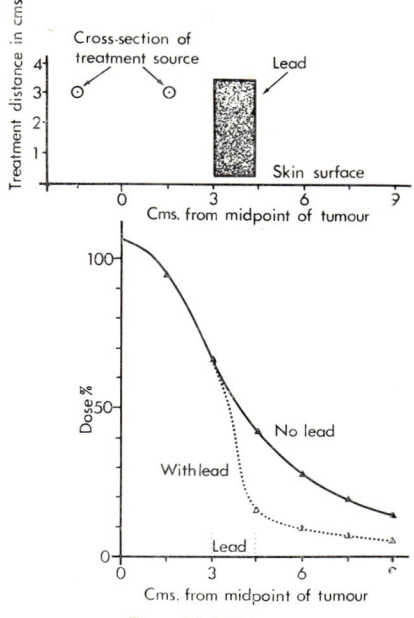

FIG. 12.14(b).

FIG. 12.14(a) In order to protect adjacent tissues a lead surround is used. The penumbra is reduced but is still much wider than that for conventional beam-directed treatment. (b) The fall-off in dose beyond the treatment area can be greatly increased by lead protection. (By courtesy of C. Smith, Velindre Hospital, Cardiff.)

exposure are over-stressed. However, there are the added advantages of reducing inconvenience to the patient, particularly when high activity sources are used. In addition, it becomes practical to introduce fractionation techniques and to combine intracavitary treatment better with external beam therapy.

Combined therapy allows high doses of radiation to be delivered to selective portions of the overall treatment volume. The importance of being able to control isodose distribution in this manner is that it then becomes possible to think in terms of homogeneous radiobiological iso-effect rather than homogeneous isodose (Ellis, 1969; Kirk, Gray and Watson, 1971). A possible way in which this radiobiological iso-effect may be improved is to consider the use of neutron emitters such as Californium-252 (see Chapter 9).

Much radiobiological investigation and clinical assessment is required before these more advanced techniques are likely to be put into everyday use. Although there are many who defend well tried and proven methods, these themselves were a few years ago considered revolutionary. This chapter has attempted to review the progressive improvements in the handling of radioactive materials for the treatment of malignancy and some of the problems encountered. It is suggested that afterloading is becoming accepted as a necessary method with advantages for both patients and staff and that these developments will continue.

REFERENCES

ABBE, R. (1910/11). Scientific report. *Archs. Roentg. Ray*, **15**, 74.

BRASFIELD, R. D., & HENSCHKE, U. K. (1958). Treatment of internal mammary lymph nodes by implantation of radioisotopes into internal mammary artery. *Radiology*, **70**, 259.

BRASFIELD, R. D., & HENSCHKE, U. K. (1961). Intravascular irradiation of internal mammary lymph nodes in breast cancer. *Am. J. Roentg.*, **85**, 849.

CARDIS, R., & KJELLMAN, J. (1968). *A New Apparatus for Intracavitary Radiotherapy —Cervitron II*. Geneva: Industries Atomiques.

CHASSAGNE, D., DELOUCHE, G., ROCOPLAN, J. A., PIERQUIN, B., & GEST, J. (1969). Description et premiers essais du Curietron. *J. Radiol. Electrol. Méd. nucl.*, **50** (12), 910.

DOBBIE, B. M. W. (1953). Vaginal recurrences in carcinoma of the body of the uterus and their prevention by radium therapy. *J. Obstet. Gynaec. Br. Commonw.*, **60**, 702.

DUTREIX, A., WAMBERSIE, A., & PIERQUIN, B. (1968). Étude de la répartition des doses autour de sources ponctuelles alignées. *Acta radiol.*, **7**, 389.

ELLIS, F. (1961). Reduction of radiation hazards in use of radium and similar sources. *Br. J. Radiol.*, **34**, 408.

ELLIS, F. (1969). Dose, Time and Fractionation. *Clin. Radiol.*, **20**, 1.

ELLIS, F. (1970). Afterloading techniques. *Proc. R. Soc. Med.*, **63**, 1034.

ELLIS, F., *et al.* (1970). Publication pending.

FALLON, R. J. (1960). Sterilisation of radium needles and gynaecological applicators. *Lancet*, **ii**, 1133.

FEINE, U., & KOBURG, E. (1969). *Tumoren der Mundhöhle, des Rachens und des Kehlkopfes. Die Bestrahlung von malignen Tumoren im Hals-Nasen-Ohren-Bereich mit ferngesteuerter Iridium-192-Kontaktbestrahlung.* Interdisziplinare Diskussione Deutschen Röntgenkongress 1968, pp. 178–82. Munchen-Berlin-Wein: Urban & Schwarzenberg.

GALLAGHER, R. G., & SAENGER, E. L. (1957). Radium capsules and their associated hazards. *Am. J. Roentg.*, **77**, 511.

GREEN, A., & JENNINGS, W. A. (1951). New techniques in radium and radon therapy. *J. Fac. Radiol.*, **2**, 206.

GREEN, A. (1970). Personal communication.

HARPER, P. V., & LATHROP, K. A. (1954). Isotope Therapy for Carcinoma of Pancreas. Clinical Congress Am. College Surgeons, Philadelphia, *Surg. Forum*, **5**, 650.

HENSCHKE, U. K. (1960). 'Afterloading' application for radiation therapy of carcinoma of uterus. *Radiology*, **74**, 834.

HENSCHKE, U. K., HILARIS, B. S., & MAHAN, G. D. (1963). Afterloading in interstitial and intracavitary radiation therapy. *Am. J. Roentg.*, **90**, 386.

HENSCHKE, U. K., HILARIS, B. S., & MAHAN, G. D. (1964). Remote afterloading with intracavitary applicators. *Radiology*, **83**, 344.

HENSCHKE, U. K., HILARIS, B. S., & MAHAN, G. D. (1966). Intracavitary radiation therapy of cancer of the uterine cervix by remote afterloading with cycling sources. *Am. J. Roentg.*, **96**, 45.

HORWITZ, H., KEREIAKES, J. G., BAHR, G. K., CLUXTON, S. E., & BARRETT, C. M. (1964). Afterloading system utilizing caesium-137 for treatment of carcinoma of cervix. *Am. J. Roentg.*, **91**, 176.

INTERNATIONAL ATOMIC ENERGY AGENCY, VIENNA. (1967). *Technical Reports Series No. 75, Physical Aspects of Radio-isotope Brachytherapy.* Vienna: I.A.E.A.

JOELSSON, I., & BÄCKSTRÖM, A. (1970). Applicators for remote afterloading technique for optimum pelvic dose distribution in carcinoma of the uterine cervix. *Acta radiol. ther. phys. biol.*, **9**, 233.

JOSLIN, C. A., LIVERSAGE, W. E., & RAMSEY, N. W. (1969). High dose-rate treatment moulds by afterloading techniques. *Br. J. Radiol.*, **42**, 108.

JOSLIN, C. A., O'CONNELL, D., & HOWARD, N. (1967). The treatment of uterine carcinoma using the cathetron. Part III. Clinical considerations and preliminary reports on treatment results. *Br. J. Radiol.*, **40**, 895.

JOSLIN, C. A. & SMITH, C. W. (1970). Use of high activity cobalt-60 sources for intracavitary and surface mould therapy. *Proc. R. Soc. Med.*, **63**, 1029.

JOSLIN, C. A., & SMITH, C. W. (1971). Post-operative radiotherapy in the management of uterine corpus carcinoma. *Clin. Radiol.* **22**, 118.

KIRK, J., GRAY, W. M., & WATSON, E. R. (1971). Cumulative radiation effect. *Clin. Radiol.*, **22**, 145.

KOTTMEIR, H. L. (1959). Carcinoma of the corpus uteri: diagnosis and therapy. *Am. J. Obstet. Gynec.*, **78**, 1127.

KOTTMEIR, H. L., & WALSTAM, R. (1962). Caesium-137 as a Radiation Source for Intracavitary Gynaecological Application. *The Swedish Cancer Society Yearbook*, 3, p. 397. Bergstrand, H. (Ed.). Stockholm: Almqvist & Wiksell.

KUNKLER, P. B. (1968). Personal communication.

LIVERSAGE, W. E. (1966). The application of cell survival theory to high dose-rate intracavitary therapy. *Br. J. Radiol.*, **39**, 338.

LIVERSAGE, W. E., MARTIN-SMITH, P., & RAMSEY, N. W. (1967). The treatment of uterine carcinoma using the cathetron. Part II. Physical measurements. *Br. J. Radiol.*, **40**, 887.

MARTENSON, B., & VIKTERLOF, K. J. (1962). *A Modified Method for Intracavitary Irradiation of Gynaecological Cancer. Xth International Congress of Radiology, Book of Abstracts*, 178.

MCLAREN, H. C., & BLOMFIELD, G. W. (1959). *Treatment of Cancer in Clinical Practice*, pp. 664–85. Kunkler, P. B., and Rains, A. J. H. (Eds.). Edinburgh and London: E. and S. Livingstone.

MORPHIS, O. L. (1960). Teflon tube method of radium implantation. *Am. J. Roentg.*, **83**, 455.

MOWATT, K. S., & STEVENS, K. A. (1956). Afterloading—contribution to protection problem. *J. Fac. Radiol.*, **8**, 28.

MUNDINGER, F. (1964). Die interstitielle Radio-Isotopenbestrahlung bei infiltrierenden Hirntumoren, Hypophysenadenomen und zur Hypophysektomie. Technik, Dosimetrie und Ergebnisse. *Vort Societas Neurochirurgica Fennica*, Helsinki, 3. 4.

MUNDINGER, F. (1966). The Treatment of Brain Tumours with Radioisotopes. *Prog. Neurol. Surg.*, **1**, 202. Basel and New York: Karger.

MUNDINGER, F. (1969). Erfahrungen mit der stereotaktischen interstitiellen Brachytherapie mit Iridium-192 'Gamma Med' bei infiltrierenden Hirntumoren. *Fortschr. Geb. RöntgStrahl. NuklMed.*, **110**, 254.

MUNDINGER, F. (1969). Techniques and indications for the interstitial irradiation of brain and pituitary tumours with radionuclides. *Kerntechnik*, **11**, 333.

NEARY, G. J. (1947). Physical aspects of intracavitary radium treatment of carcinoma of the cervix uteri. *Br. J. Radiol.*, **20**, 454.

OLIVER, G. D., & ALMOND, P. R. (1970). *Evaluation of Calfornium-252 as a Neutron Emitter for Interstitial and Intracavitary Therapy. Xth International Cancer Congress, Book of Abstracts*, 663.

O'CONNELL, D., HOWARD, N., JOSLIN, C. A., RAMSEY, N. W., & LIVERSAGE, W. E. (1965). A new remotely-controlled unit for the treatment of uterine carcinoma. *Lancet*, **ii**, 570.

O'CONNELL, D., JOSLIN, C. A., HOWARD, N., RAMSEY, N. W., & LIVERSAGE, W. E. (1967). The treatment of uterine carcinoma using the cathetron. Part I. Technique. *Br. J. Radiol.*, **40**, 882.

O'CONNELL, D. (1970). Personal communication.

PATERSON, R., & PARKER, H. M. (1934). A dosage system for gamma ray therapy. *Br. J. Radiol.*, **7**, 592.

PIERQUIN, B. (1964). Précis de curie thérapie. Masson. Paris.

PIERQUIN, B., & CHASSAGNE, D. (1962). La préparation non radio-active et curietherapie interstitielle et de contact. *J. Radiol. Électrol. Méd. nucl.*, **43**, 65.

REICHERT, T., & MUNDINGER, F. (1959). Ein kombinierter Zielbügel mit Bohraggregat zur Vereinfachung stereotaktischer Hirnoperationen. *Arch. Psychiat. NervKrankh.*, **199**, 337.

RIDINGS, G. R. (1963). Fractionated intra-uterine radium applications: use of small-diameter afterloading intra-uterine applicator: preliminary report. *Am. J. Roentg.*, **89**, 500.

SILVERSTONE, S. M. (1963). The intra-uterine tandem technique. *Am. J. Roentg.*, **89**, 83.

STREBEL, H. (1903). Vorschläge zur Radium Therapie. *Dt. med. Ztg*, **24**, 1145.

SUIT, H. D., MOORE, E. B., FLETCHER, G. H., & WONSNOP, R. (1963). Modification of Fletcher ovoid system for afterloading using standard-sized radium tubes (milligram and microgram). *Radiology*, **81**, 126.

SUIT, H. D., SHALEK, R. J., MOORE, E. B., & ANDREWS, J. R. (1961). Afterloading technique with rigid needles in interstitial radiation therapy. *Radiology*, **76**, 431.

TAYLOR, L. S. (1958). *Radiation Protection*. Braestrup, C. B., and Wyckoff, H. O. (Eds.). Springfield, Illinois: Charles Thomas.

TOD, M. C., & MEREDITH, W. J. (1953). Treatment of cancer of the cervix uteri—a revised 'Manchester method'. *Br. J. Radiol.*, **26**, 252.

TROTT, N. G., & TAYLOR, K. W. (1961). General study of solid source handling problems. *Br. J. Radiol.*, **34**, 420.

TUDWAY, R. C. (1953). Use of radioactive isotopes in applicator for treatment of carcinoma of cervix uteri. *Acta Radiol.*, **39**, 415.

TUDWAY, R. C., FREUNDLICH, H. F., & MARSHALL, T. S. (1954). *An Applicator for Treatment of Carcinoma of Cervix Uteri Employing Radioactive Iridium*. Radio-isotope Conference, 1954. New York: Academic Press.

TWISS, D. B., & BRADSHAW, A. L. (1970). Automatic source positioning for cathetron treatments. *Br. J. Radiol.*, **43**, 48.

WALSTAM, R. (1962). Remotely-controlled afterloading radiotherapy apparatus. (A preliminary report). *Acta Radiol.*, *Suppl.* 236.

WALSTAM, R. (1965). Studies on therapeutic short-distance and intracavitary gamma beam techniques. *Physics Med. Biol.*, **7**, 225.

13 Use of Computers in Radiotherapy

J. S. ORR

Much of the organization of life today is dependent on the ways in which we use writing and mathematics, and since computers change these ways, they must also eventually change the organization. Such changes are compelled by the manner in which computers function. When properly used, computers extend human capabilities by providing much more rapid, precise and extensive processing of symbolic and numerical information. The value of this can only be realized, however, when the difficulties of feeding the information into the computer and of obtaining an output suitable for use and action, have been overcome. Most of these difficulties arise from problems of organization.

COMPONENTS

Digital computers can be considered as consisting of five parts. The most important of these is the output. The capabilities of the output limit the kind of answers which can be obtained, and therefore the kind of problems it is worth setting. Outputs are of two types; those which are intended to be used by machines and those which are intended to be used by people. The first can be magnetic tape, paper tape or punched cards. The second can be typewriter, line printer, plotter, oscilloscope visual display unit or over-printed punched cards.

The second most important part is the input. Due to the large differences in the methods of sensory perception used by machines and humans, it has been very difficult to find a common medium. The problem is still unsolved, although recent developments in document readers appear to be approaching a partial solution. There must always, therefore, be a translation step in which written data or information is translated into a machine compatible form by punching on to cards or tape. For reasons of economy, it is also usually imperative to use the layout and ordering of the data as a vital part of the information. That is to say, the meanings assigned to numbers, letters or words depend entirely on the positions they occupy. This kind of grammar imposes a strict organization on the data, which is foreign to human communication except in mathematics.

The other three parts of a computer can be classified as a memory, an arithmetic unit, and a control. The arrangement is illustrated in

Fig. 1. The memory serves to hold both data and instructions. The instructions, which make up the programme, are used by the control to determine the steps to be carried out in the processing of the data. Many of the instructions depend on the results of a comparison, so the control must feed itself both with instructions from the memory and with results from the arithmetic unit. The influence of these results in determining the alternative instructions or groups of instructions which are to be used is rather naive, simple-minded, and unsophisticated. It is due to this feature that the computer is much less flexible and subtle than the human mind.

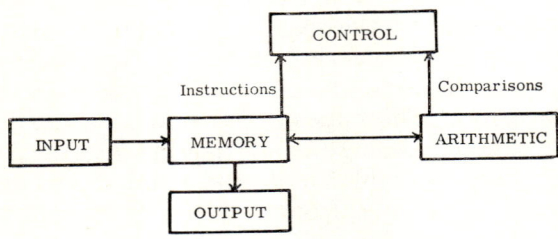

FIG. 13.1. The basic functional parts of a computer.

PROCESSING AND ORGANIZATION

The first phase of any computer application is usually concerned with the purely technical problems of information processing within the computer. In radiotherapy this phase is virtually complete. The second phase is the organization of the use made of the output, which dictates its form and also the form of the input. This enforced continuous reorganization is the theme of recent progress and current activities in the applications of computers in radiotherapy (Orr, Cain, Etchells, Halnan and Hope, 1970).

Fig. 2 shows the number of papers on computers in radiotherapy which have been published each year in the most relevant journals. It is apparent that after the few pioneering papers of the fifties came a steep rise in the early sixties which has been followed by a plateau. The number of papers in the regular periodicals has in fact declined, but this fall has been roughly balanced by the papers presented at the two I.A.E.A. meetings in Vienna and at the International Conferences (I.A.E.A., 1966 and 1968; British Institute of Radiology, 1967, 1971; Cohen, 1970; Computers in Radiology, 1970).

Most of the papers are concerned with the calculation of dose distributions from multiple external or internal radiation sources as a part of treatment planning. The processes of treatment planning included in Fig. 3 consist of: the delineation and location of the tumour; the

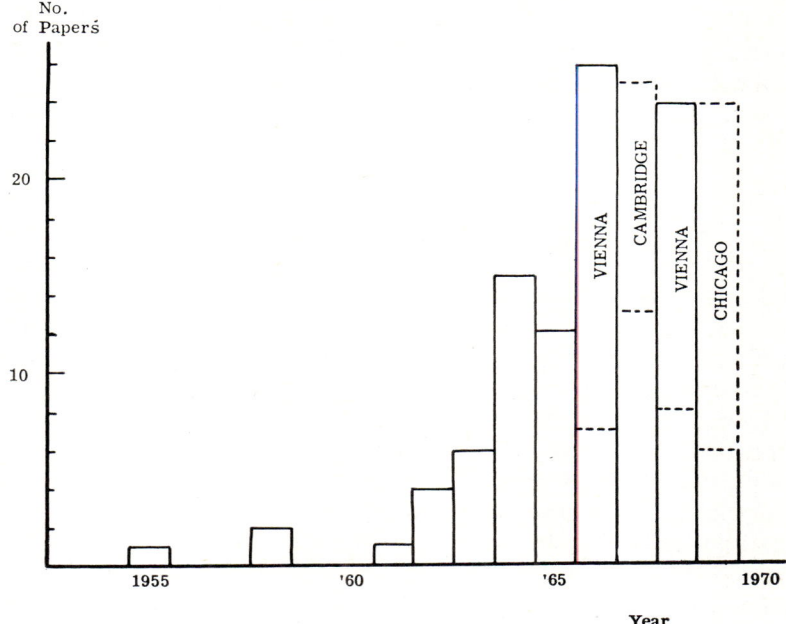

FIG. 13.2. Histogram of published papers on the use of computers in radiotherapy. The two parts labelled Vienna represent references (1) and (2). The two parts labelled Cambridge and Chicago are estimates.

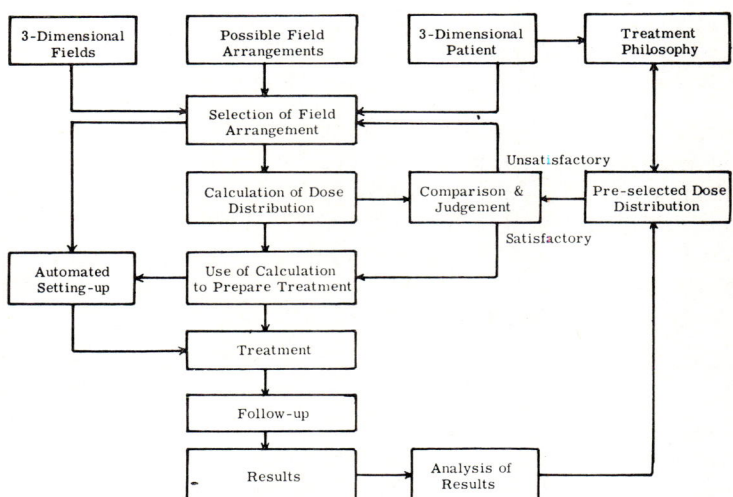

FIG. 13.3. Analysis of the system of radiotherapy treatment planning and implementation.

selection of a field arrangement which could be expected to give a satisfactory dose distribution; the calculation of the actual dose distribution to check the selected field arrangement; and the calculation of actual treatment times using the results of the calculated dose distribution.

DOSE DISTRIBUTION

The process which is most tedious, repetitive and time consuming to do by hand is the calculation of dose distributions. It is a process for which every step has been well defined in a simple logical sequence and for which all the rules required for adequate accuracy have been established. Dose distribution from single beams or fields of radiation are measured in a tank of water which simulates an idealized patient. Since the doses from several fields to any one point can simply be added to give the total dose, the only difficulties arise from the ways in which the real patient differs from the idealized one. Differences occur at the surface which is not usually flat in practice, and where there are inhomogeneities such as lung, air cavities, or bone. For every point in the patient at which the total dose is to be calculated, all these factors must be taken into account for each field. The manual methods have proved readily adaptable to the computer, and there is general agreement that the results produced by the computer can be quite satisfactory. Usually there has been some compromise in the computer work between speed and completeness, but nearly all requirements can be met.

Although there are four topics in the calculation of dose distributions, attention has been concentrated on the first three, which is typical of the early phase of computer application. The four topics are:

1. Organization of data on radiation fields from single sources, external or internal, in a form suitable for the computer.
2. Organization of data on the spatial relationship of these sources to each other and to the anatomical features of the patient.
3. Details of the simple mathematical procedures carried out on these data.
4. Presentation of the results.

Although much of the investigative work on the first three topics can now be regarded as complete, a brief review will be helpful towards appreciation of later developments.

Most of the radiation field data for the computer have been prepared from isodose data originally collected for manual use. These data are presented for manual use as isodose charts, consisting of a series of curves joining points of equal dose. From these charts the dose to any point can be read by interpolation between the isodose curves. The earliest direct digitizations of isodose charts have been superseded by analyses of the data to produce semi-empirical tables or formulae, or a separation of the scattered radiation. The most important aspect of these methods of describing single fields, although it was not always realized at the time, was their suitability for being adapted to take account of modifications due to wedges, patient curvature and hetero-geneities. These factors cause the shapes of the isodose curves to be distorted from the almost flat shapes produced by a beam of radiation normally on a tank of water (Fig. 4). Some descriptions of single fields which are based on the almost flat isodose curves are not suitable for adaptation to take account of the distortions. Even yet, methods of measuring radiation dose which have been designed specifically for computer use are relatively rare.

The description of the field arrangement and the contour and other features of the patient have usually used whichever co-ordinate system or systems minimized the manual effort required to input the data. A polar co-ordinate system at preset radial intervals requires half the data required by a cartesian system, but electro-mechanical transducers are the most attractive (Fig. 5). Once the description is in the computer it can be processed in any way convenient before being combined with the radiation field data. The combination of the field data is always based on a simple change of axes where the ultimate co-ordinate system is that which will be used in the presentation of the results. The changes of axes involve interpolation or calculation, and the field data must be modified to take account of the patient's features. All these steps in the case of external beams mimic the original hand methods of calculation. For internal sources the position is slightly different, because hand methods of producing full dose distributions are not feasible on a routine basis, and because measurement of the radiation fields from individual sources is difficult. The basic steps used in the computer are still similar to the manual methods of obtaining doses at a few selected points.

PRESENTATION AND COMPARISON

For both internal and external sources the primary purpose of cal-culated dose distributions for individual patients is to allow a compari-son with idealized dose distributions which have never been presented explicitly in pictorial form. This comparison and the changes and modi-fications required to reduce the differences between actual and ideal comprise the process of optimization. The way in which the results of a dose calculation are presented should therefore be dictated by the requirements of the comparison. In almost all cases, however, the computer output and presentation of results has slavishly copied the

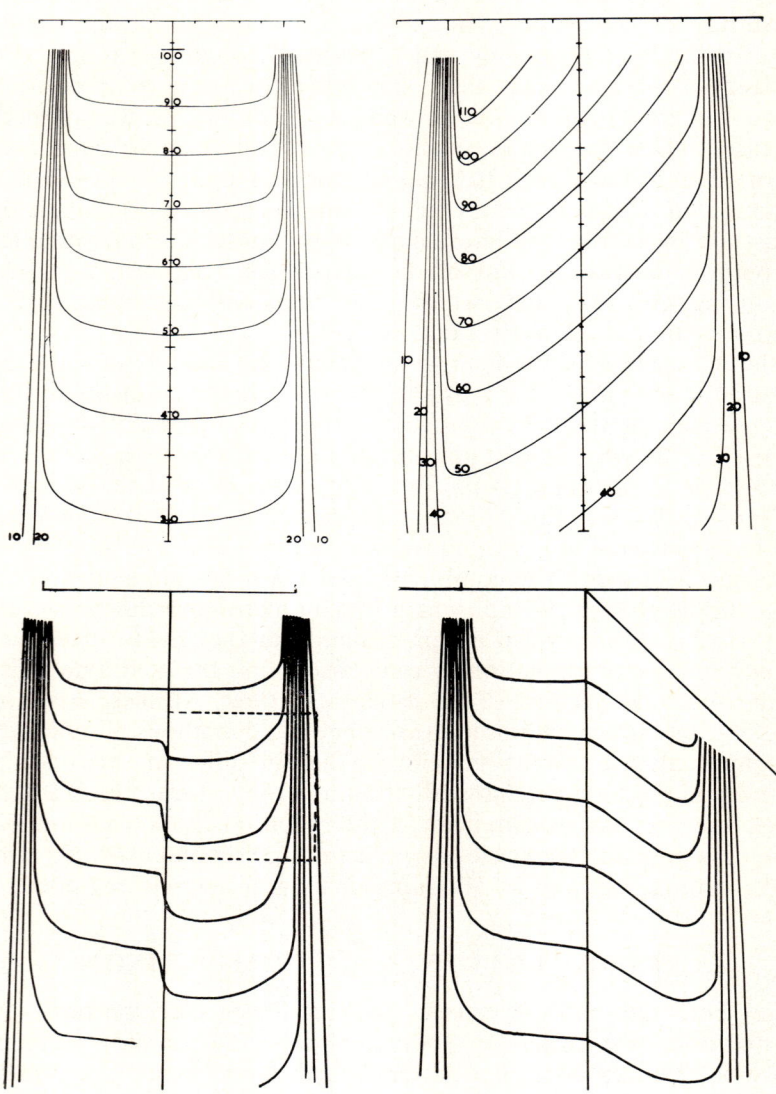

FIG. 13.4. Isodose charts for a plain field, a wedged field, a plain field distorted by
oblique incidence, and a plain field distorted by a heterogeneity.

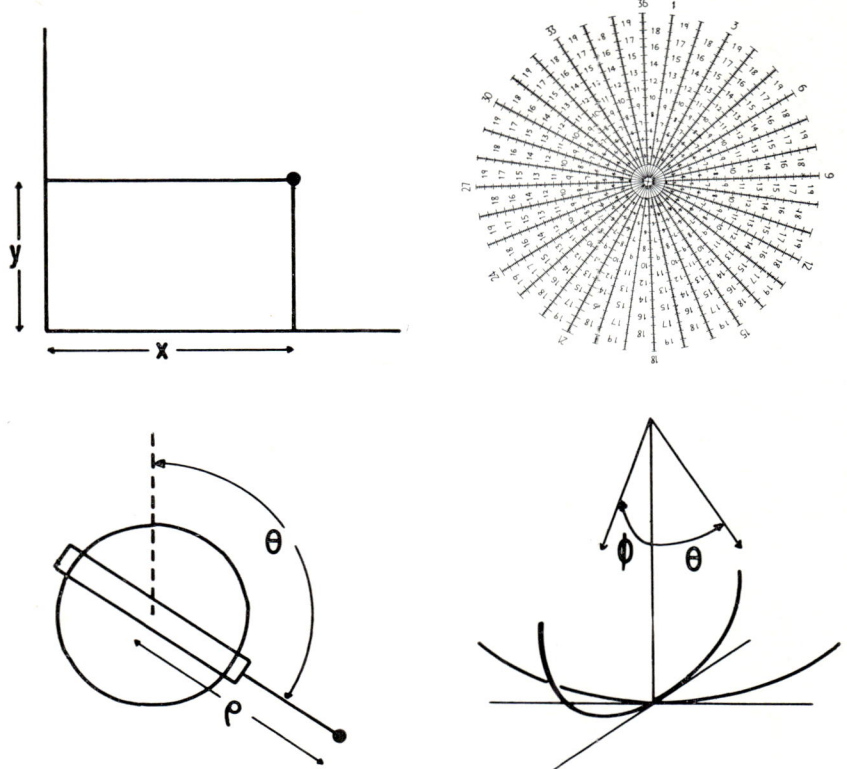

FIG. 13.5. Some methods of deriving and expressing graphical input data.

old-established manual methods (Fig. 6). No scientific attempts have been made to study, in this context, the human processes of visual perception or image analysis on which the comparison is based. In fact, some of the computer presentations, for example, the representation of isodose lines by widely spaced characters, or the unbroken array of variegated characters, are manifestly worse than the manual presentation (Fig. 7).

Important deficiences in the process of comparison of hand calculated dose distributions with idealized distributions arise from the slow rate at which they can be produced and assimilated, and the relatively few distributions, usually one, which are in fact produced. Thus most of the calculation and comparison is done mentally and the paper version is only a final check. This rather primitive situation is mimicked by a single computer calculated dose distribution, no matter how accurate or extensive it may be, unless some re-organization of the use of the dose distribution is attempted. Current progress is largely bound up with the attempt to break out of this position.

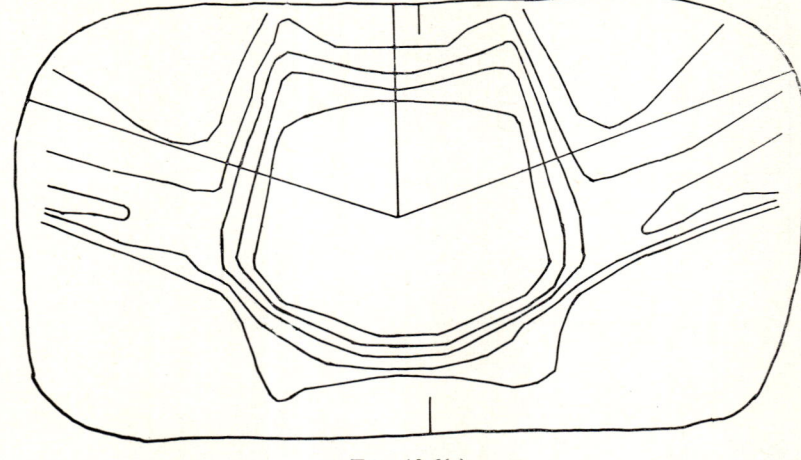

FIG. 13.6(a).

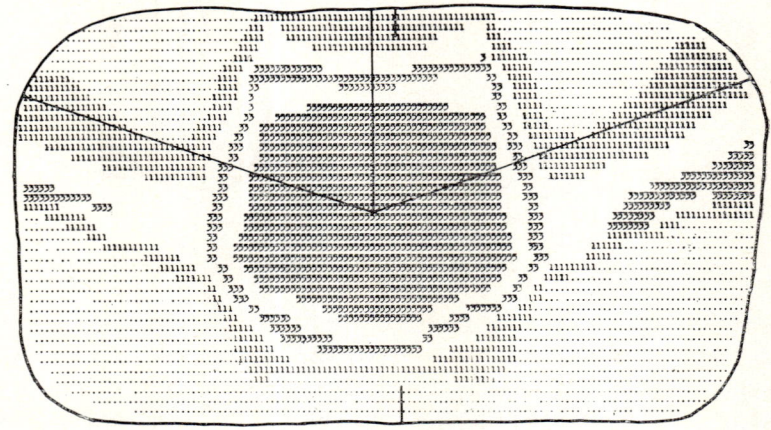

FIG. 13.6(b).

FIG. 13.6 (a) and (b). Illustrating computer outputs which simulate and are as good as manual representations.

PROGRAMMING IN PRACTICE

There has been a rapid and widespread increase in the number of radiotherapy centres routinely computing dose distributions. These computed distributions can have advantages of accuracy, completeness, consistency and speed, with less manual effort. They also form the starting point for applications of computers to optimization. Many radiotherapy centres routinely use programmes and procedures developed elsewhere with minor modifications to suit local conditions.

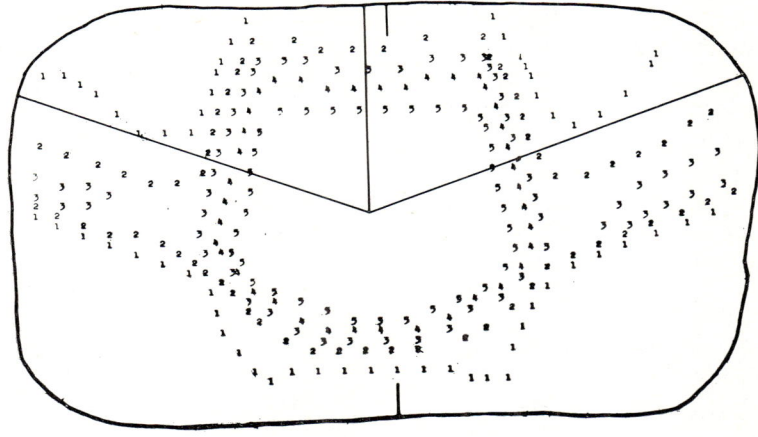

FIG. 13.7(a).

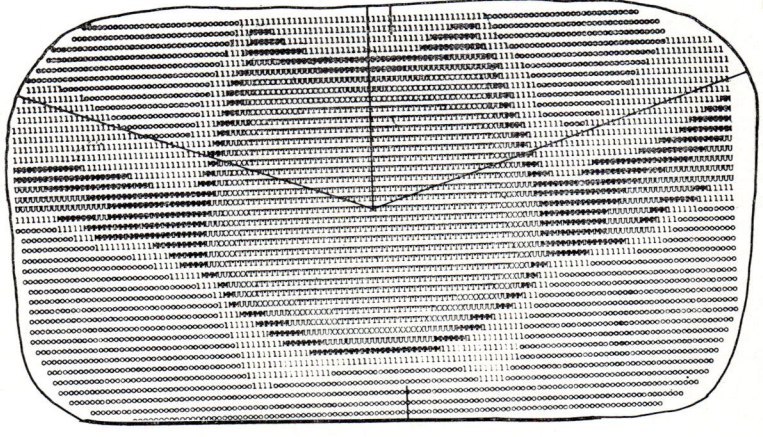

FIG. 13.7(b).

FIG.13.7. Illustrating computer outputs which do not convey information as well as manual representations.

Such centres are motivated by the desire to put these programmes into practical use and not by the satisfaction of creating them, which is at least part of the motivation of the originating centres. This is a very healthy situation since the organization of the output can be planned on the basis of an existing package, and this allows much more attention to be given to the most important part of the system—the use of the output. Some programming changes are usually required, but if the programmes have been written in a high level language, preferably Fortran, and in some approach to a modular form, no difficulties arise.

It is essential that the recipients should be adequately versed in the radiotherapy physics of the methods used, and be familiar with the programmes, so that they can take responsibility for monitoring performance and detecting discrepancies.

There are a number of examples of the ways in which programmes for calculating dose distributions can be adapted to extend their usefulness. Integral doses or indices of integral doses can be calculated to take account of the volumes of tissue receiving radiation. The volumes involved influence the dose which can be given and the response. Modal

MODAL DOSE = 159
MODAL DOSE HISTOGRAM
OF TUMOUR AREA
144–146:**
146–148:**
148–150:***
150–152:****
152–154:*****
154–156:******
156–158:*******
158–160:**********
160–162:****

MODAL DOSE = 139
MODAL DOSE HISTOGRAM
OF TUMOUR AREA
122–124:**
124–126:**
126–128:**
128–130:**
130–132:***
132–134:***
134–136:**
136–138:***
138–140:******

MODAL DOSE = 157
MODAL DOSE HISTOGRAM
OF TUMOUR AREA
148–150:*
150–152:**
152–154:****
154–156:*****
156–158:*******
158–160:*****
160–162:***
162–164:***
164–166:**

MODAL DOSE = 143
MODAL DOSE HISTOGRAM
OF TUMOUR AREA
136–138:**
138–140:***
140–142:***
142–144:****
144–146:***
146–148:***
148–150:****
150–152:***
152–154:***

FIG. 13.8. Histograms obtained by computer of the doses within the tumour area. Although these histograms do not take account of position within the tumour area, this kind of information may be a useful bonus when dose distributions are computed.

doses can be found and the distribution over the tumour area presented as a histogram so that uniformity or non-uniformity can be quantitated (Fig. 8). Outputs of the treatment units can be included so that time per field per treatment can be provided. The aspects of treatment which are to be recorded for a computer based record system can be supplied directly thus avoiding manual transcription.

It is more difficult to improve the ways in which programmes for calculating dose distributions in three dimensions can be used, because of the problems of presentation. While dose distributions in two dimensions can be fully expressed by lines, in three dimensions distributions require a series of surfaces within one another (Fig. 9). Such series of surfaces are difficult to present even when three dimensions are actually available, and it may be that in practice only one surface can be presented at a time. The separate presentation of the distributions in a series of sections is barely suitable for routine use, even for interstitial radiation sources. Although holography has been suggested, more practical possibilities are the use of stereo systems or an oscilloscope display in which the illusion of depth is created by a

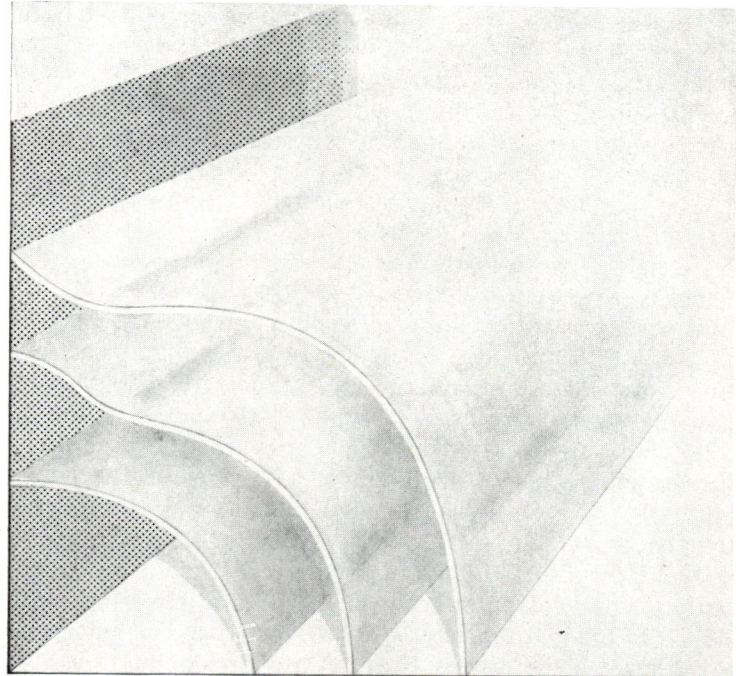

FIG. 13.9. Illustrating the difficulties of representing a series of surfaces within one another in three dimensions.

combination of movement and the shape of the symbols. While stereoscopy is excellent for visualizing lines in three dimensions it is much less satisfactory for presenting surfaces. Stereo pairs can easily be produced by computer by a simple change of co-ordinates. In fact, once a three dimensional distribution has been calculated, a computer can easily determine how it would appear when viewed for any desired direction. The best solution probably lies in some such computer application, but the presentation must be oriented to the faculties of the human user, and the problem requires extensive investigation.

Possibly the most important factors affecting the use of computed dose distributions are the speeds with which input data can be prepared and output returned to the user, and delays at the computer before computation. If these procedures are grossly out of keeping with the speed of the actual computation then the system must be regarded as being only partially implemented.

The problem of delay at the computer is solving itself as the typical processor available for radiotherapy use becomes large enough to deal immediately with radiotherapy problems which are relatively small-scale. When a line printer or incremental plotter output is required the problem of the return of the output to the user has not yet been satisfactorily overcome. The use of a remote teletype terminal tends to reduce the attractiveness of the layout of the output, although it does enhance the directness (Haybittle and Houston, 1968).

An increasing number of medical physics departments and radiotherapy centres are finding it worthwhile to have their own small computer. If an oscilloscope display is required there is no alternative. If a variety of other services, such as isotope work or statistical analyses form a substantial work load, then a small computer can be well justified. There is no general solution as yet to the problem of combining speed and service, but for reasons of economy it is best to put as much of the work load as possible on to the largest available well-managed computer from which a reasonably expeditious return can be obtained.

The availability and use of a small local computer is intimately bound up with one of the currently active approaches to optimization. This involves the rapid presentation of a number of alternative dose distributions. These may be presented sequentially or together. It is essential that the input, calculation and presentation should be sufficiently rapid for direct interaction between the person judging the distributions and the computer. The deficiences of one distribution must be the basis of the modifications used for the next. This interaction can best be achieved if the display is on an oscilloscope and the computer input must be immediately accessible. The most dedicated workers on this method of optimization have been Bentley at the Royal Marsden Hospital, and the group working on the programmed console at St. Louis under Cox (Holmes, 1970). Whether a good compromise between speed and detail has been reached with the computers now becoming available has not yet been reported. Where the output is on a teletype or a plotter, the disadvantage of less speed is at least partially balanced by the advantage of a hard copy.

The other currently active approach to optimization does not depend on the on-line use of a computer. Instead of the human observer judging the dose distributions, the computer is given some expression of the criteria used and it carries out the judging itself. The most practical realizations of this approach have been those of Hope and colleagues (1967) and Jamieson and Trevelyan (1969). It has been shown that for supervoltage units with narrow beam penumbras, it is possible for the computer to select field arrangements which produce dose distributions recognized by the therapist as being the best obtainable. Criteria taken into account have been: skin or subcutaneous dose, uniformity of tumour dose, integral dose, dose to vulnerable regions, dose to regions of probable lymphatic spread, and minimum normal tissue treated unnecessarily to tumour dose (Fig. 10).

The present position is that both of the above approaches are ready to be brought into routine use. To some extent they are complementary,

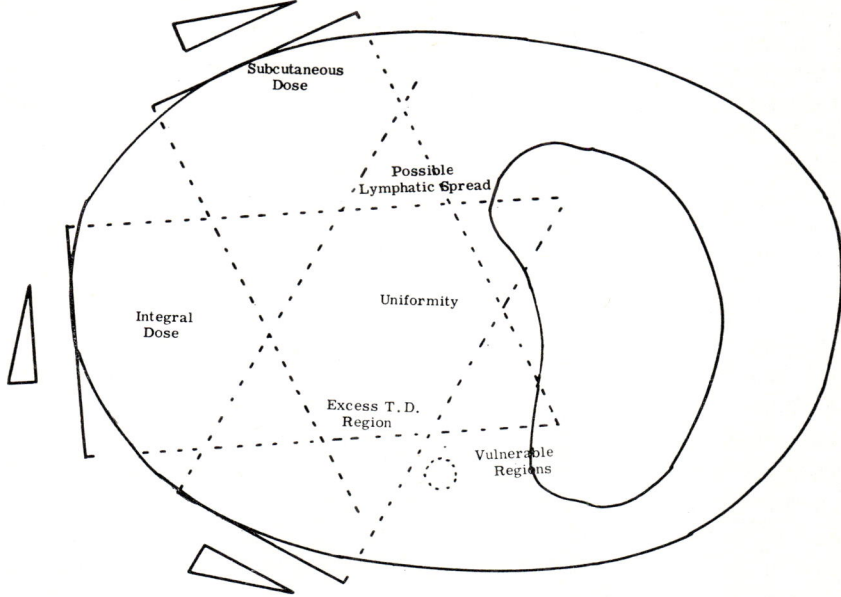

FIG. 13.10. Illustrating some of the features of a dose distribution which are taken into account in judging its merits.

as the continuous development of quantitated criteria is dependent on a detailed study of the changing features of distributions as the field arrangement is varied. The routine use of these optimization methods involves a reorganization which depends on the use envisaged. The input data need only be the patient and tumour description, and the output need only be the field arrangement details with modal, maximum and minimum tumour dose, and the dose to vulnerable regions. Standard field arrangements could be permitted unless the distribution was worse than a specified level of acceptability. The full dose distribution would simply be a check on the working of the system and in the normal course of events would not need to be used in the treatment planning process.

It is necessary to emphasise again that optimization in this special sense means comparison with an idealized dose distribution. The easier the process of optimization becomes, the more attention can be paid to the properties of the idealized distribution. This distribution is based on the analyses of clinical observation of the results of treatment and on the influence of experimental radiobiological findings and their interpretation. The computer is now starting to play a part in both of these subjects, but in so far as outputs useful in practical radiotherapy are concerned, these applications are in a very early phase, and are perhaps ten years behind the application to treatment planning. One important exception is the work at Houston (Castro, Lindberg and Fletcher, 1969; Fletcher and Stovall, 1962) on the use of computed dose distributions from interstitial implants in a study of correlations between computed dose and local result, in terms of recurrence or necrosis. This kind of work illustrates the problems of applying full dose distributions from implants in clinical practice (Fig. 11). No such study of correlations has been published on the use of computed dose distributions for external beams in an analysis of clinical results.

OPERATION OF EQUIPMENT AND RECORDS

All the work described above has the double objective of improving the results obtained and saving the time and effort of radiotherapists, physicists, and planning room staff. The application of automation to the actual administration of treatment by the radiographers has had a relatively late start. Several advantages are claimed for equipment capable of providing automatic positioning of the treatment unit and control of the exposure time by means of punched cards. These advantages include a reduction in the work load for the operating staff, exact reproducibility of all setting data, more economic use of the treatment unit, and automatic documentation of all treatments. This is an interesting development, but major benefits will result only if it is accompanied by an extensive reorganization of all associated factors, such as the arrival of patients, the fractionation of treatment, the arrangement of fields and the handling of records. Many centres will be reluctant to undertake such a reorganization until much more development work has been carried out.

Many computer based record systems are now being introduced to deal with a relatively small amount of administrative, clinical, and treatment information about large numbers of patients. These are at a very early stage of development towards fulfilling possible roles of giving early warning of exceptionally good or bad treatments, or providing

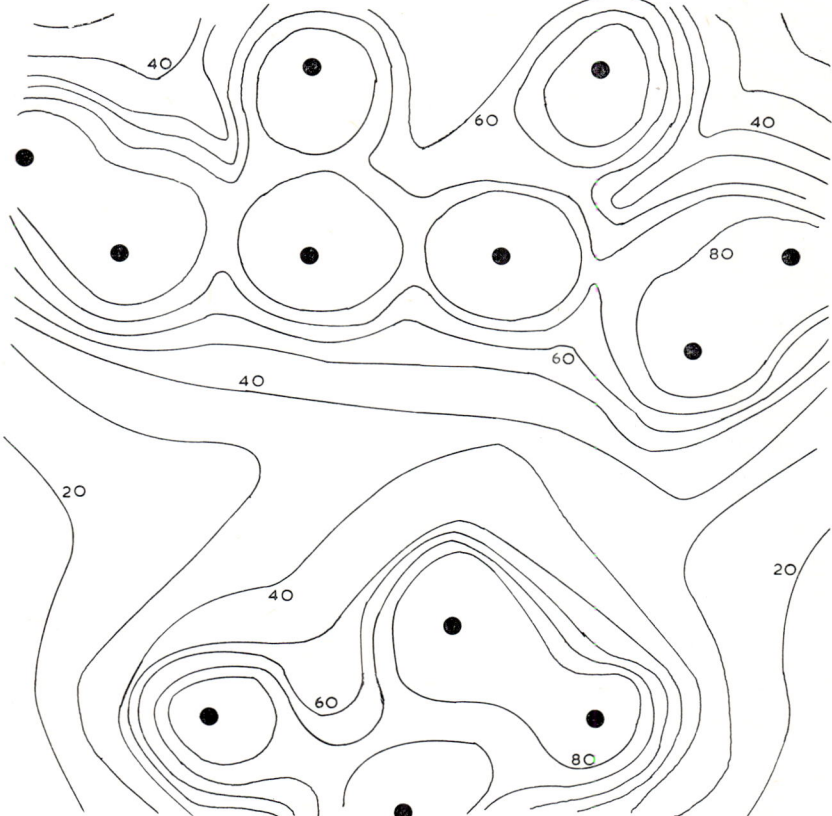

FIG. 13.11. Illustrating the problems raised when full dose distributions are available for interstitial implants. No single representative figure for dose-rate is provided.

suggestive correlations between some of the data stored. It is, therefore, not yet possible to assess their suitability for these purposes. None of the previously well established and maintained manual record systems have been changed to full computerisation, so new computer systems have double problems both of a technical and a use and organization nature.

Published work on computerized radiotherapy records is largely confined to discussions of input methods. A wide variety of forms of input have been devised and tested. These range from a simple arrangement with completely defined procedures, suitable for secretarial assistants, to an input providing considerable freedom to the therapist but requiring proportionally greater attention, supervision and processing before it is ready for storing. The systems which are being introduced in practice appear to favour the simple rigid inputs. Where such a system has been in regular use on a hospital or group scale, while it does not directly provide more than a clinical index (which in itself is useful), it has encouraged the inception of prospective clinical trials using the machinery of the routine records system.

RADIOBIOLOGICAL MODELS

Radiobiological models have had a strong influence on radiotherapeutic rationalization, although they have not so far had much influence on actual practice. Radiobiological data which are to be interpreted in terms of more than the simplest and most naive model require mathematical techniques which usually involve computers. Useful models must be based on a mechanism and mechanisms and responses can be tested, thus providing more data. This interaction is the essential process leading to understanding and for this kind of research the use of computer facilities is necessary. At all levels of biology, current concepts of organization lead to models whose behaviour cannot be followed and understood without the help of a computer. This computer work, although related to radiotherapy, and probably the most hopeful long term research, is far from being applicable to clinical use. Interesting and stimulating suggestions can arise (Cohen and Scott, 1968; Fischer, 1969), but their limitations must always be borne in mind (Fig. 12).

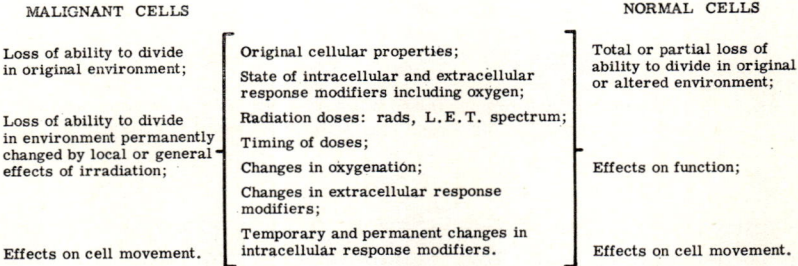

FIG. 13.12. Some of the factors which may be necessary for a computer model of the effects of radiotherapy.

CONCLUSION

From an overall viewpoint of current uses of the computer in radiotherapy, the key concept is organization. Organization is an investment and must eventually pay a dividend. Where an organization has already been established and is functioning smoothly and well, the tendency is to delay reorganization in the face of changing circumstances as long as possible. However, plans for eventual reorganization and preparatory work must be instituted in good time before obsolescence sets in. Since the computer is synonymous with reorganization if actually used, the computer can be one of the catalysts which help precipitate the reorganization.

In the nature of things it is to be expected that the proper and successful use of the computer should eventually lead to its discontinuance in the original fields of effort. Then the reorganization will be within the computer group enforced by the demands of radiotherapy. However, as automatic data processing is an extension of human capability comparable with the inventions of writing, mathematics and telecommunications, it will be with us for a long time.

REFERENCES

CASTRO, J. R., LINDBERG, R. D., & FLETCHER, G. H. (1969). Clinical application of computer dosimetry in interstitial radium therapy. *Am. J. Roentg.*, **105**, 165.

COHEN, L., & SCOTT, M. J. (1968). Fractionation procedures in radiation therapy: a computerised approach to evaluation. *Br. J. Radiol.*, **41**, 529.

COHEN, M. (1970). Special Report No. 4. Computers in radiotherapy. *Br. J. Radiol.*, **43**, 658.

Computer Calculation of Dose Distribution in Radiotherapy (1966). Technical Reports Series No. 57. Vienna: I.A.E.A.

Computers in Radiology (1970). Basel: Karger.

FISCHER, J. J. (1969). Theoretical considerations in the optimisation of dose distribution in radiation therapy. *Br. J. Radiol.*, **42**, 925.

FLETCHER, G. H., & STOVALL, M. (1962). Study of explicit distribution of radiation in interstitial implantations. II. Correlation with clinical results in squamous cell carcinoma of anterior two-thirds of tongue and floor of mouth. *Radiology*, **78**, 766.

HAYBITTLE, J. L., & HOUSTON, A. A. (1968). The use of a multi-access computer for radiation treatment planning. *Br. J. Radiol.*, **41**, 927.

HOLMES, W. F. (1970). External beam treatment—planning with the programmed console. *Radiology*, **94**, 391.

HOPE, C. S., ORR, J. S., LAURIE, J., & HALNAN, K. E. (1967). Optimisation of X-ray treatment planning by computer judgement. *Physics Med. Biol.*, **12**, 531.

JAMIESON, D. G., & TREVELYAN, ANNE (1969). A computer approach to dose calculation for supplementary beam therapy. *Br. J. Radiol.*, **42**, 57.

ORR, J. S., CAIN, OLIVE, ETCHELLS, A. H., HALNAN, K. E., & HOPE, C. S. (1970). Computing in radiotherapy. *Scott. med. J.*, **15**, 370.

The Role of Computers in Radiotherapy (1968). STI/PUB/203. Vienna: I.A.E.A.

The Use of Computers in Therapeutic Radiology (1967). British Institute of Radiology, Special Report No. 1, and 1971, in press.

Index